The Concise Handbook of
Human Anatomy

Manson Publishing Ltd
73 Corringham Road
London NW11 7DL, UK

Copyright © 1998 Manson Publishing Ltd

All rights reserved. No part of this publication may be reproduced, stored in a retrieval system or transmitted in any form or by any means, electronic, mechanical, photocopying, recording, or otherwise without either prior permission in writing from the publisher or a licence permitting restricted copying issued in the United Kingdom by the Copyright Licensing Agency, 90 Tottenham Court Road, London W1P 9HE.

First published 1998

BookPower edition first published 2003

ISBN 1–84076–042–7

Printed in Spain

BookPower (formerly ELST) is a registered charity which makes available low-priced, unabridged editions of British publishers' textbooks to students in developing countries.

BookPower is grateful to the many inidividuals, trusts and organisations who have provided funding to cover the cost of its operation. These include:

Barclays Bank
CfBT
Grocers Company
Haberdashers Company
The Tanner Trust
The Mary Webb Trust

Below is a list of some other medical books published under the BookPower/ELST imprint:

Adler
ABC of Aids
BMJ Books

Browse
An Introduction to the Symptoms and Signs of Surgical Disease
Arnold

Buxton
ABC of Dermatology
BMJ Books

Campbell and Lees (eds.)
Obstetrics by Ten Teachers
Arnold

Campbell and Monga (eds.)
Gynaecology by Ten Teachers
Arnold

Child Advocacy International
International Child Health Care
BMJ Books

Cook and Zumla
Manson's Tropical Diseases 21 e
Saunders

Mayne
Clinical Chemistry in Diagnosis and Treatment
Arnold

The Concise Handbook of
Human Anatomy

R.M.H. MCMINN, MD, PhD, FRCS (Eng)
Emeritus Professor of Anatomy, Royal College of Surgeons of England
and University of London, UK

R.T. HUTCHINGS
Formerly Chief Medical Laboratory Scientific Officer,
Royal College of Surgeons of England, UK

B.M. LOGAN, MA, FMA, Hon. MBIE, MAMAA
University Prosector, University of Cambridge, UK

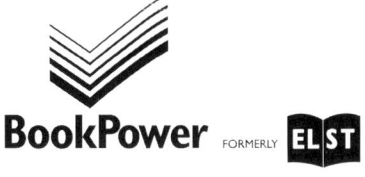

with Manson Publishing
in co-operation with the
British Council

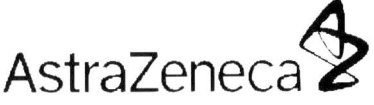

Sponsored by AstraZeneca PLC

Contents

Preface   6

Acknowledgements   6

1. Body form and function   7
   Systems   8
   Anatomical terms   15

2. Bones and joints   17
   Axial skeleton   20
      Skull   20
      Hyoid bone   21
      Vertebrae   21
      Ribs and sternum   25
   Appendicular skeleton   25
      Upper limb bones   25
      Lower limb bones   29
   Summary   34

3. Head, neck and vertebral column   35
   Cranial cavity   36
   Skull foramina   41
   Head and neck in sagittal section   41
   Brain, spinal cord, and nerves   44
      Brain   44
      Cranial nerves   50
      Spinal cord   53
      Spinal nerves   56
   Face and scalp   60
      Mouth   65
      Nose and paranasal sinuses   67
      Eye and lacrimal apparatus   69
      Ear   74
   Neck and vertebral column   77
      Thyroid and parathyroid glands   82
      Larynx   83
      Pharynx   84
   Summary   88

4.	**Upper limb**	89
	Shoulder, axilla and arm	90
	Elbow, forearm and hand	97
	Summary	108
5.	**Thorax**	109
	Breasts	110
	Diaphragm	112
	Mediastinum	112
	Heart	116
	Lungs and pleura	123
	Summary	125
6.	**Abdomen**	127
	Anterior abdominal wall	128
	Surface features	129
	Posterior abdominal wall	131
	Abdominal vessels and nerves	133
	Abdominal viscera	136
	Stomach	137
	Small intestine	138
	Large intestine	139
	Liver	141
	Gall bladder and biliary tract	142
	Pancreas	144
	Kidneys and ureters	145
	Adrenal glands	145
	Spleen	146
	Summary	147
7.	**Pelvis and perineum**	149
	Male pelvic and genital organs	155
	Female pelvic and genital organs	158
	Summary	161
8.	**Lower limb**	163
	Hip and thigh	164
	Knee, leg and foot	171
	Summary	185
	Glossary	187
	Index	190

Preface

Despite all the wonders of 'microchippery', there will always be a need for books that can be perused and provide a welcome relief from staring at a rectangular screen. This short synopsis is intended for those who need the essential facts of Human Anatomy without becoming lost in the mass of detail that occupies so much of most anatomical texts. We have attempted to sort out the wood from the trees and to give a concise account of the more important anatomical facts, without becoming bogged down in academic details which, although necessary for some, only hinder the understanding of the things that really matter for most people beginning the study of anatomy. Of course, there are endless arguments as to what is regarded as essential or basic, but we offer this as a presentation based on long experience of teaching at medical and paramedical levels.

The surface of the body is all that most people (except surgeons!) ever see of it, and much of 'learning anatomy' is really an exercise in being able to visualise exactly what is below each part of the surface, and then to think of the practical implications; there are numerous illustrations of surface anatomy in this book. When looking at the surface it is necessary to be able to 'mentally X-ray' every bit of the body, especially the chest and abdomen. Conventional radiology and modern imaging techniques are powerful aids to 'looking below the surface', and selected examples are included here to supplement dissections and explanatory drawings.

We hope this small volume will be helpful to all who are seeking a concise account of Human Anatomy as a basis for medical and paramedical studies.

R.M.H. McMinn
R.T. Hutchings
B.M. Logan

Acknowledgements

We are much indebted to Lynette Nearn for assistance with the preparation of dissections, to Rosie Watts for all artwork apart from that in Part 1, to Dr Kate Stevens for the provision of radiographs and images and to our models for surface anatomy. The artwork in Part 1 is the copyright of Anejo SA, Argentina, and the model in Figure 1.2 on page 9 is the copyright of the Denoyer-Geppert Company, Chicago, USA.

We would also like to thank Pat Daly and John Ormiston for their editorial skills and Michael Manson for embracing our project so enthusiastically.

Part 1

Body form and function

The study of anatomy, from the Greek meaning to cut up, refers to the study of the structure of the body allied to its function, and as seen with the naked eye (in contrast to various kinds of microscopy) is often referred to as gross or topographical anatomy – the geography of the body.

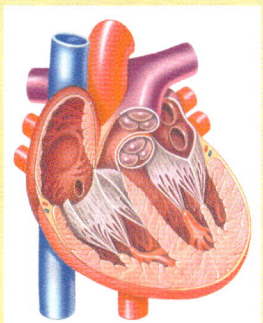

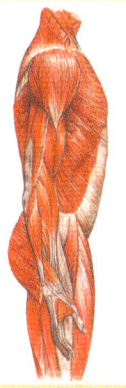

Dissection, the Latin equivalent of the Greek for cutting, has been the traditional way of learning gross anatomy, and although many present-day students do not carry out dissections themselves, they are usually able to see appropriate specimens prepared by their teachers.

Modern imaging techniques allow all parts of the body to be examined without a knife or even a finger being laid upon the body. The names of most structures are Greek or Latin in origin.

Human Anatomy

IN THE MAIN part of this book the anatomy of the body is considered according to its various parts or regions, e.g. head, hand, thorax, pelvis, etc. (regional anatomy), but the various structures of the body can also be grouped together according to their common function, to make up what are commonly called systems (systematic anatomy). Thus, the heart and blood vessels form the cardiovascular system (or circulatory system), the air passages and lungs form the respiratory system, and so on; these and the other systems are summarized briefly below, although the nervous system has a rather longer explanation to provide an adequate background to the later descriptions of the brain and spinal cord.

Systems

Skeleton and muscular system – the skeleton, consisting of bones and cartilages, gives support to the body and provides protection for some organs, especially the brain and spinal cord. It also acts as a storehouse for minerals, and the marrow cavities of some bones are the site of formation of blood cells. The voluntary or skeletal muscles that move the skeleton form the muscular system; the term skeletomuscular system is sometimes given to the bones and cartilages of the skeleton, the joints connecting them, and the muscles that move them (**1.1**). The parts of the skeleton and individual bones are described in Part 2 (p. 17).

Skin – properly, but not commonly, called the integument or integumentary system, it forms the protective outer covering of the body, and includes specialized derivatives – nails, hair, sebaceous glands (which lubricate the surface), and sweat glands (**1.2**) which, in association with the bloodflow through the skin, play a vital part in the control of body temperature (by surface evaporation). The breasts (mammary glands), which are modified sweat glands, secrete milk for the newborn, and are described in the chapter on the thorax (p. 110). Through its sensory nerve supply (cutaneous nerves, with specialized endings or receptors) the skin assesses the body's environment; certain kinds of skin cells are concerned with pigmentation, immune responses, and the synthesis of vitamin D.

Cardiovascular system – otherwise known as the circulatory system, it includes the heart as a muscular

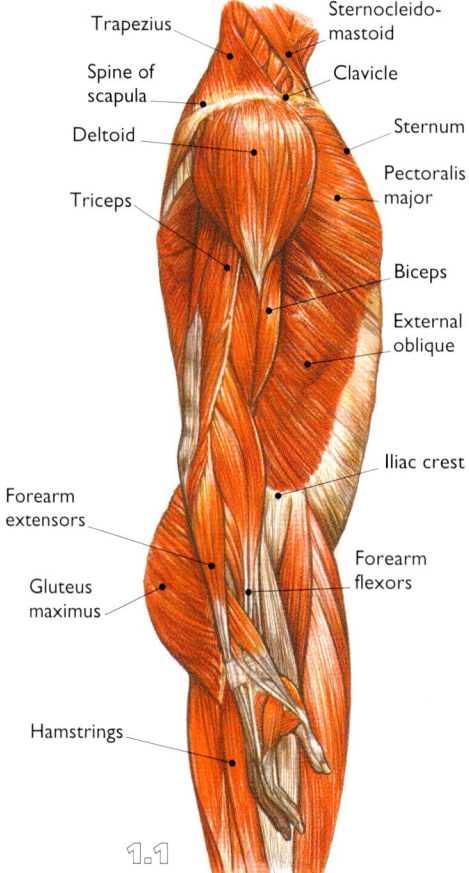

1.1. Some muscles and bony landmarks, from the right

Body form and function

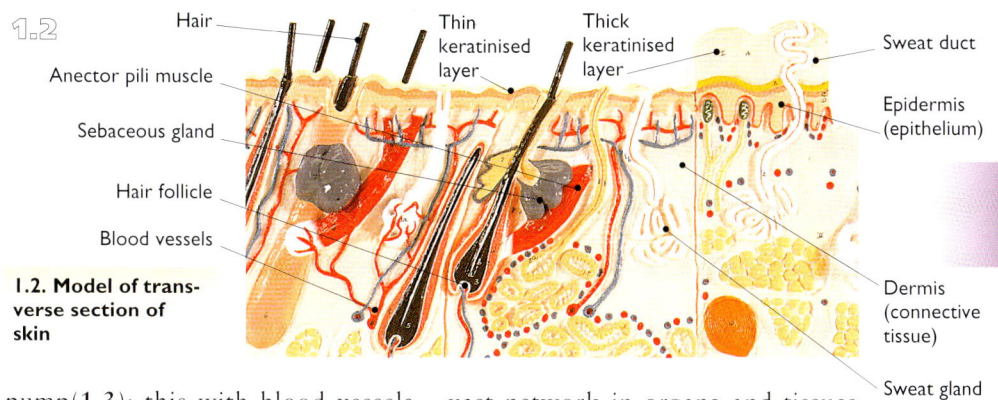

1.2. Model of transverse section of skin

pump(**1.3**); this with blood vessels and the blood that circulates through them forms a transport system for many substances. Arteries conduct blood away from the heart and veins conduct it back to the heart. Through branches of ever-decreasing size, blood reaches the blood capillaries, the microscopic vessels which form a vast network in organs and tissues and through which fluid and many substances, including blood gases (oxygen and carbon dioxide) can be exchanged. From the capillaries blood is gathered into veins of ever-increasing size to be returned to the heart. Blood consists of a fluid (plasma) containing red cells (erythrocytes, for

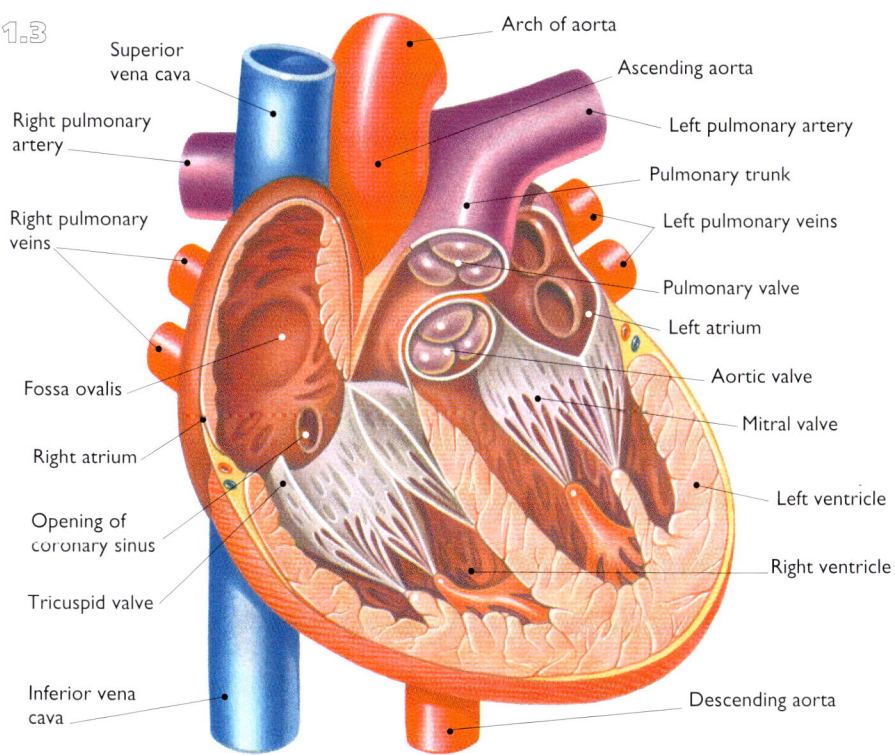

1.3. Heart and great vessels, opened up from the front

9

Human Anatomy

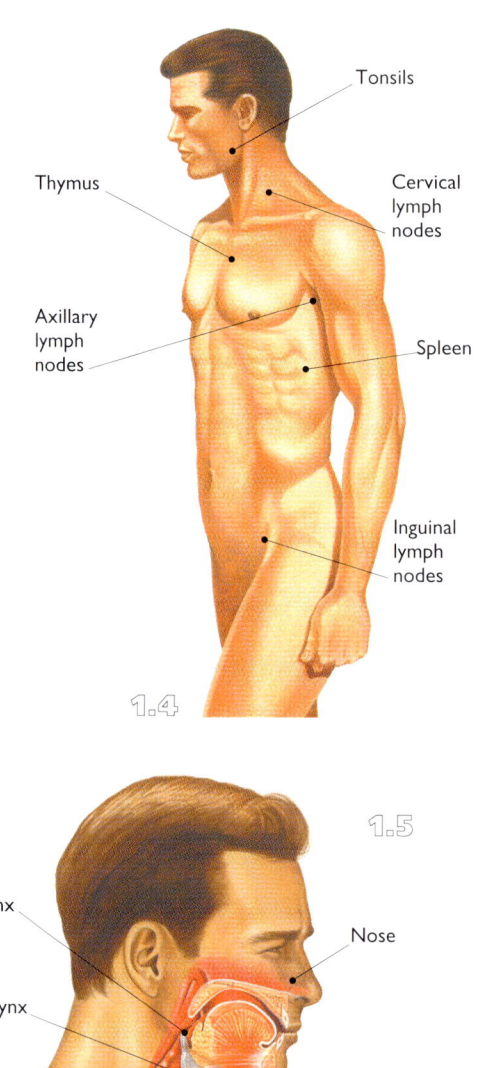

1.4. Position of principal lymphoid organs and palpable lymph nodes

1.5. Parts of the respiratory system

the transport of blood gases), various types of white cells (leucocytes, for body defences, including lymphocytes –see below) and platelets (thrombocytes, concerned with blood clotting).

Lymphatic system – closely allied to the cardiovascular system, the lymphatic system consists of the lymphoid organs (thymus, spleen, tonsils, and lymph nodes, **1.4**), lymphoid follicles scattered in certain non-lymphoid organs (especially in parts of the digestive tract), and lymphatic channels (lymphatics) which drain lymphocytes and fluid from the lymphoid organs and follicles, as well as tissue fluid from other components of the body. Lymph is the fluid within lymphatics. Nodes may become the sites for infections or cancerous deposits derived from any part of the drainage area. The cervical, axillary, and inguinal nodes are those most readily palpable and routinely examined. Apart from drainage, the system is concerned with the manufacture and transport of lymphocytes for the body's immune responses. Part of it also transports fat absorbed from the intestine.

Respiratory system – concerned with the exchange of oxygen and carbon dioxide between blood and air. These exchanges take place in the lungs (**1.5**); the rest of the respiratory system is the respiratory tract, which is simply a conducting pathway for air and includes the nose and paranasal sinuses, pharynx, larynx, trachea, and bronchi. Part of the larynx acts as a respiratory sphincter, concerned with the production of voice.

Body form and function

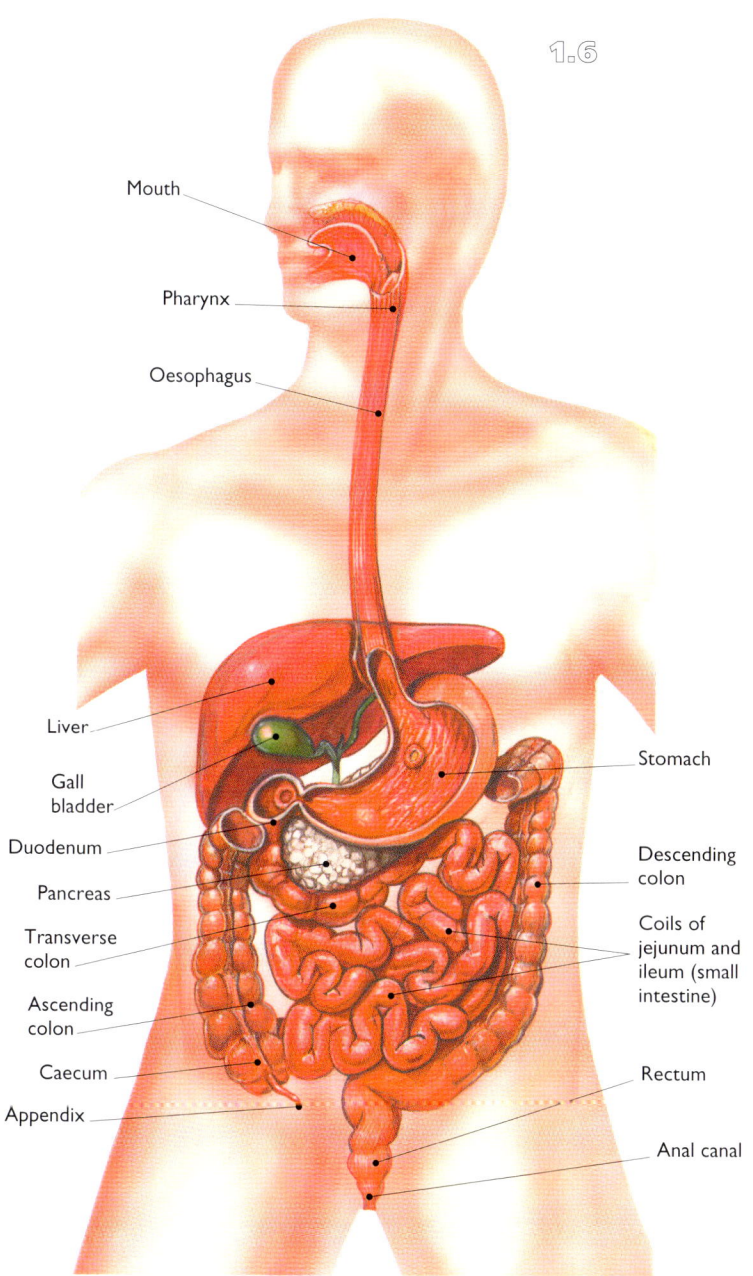

1.6. Parts of the digestive system

Digestive system – concerned with the digestion and absorption of the foodstuffs necessary to provide the chemical energy for all body functions. The digestive or alimentary tract (**1.6**) is composed of the mouth, pharynx, oesophagus, stomach, small intestine (duodenum, jejunum, and ileum), and large intestine (caecum and appendix, colon, rectum, and

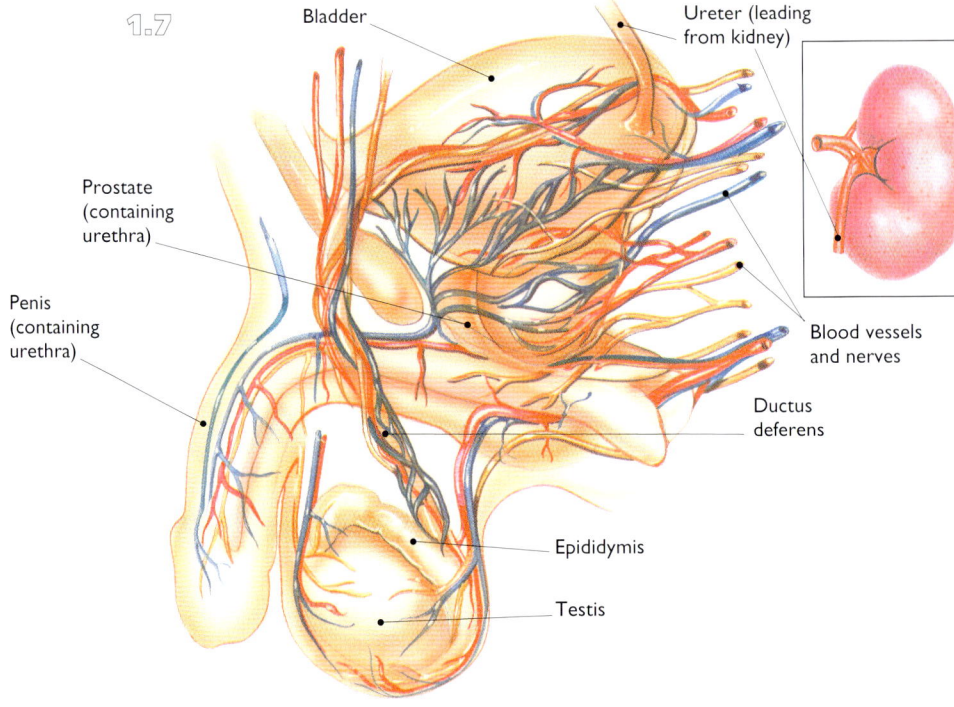

1.7. **Male genito-urinary organs** (inset: the kidney)

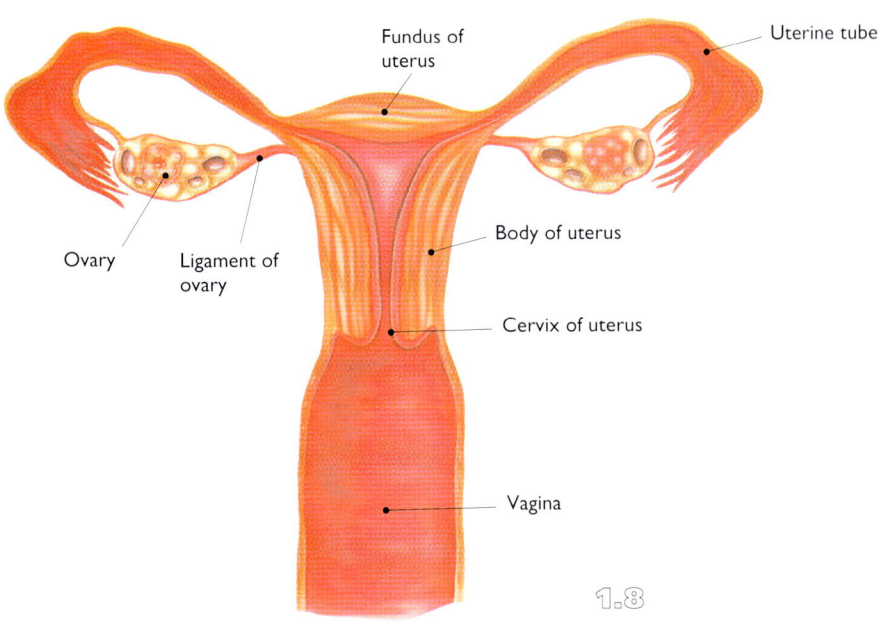

1.8. **Female genital organs**

Body form and function

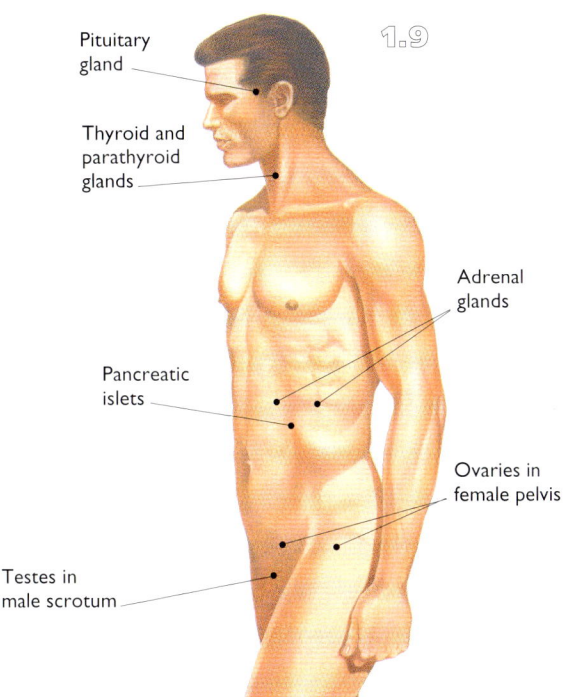

1.9. Postion of principal endocrine organs

anal canal). The digestive processes of the stomach and intestines are assisted by the secretions of the major digestive glands – the liver (with the gallbladder) and pancreas.

Urinary system – in both sexes consists of the paired kidneys and ureters, and the single urinary bladder and urethra (**1.7**). It is concerned with the production, storage, and elimination of urine in order to maintain the body's proper content of water and dissolved substances.

Reproductive system – in the female provides the female germ cells [ova (singular, ovum)] from the paired ovaries, while the uterus and vagina are organs for the conception, development, and birth of a new individual (**1.8**). In the male reproductive system the paired testes provide the male germ cells [sperm or spermatozoa (singular, spermatozoon)]. Since some of the male genital organs are shared with some urinary organs, the combined systems are often called the genito-urinary system (**1.7**).

Endocrine system – like the nervous system, the endocrine system is for communication, but it acts at a much slower rate via the hormones secreted by its various components and mostly distributed by the bloodstream. It consists of the main endocrine organs (the pituitary gland and the adjacent part of the brain, the adrenal, thyroid, and parathyroid glands) and various other groups of endocrine cells that are found in other organs, especially in the pancreas (where they form the islets of Langerhans), testis, ovary, and digestive tract (**1.9**).

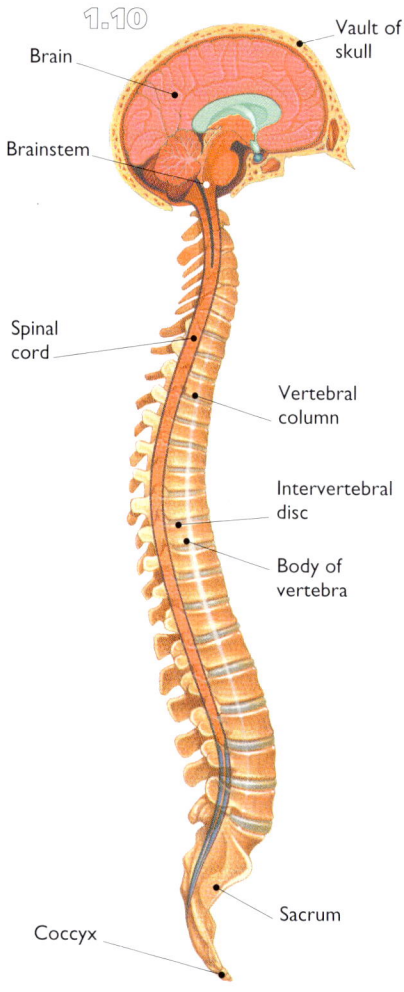

1.10. Left half of brain and spinal cord, within part of the skull and vertebral column

Nervous system – a communication system the purpose of which is to receive information from the outside world and from the body itself, and to make appropriate responses. It is divided into the central nervous system (CNS), composed of the brain and spinal cord (**1.10**), and the peripheral nervous system (PNS), composed of cranial nerves attached to the brain and spinal nerves attached to the spinal cord. Motor nerves that supply skeletal (voluntary) muscle constitute the voluntary or somatic nervous system, while others supply cardiac muscle, smooth (involuntary) muscle, and glands to form the autonomic nervous system (ANS), which is concerned with automatic or involuntary activities, such as heart rate, constriction of blood vessels, sweating, secretion in the stomach, and the size of the pupil.

Nerve cells (neurons) have filamentous processes (nerve fibres) that are collected into bundles to form the nerves of the PNS and the various tracts in the brain and spinal cord. Fibres that convey nerve impulses away from their own cell bodies (the part of the nerve cell containing the nucleus) or from the CNS are efferent fibres; these include the motor fibres that supply muscles and glands. Those that convey impulses towards their own cell bodies or to the CNS are afferent fibres; these include the sensory fibres that convey general or special types of sensation, as well as those unconscious impulses concerned with reflexes. General sensations are those of touch, pain, pressure, temperature, and proprioception (muscle–joint sense, which gives information on position and movement) and the special sensations are vision, smell, taste, hearing, and balance (equilibrium).

The transmission of nerve impulses from one neuron to another occurs at specialized sites, known as synapses, and depends on the release of a transmitter substance which sets off an impulse in the receiving cell. The synaptic connections between neurons complete the neuronal pathways that control bodily activities. Neuromuscular junctions are sites on skeletal muscle fibres that are similar to synapses; at these sites the impulse for contraction is passed on from nerve to muscle, again by a transmitter substance. At these junctions and at parasympathetic synapses the transmitter is acetylcholine; at sympathetic synapses it is noradrenaline. Elsewhere there may be other transmitters.

The majority of neurons within the CNS have microscopically short processes and are collectively called interneurons. They vastly outnumber the main motor and sensory neurons, and form intercommunicating networks between themselves and the larger neurons.

As far as motor activity is concerned it is essential to understand the difference between somatic and autonomic innervation. In somatic motor nerves the fibres run directly from their cells of origin in the CNS to skeletal muscle fibres, without interruption. In autonomic innervation there are two sets of neurons:

Preganglionic, with cell bodies in the CNS whose fibres run to ganglion cells outside the CNS.
Postganglionic, with ganglion cells whose fibres run to the target organ.

If sympathetic, the preganglionic cell bodies are in the thoracic and upper lumbar parts of the spinal cord. Their fibres run out in the thoracic and upper lumbar spinal nerves to synapse with the postganglionic cells, which are either in the ganglia of the sympathetic trunks lying beside the vertebral column or in other ganglia connected to the trunks that are collectively called collateral ganglia. (A few fibres pass directly to cells of the medulla of the adrenal glands.) The postganglionic fibres are widely distributed to all parts of the body by peripheral nerves and/or blood vessels; for the body surface they supply blood vessels, sweat glands, and the arrector pili muscles (the ones attached to hair follicles that cause 'goose pimples' on a cold day).

If parasympathetic, the preganglionic cells are in certain cell groups in the brainstem and the sacral part of the spinal cord. Their fibres run out in cranial or sacral nerves to postganglionic cells which are within or very near the walls of some organs (in particular the heart, stomach, and pelvic viscera), or in the head and neck in four small discrete ganglia (ciliary, otic, pterygopalatine, and submandibular) to supply the pupil or salivary and lacrimal glands. Parasympathetic nerves are more localized in their distribution than are sympathetic, and do not supply any part of the limbs or body surface.

Anatomical terms

Like any other subject, anatomy has its own jargon to describe how structures lie in relation to one another when the body is in a standard position, the anatomical position. This is the body standing upright with the feet together, the head and eyes facing forwards, and the arms straight at the sides with the palms of the hands facing forwards. It does not matter whether you are standing up, lying down, or standing on your head – the terms are always used to refer to this standard anatomical position.

Superior and inferior – towards the upper and lower ends of the body; e.g. the head is superior to the neck, the knee is inferior to the hip.

Anterior (ventral) and posterior (dorsal) – nearer the front and back of the body; e.g. the eyes are anterior to the ears, the ears are posterior to the eyes.

Proximal and distal – nearer to and further from the root of the structure; e.g. the elbow is proximal to the forearm, the hand is distal to the forearm.

Medial and lateral – nearer to and further from the median plane; e.g. the great toe is on the medial side of the foot, the little toe on the lateral side.

Superficial and deep – nearer to and further from the skin surface.

Some special terms apply to the hand and foot. In the hand the palm is the anterior (palmar) surface and the dorsum is the posterior (dorsal) surface. In the foot the upper surface is the dorsum (dorsal surface) and the lower surface is the sole or plantar surface.

For joints of the limbs, flexion means bending and extension means straightening out. Special terms are used for certain forearm movements. Flex your elbow to a right angle and look at the palm of the hand, then turn the hand over so that you are looking at the dorsum of the hand. This is the movement of pronation, where the lower end of the radius (the lateral bone of the forearm) rotates round the lower end of the ulna (the medial bone of the forearm), carrying the hand with it. Now turn the hand over so that you are looking at the palm again; this is the movement of supination. For many common actions, like holding a glass, the forearm and hand are used in the midprone position, somewhere between full pronation and full supination. The ligaments of the radio-ulnar joints (p. 106) and the fibrous interosseous membrane stretching between the radius and ulna keep the two bones together during these movements.

Flexion and extension are also used for movements of the head and trunk. Bending the head or trunk forwards is flexion and the opposite is extension. Bending sideways (but still looking straight ahead) is lateral flexion.

Medial and lateral rotation applied to the limbs means rotation in the long axis of the limb. Putting a hand behind your back involves medial rotation of the arm, while putting it behind your head involves lateral rotation of the arm.

The Glossary (p. 187) explains the derivation of these and other terms.

Part 2

Bones and joints

Without the support given by its bones and cartilages, the body would collapse like a jellyfish out of water. Most of the joints between bones are mobile, so enabling the whole or selected parts of the body to move as required by the muscles acting upon them.

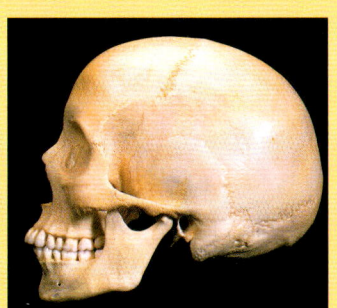

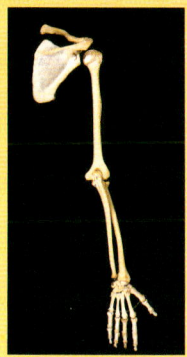

The common diseases of joints (arthritis) are not life-threatening but can result in varying degrees of disability, ranging from interference with the commonplace hand movements that are so essential for everyday life to severe mobility problems that prevent people from getting about in the normal way.

In the course of human evolution the more general four-legged support of the mammalian body which was concerned entirely with locomotion has given place to locomotion confined to the lower limbs, with the upper limbs becoming specialised for prehensile activities.

THE BONES of the body (**2.1–2.4**) make up its internal supporting framework or skeleton, and can be classified as those of the axial skeleton (head, neck, and trunk) and those of the appendicular skeleton (limbs). Bones can also be classified according to their shapes, as long (the main limb bones), short (as in fingers and toes), flat (like the scapula or shoulderblade), irregular (as in the skull, vertebral column, hand, and foot), and sesamoid (found in some tendons; the largest is the patella or kneecap).

A few bones (clavicle, mandible, and some other skull bones) develop in fetal life by groups of connective-tissue cells becoming transformed into bone-forming cells (osteoblasts); this is 'ossification in membrane', or intramembranous ossification, and the site where the bone is first formed is a primary centre of ossification. However, most bones are formed first as cartilage which is later destroyed and then replaced by bone in the process known as endochondral ossification ('ossification in cartilage'). The cartilaginous shaft of a long bone, for example, develops in early fetal life a primary ossification centre from which bone formation spreads throughout the length of the shaft, but the ends of the bone remain cartilaginous until about the time of birth or later; only then do the ends (called epiphyses) develop their own or secondary centres of ossification. Although subject to some variation, each bone has its own characteristic time pattern for the appearance of ossification centres. Radiographs in children and adolescents show that epiphyses are separated from the shaft by a gap, the epiphyseal line (see **4.13B**) which is due to the remaining plate of cartilage (the epiphyseal plate, which is radiolucent, not radiopaque like bone, and must not be mistaken for a fracture line). It is the site where much of the growth in length of the bone occurs. When growth is complete, the epiphyseal cartilage disappears.

The sites at which bones are held to one another are the joints or articulations; they are of three types – fibrous, cartilaginous, and synovial.

Fibrous joints – bones united by fibrous tissue, allowing no movement, as in skull sutures.

Cartilaginous joints – bones united by plates of cartilage, sometimes allowing limited movement, as at intervertebral discs between the bodies of vertebrae and the pubic symphysis between the front ends of the two hip bones. The junctions between the shafts and epiphyses of developing bones are also a type of cartilaginous joint, although they disappear as growth ceases.

Synovial joints – typical joints of the limbs, and what most people understand by the word joint. The bone ends are covered by cartilage and surrounded by a fibrous capsule that encloses a joint cavity. The capsule is reinforced by ligaments on the outside and sometimes has other ligaments inside. The inside of the capsule is lined by synovial membrane, which secretes a minute amount of synovial fluid (the knee joint, the largest, has only 0.5 ml). Synovial joints allow varying degrees of movement and, depending on the shapes of the articulating surfaces, can be classified into various types: ball-and-socket (hip, shoulder), hinge (elbow, interphalangeal joints of fingers and toes), condylar (modified hinge, as at the knee and temporomandibular, or jaw, joint), ellipsoid (modified ball-and-socket, as at the wrist), saddle (saddle-shaped surfaces, as at the base of the thumb), and plane (rather flat surfaces, as between some wrist and foot bones).

The details of individual joints are considered in the chapters for the appropriate regions.

Bones and joints

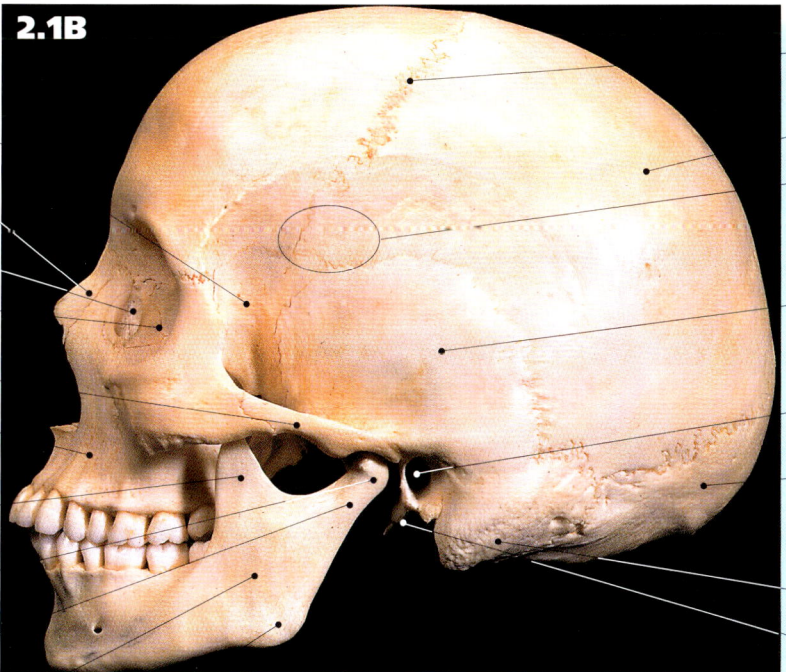

2.1. **Skull.**
A from the front
B From the left
C External surface of the base

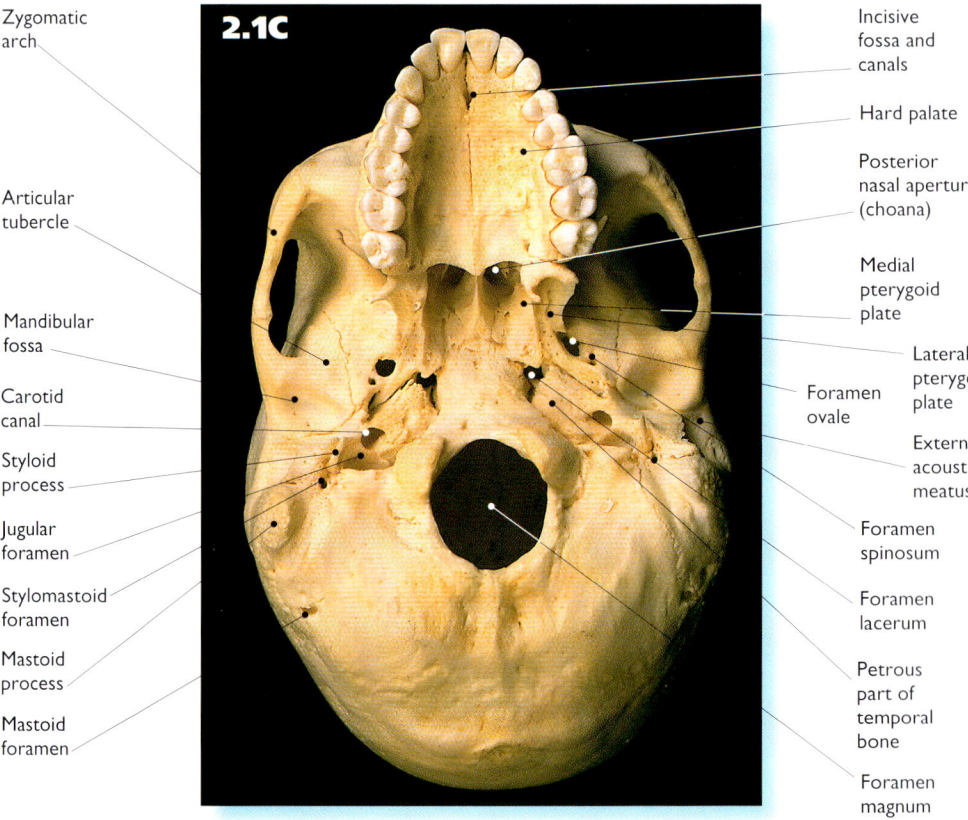

Axial skeleton

The axial skeleton consists of the skull, hyoid bone, vertebrae, ribs and costal cartilages, and the sternum (2.1–2.2).

Skull

The skull (2.1) consists of paired and unpaired bones (a total of 22), most of which are firmly connected by sutures (fibrous joints), except for the mandible, which makes the movable temporomandibular joint (jaw joint, synovial) on each side with the temporal bone. In radiographs, suture lines must not be mistaken for fracture lines.

Cranium – strictly means the skull without the mandible, but is often used to mean the upper part of the skull that encloses the brain; it is made up of paired parietal and temporal bones and of single occipital, sphenoid, ethmoid, and frontal bones. The uppermost part is the cranial vault, the rest is the base of the skull. External features are considered below, and internal features on p. 38.

Pterion – region where parietal, frontal, sphenoid, and temporal bones meet to give an H-shaped pattern of suture lines (2.1B). It lies about 5 cm above the midpoint of the zygomatic arch. Underlying it on the inside is a branch of the middle meningeal artery, liable to be damaged in skull fractures and cause haemorrhage, with resulting pressure on the brain. Bone can be drilled away to ligate the damaged vessel.

Facial skeleton – the front part of the skull, containing the orbital and nasal cavities. The principal bones are the single mandible (lower jaw, with lower teeth) and paired zygomatic bones and maxillae (forming the upper jaw with upper teeth), with the frontal bone forming the forehead. The margins of each orbit are formed by the frontal and zygomatic bones and maxilla. The zygomatic bone is often called the cheek bone. The frontal, ethmoid, and sphenoid bones and the maxillae contain the paranasal air sinuses (p. 67).

External surface of the base
Hard palate – forms the floor of the nose and roof of the mouth (**2.1C**).

Posterior nasal apertures (choanae) – above the back of the hard palate, opening into the nasal part of the pharynx.

Mandibular fossa – in the temporal bone, making the temporomandibular joint (jaw joint) with the head of the mandible.

Occipital condyles – at the side of the foramen magnum, making atlanto-occipital joints with C1 vertebra (atlas).

Mastoid process – part of the temporal bone, forming the bony prominence behind the ear, and containing mastoid air cells which communicate with the middle ear (p. 74).

Hyoid bone
A small U-shaped bone in the front of the neck below the mandible and above the thyroid cartilage of the larynx (see **3.39**), it consists of a central body and a greater horn on each side, with a much smaller lesser horn projecting up from the junction between body and greater horn. Various muscles and ligaments are attached to it but it is unique in that it makes no joint with any other bone.

Vertebrae
There are normally 33 vertebrae – seven cervical, twelve thoracic, five lumbar, five sacral (fused as the sacrum), and four coccygeal (fused as the coccyx), all linked to form the vertebral column (spinal column, spine, or backbone, 'the back') (**2.2**).

Each vertebra typically consists of a body at the front, with at the sides and back a vertebral (neural) arch. The space between the body and arch is the vertebral foramen; in the articulated vertebral column the foramina collectively form the vertebral canal, which contains the spinal cord and the surrounding membranes (p. 53). The arch is made up of a pedicle (attached to the body) on each side and a lamina at the back; two laminae unite to form the spine. From the junction of the pedicle and lamina a transverse process projects laterally, and also superior and inferior articular processes project upwards and downwards. When articulated, the gap between the pedicles of adjacent vertebrae forms the intervertebral foramen, the important opening through which spinal nerves emerge (p. 56).

The first cervical vertebra is the atlas (unique in having no body), which makes joints on each side with the skull above (atlanto-occipital joints) and with the second cervical vertebra, the axis, below (lateral atlanto-axial joints). The unique feature of the axis is the dens (odontoid process), projecting upwards from the body to articulate with the anterior arch of the atlas (median atlanto-axial joint, see **3.5**).

The remaining cervical vertebrae and the thoracic and lumbar vertebrae are united by various ligaments, in particular the anterior and posterior longitudinal ligaments (each of which is a long continuous band on the front and back surfaces, respectively,

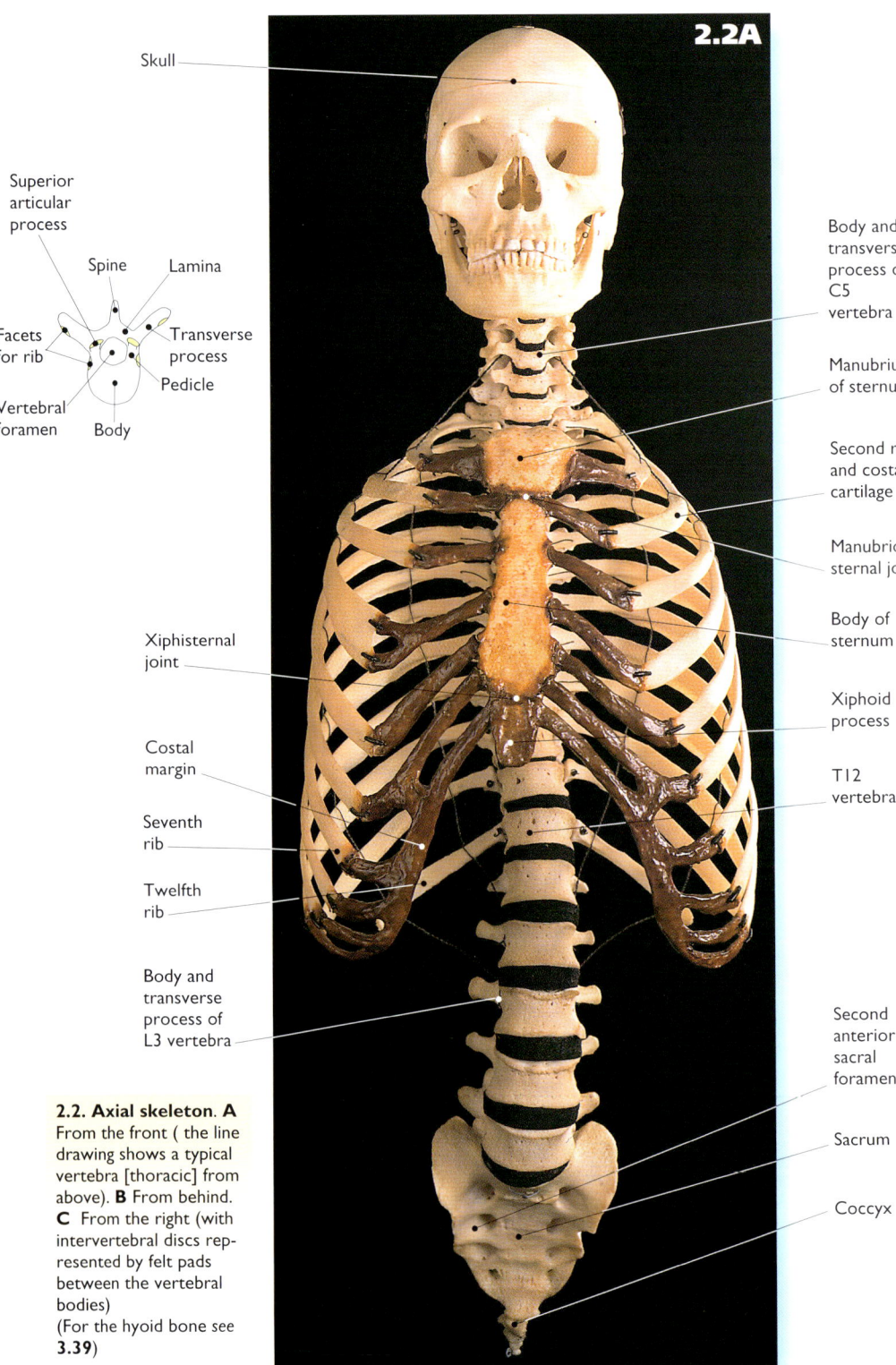

2.2. Axial skeleton. A From the front (the line drawing shows a typical vertebra [thoracic] from above). **B** From behind. **C** From the right (with intervertebral discs represented by felt pads between the vertebral bodies)
(For the hyoid bone see **3.39**)

Bones and joints

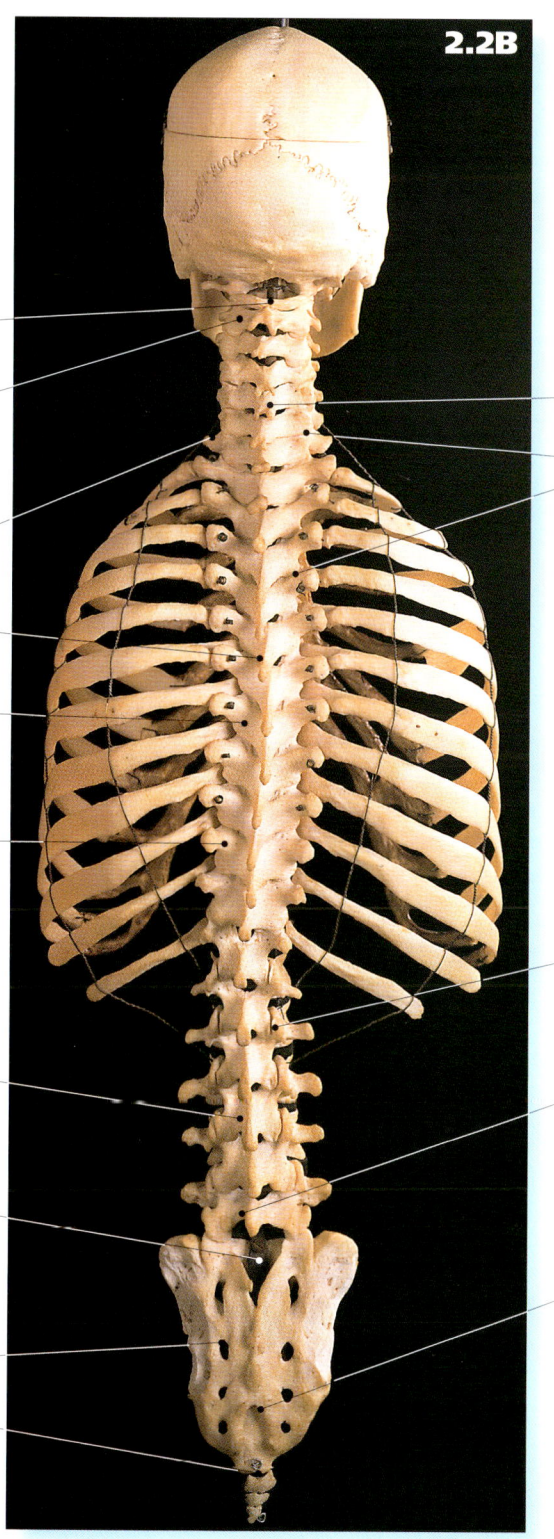

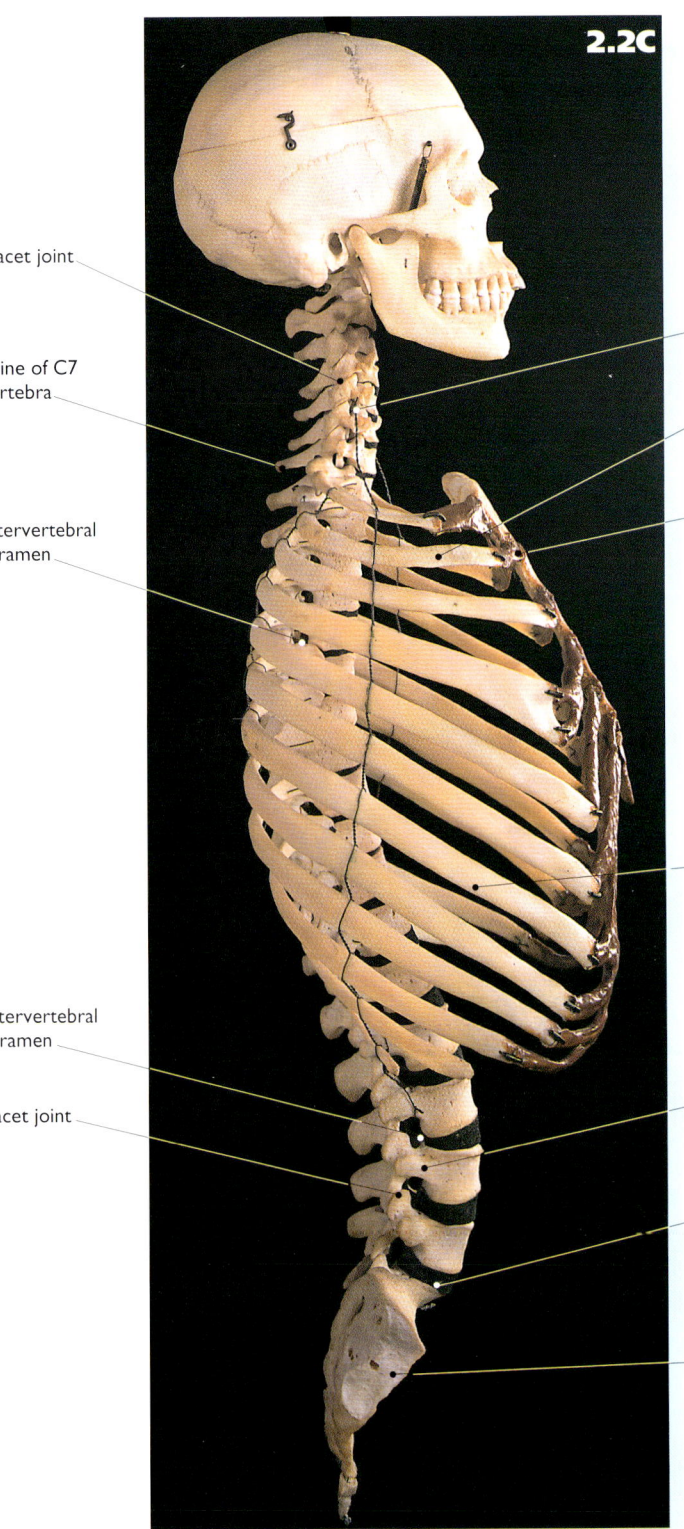

of vertebral bodies) and small joints between the adjacent articular processes (zygapophyseal joints, commonly called facet joints). Ligaments with a high content of elastic tissue, the ligamenta flava ('yellow ligaments'), unite adjacent laminae. Perhaps the most important connections between vertebrae are the intervertebral discs, which act like slightly compressible rubber washers between adjacent vertebral bodies. Each consists of outer concentric rings of fibrocartilage that form the annulus fibrosus, with a central gelatinous mass, the nucleus pulposus. In a prolapsed or 'slipped' disc the nucleus becomes displaced backwards through part of the annulus and may impinge on nerve roots in the vertebral canal. The highest disc is the one between the axis C2 and the C3 vertebra; the lowest (the one most commonly prolapsed) is between the L5 vertebra and the sacrum.

The sacrum consists of the five fused sacral vertebrae, and has four pairs of anterior and posterior sacral foramina (corresponding to the intervertebral foramina in other regions). It is joined to the fifth lumbar vertebra by an intervertebral disc and ligaments, and at the side to hip bones at the sacroiliac joints, forming the bony pelvis, with the coccyx (of four rudimentary coccygeal vertebrae) joined to the lower end of the sacrum at the sacrococcygeal joint.

Ribs and sternum

There are 12 pairs of ribs (**2.2**), articulating with vertebrae behind and with costal cartilage at their front ends. Each rib has a head, which typically articulates with the bodies of two vertebrae, a neck, a tubercle (which articulates with the transverse process of its own vertebra), and a body or shaft of variable length that forms the curved chest wall. The first seven pairs of ribs (true ribs) are joined to the sternum by their costal cartilages. The next three pairs (false ribs) are joined by their cartilages to the cartilage above. The last two pairs (floating ribs) are short and not joined to others.

The sternum consists of the manubrium (at the top), body, and xiphoid process (at the lower end). Along with the ribs, costal cartilages, and the 12 thoracic vertebrae it forms the skeleton of the thorax. The manubrium and body are not quite in line, but unite at a slight angle, the manubriosternal joint (which is cartilaginous, although it may become ossified in later life).

Appendicular skeleton

The appendicular skeleton consists of bones of the upper limbs (**2.3**) and lower limbs (**2.4**), including those of the limb girdles, which are the bones that attach the limb to the axial skeleton (clavicle and scapula, forming the pectoral or shoulder girdle, and the hip bone, consisting of the ilium, ischium, and pubis fused together to form the pelvic or hip girdle).

Upper limb bones

Clavicle – rather S-shaped, with a bulbous medial end for the sternoclavicular joint and a flattened lateral end for the acromioclavicular joint, and a groove on the under surface. The clavicle is the first bone to begin to ossify, between the fifth and sixth week of embryonic life, by intramembranous ossification.

Scapula – roughly like an upside-down triangle, with a prominent spine projecting from the dorsal surface that ends in the acromion, the flattened lateral end of the spine. The upper outer angle is expanded to form the glenoid cavity for the shoul-

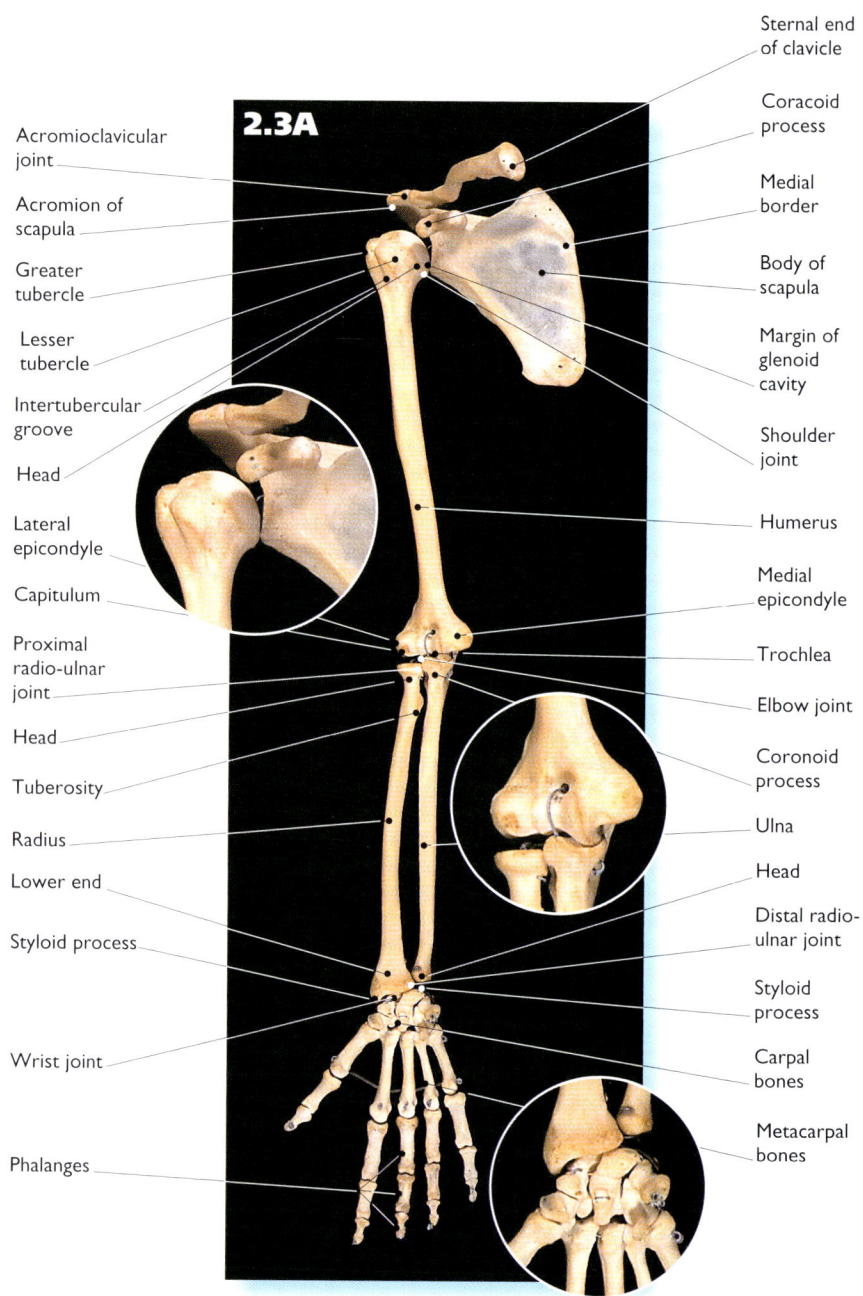

2.3. Bones of the right upper limb. A From the front. **B** From behind. **C** From the right

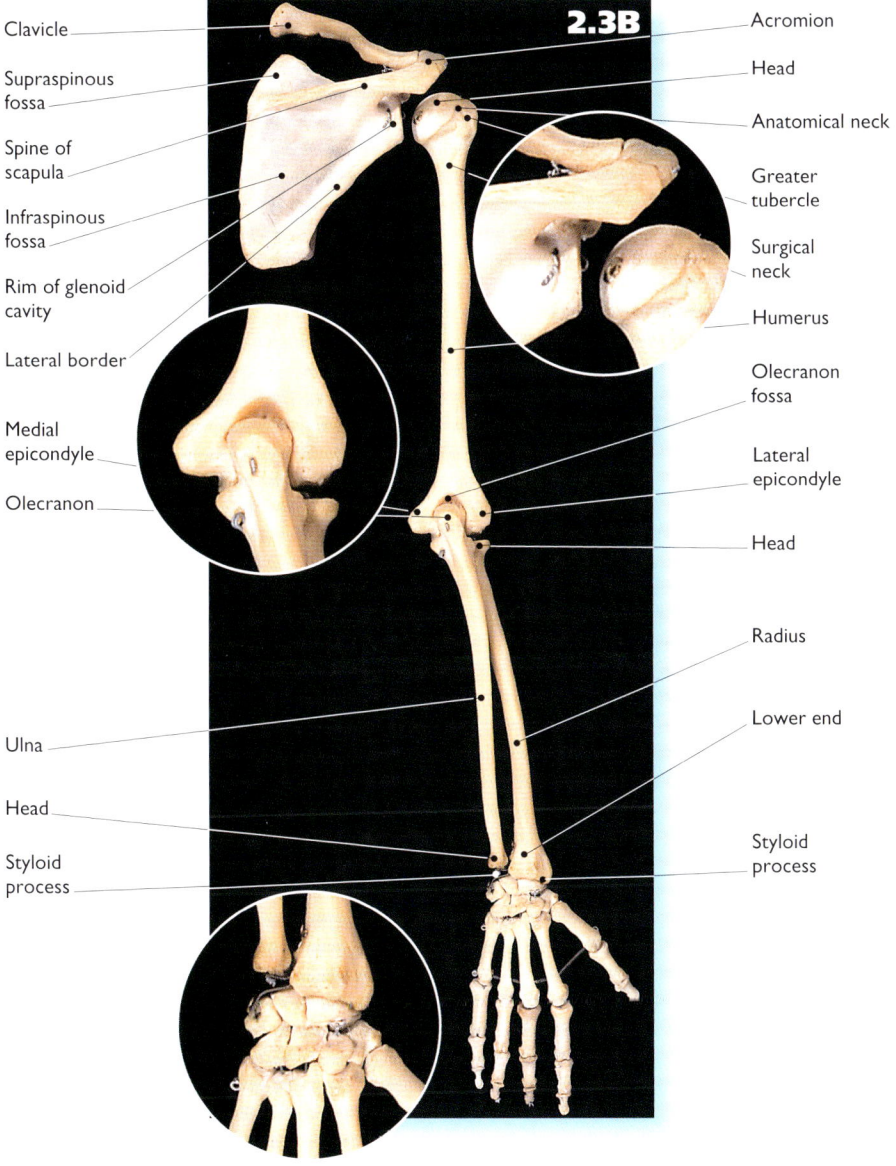

Human Anatomy

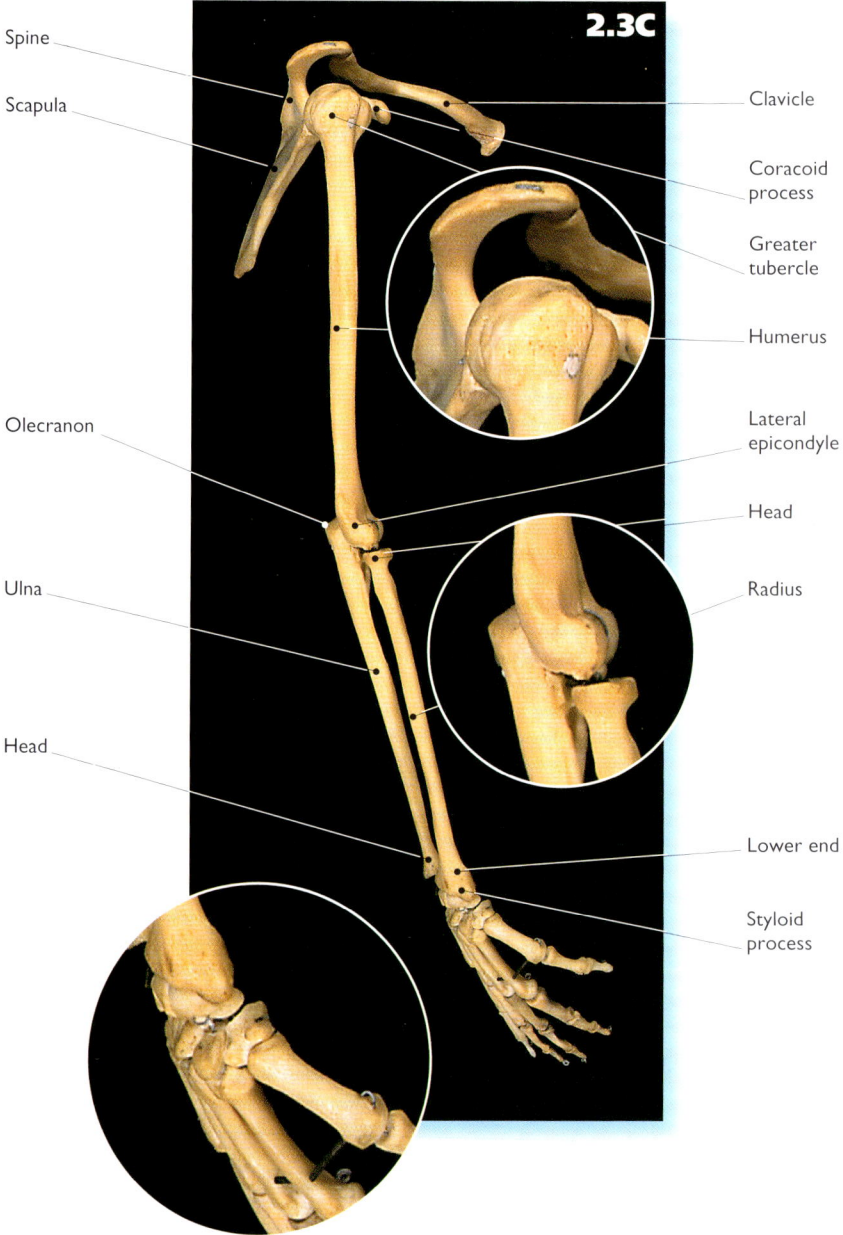

der joint. Projecting forwards above the glenoid cavity is the coracoid process.

Humerus – bone of the arm (upper arm), with a rounded head at the upper end, for the shoulder joint, greater tubercle (tuberosity) at the outer side of the head, lesser tubercle (tuberosity) below the head at the front, with the intertubercular groove (bicipital groove) between them on the front of the upper end of the shaft. The margin of the smooth head is the anatomical neck; the upper part of the shaft below the head is the surgical neck. At the lower end there is a prominent medial epicondyle and a less obvious lateral epicondyle. Between the two are the smooth articular surfaces for the elbow joint: medially, the pulley-shaped trochlea (for the ulna) with a prominent medial lip and, laterally, the rounded capitulum (for the radius). At the back of the lower end is the deep olecranon fossa which accommodates the olecranon of the ulna.

Radius – lateral bone of the forearm, with a rounded upper end which is the head for articulating with the capitulum of the humerus. The shaft immediately below the head is the neck, below which, on the medial side, is the radial tuberosity (for attachment of the biceps tendon). The lowest lateral part of the expanded lower end, which takes part in the wrist joint, is the styloid process.

Ulna – medial bone of the forearm, with the upper end deeply depressed at the front as the trochlear notch (whose posterior boundary is the olecranon) for articulation with the trochlea of the humerus. The small rounded lower end is the head, with the styloid process on its medial side. (Note: the head of the radius is its upper end; the head of the ulna is its lower end.)

Carpal bones – bones of the wrist. The eight small carpal bones each have their own characteristic sizes and shapes, details of which need not be learned. The important point is to remember the order of the bones in the two rows of four from the lateral to the medial side – in the proximal row, the scaphoid, lunate, triquetral, and pisiform bones; and in the distal row, the trapezium, trapezoid, capitate, and hamate bones. The scaphoid, lunate, and triquetral bones take part in the wrist joint. The most important carpal bones are the scaphoid (commonly fractured) and the lunate (uncommonly dislocated). The trapezium and the base of the first metacarpal make the carpometacarpal joint of the thumb, the most important of the carpometacarpal joints.

Metacarpal bones and phalanges – bones of the hand and fingers. Each has a shaft with a base at the proximal end and a head at the distal end, so that the heads and bases of adjacent bones make carpometacarpal, metacarpophalangeal, and interphalangeal joints for each digit.

Lower limb bones

Hip bone – three bones fused together, the ilium, ischium, and pubis. Parts of all three form the cup-shaped acetabulum on the outer surface, for the hip joint. The upper part is the ilium, whose upper margin is the iliac crest, ending at the front at the anterior superior iliac spine. The medial surface forms the sacroiliac joint with the sacrum. The rough lower part of the hip bone is the tuberosity of the ischium, and the front part is the body of the pubis (which in the whole pelvis unites with its fellow at the pubic symphysis). The large hole in the lower part is the obturator foramen. The ischial spine projects between the greater and lesser sciatic notches,

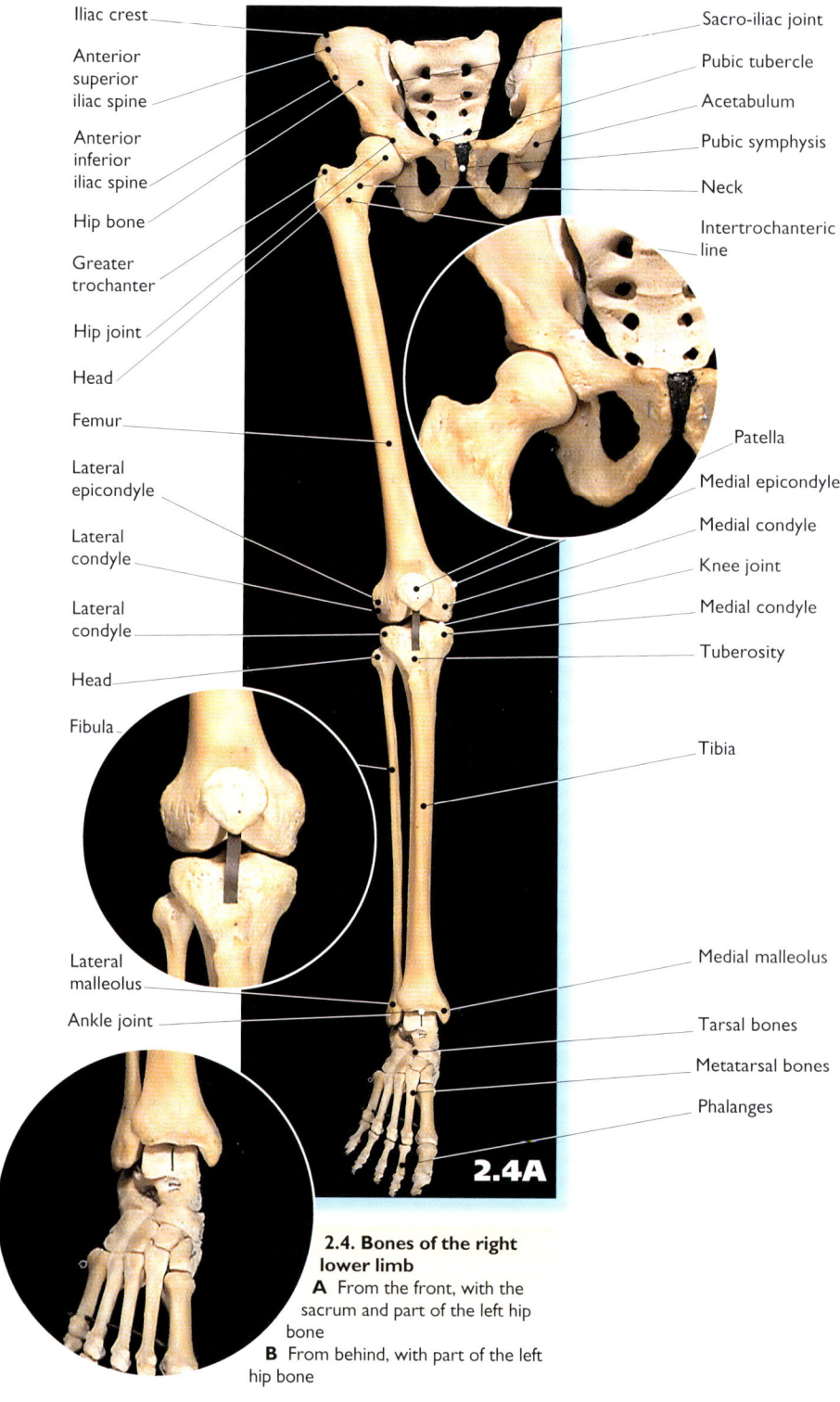

2.4. Bones of the right lower limb
 A From the front, with the sacrum and part of the left hip bone
 B From behind, with part of the left hip bone

Bones and joints

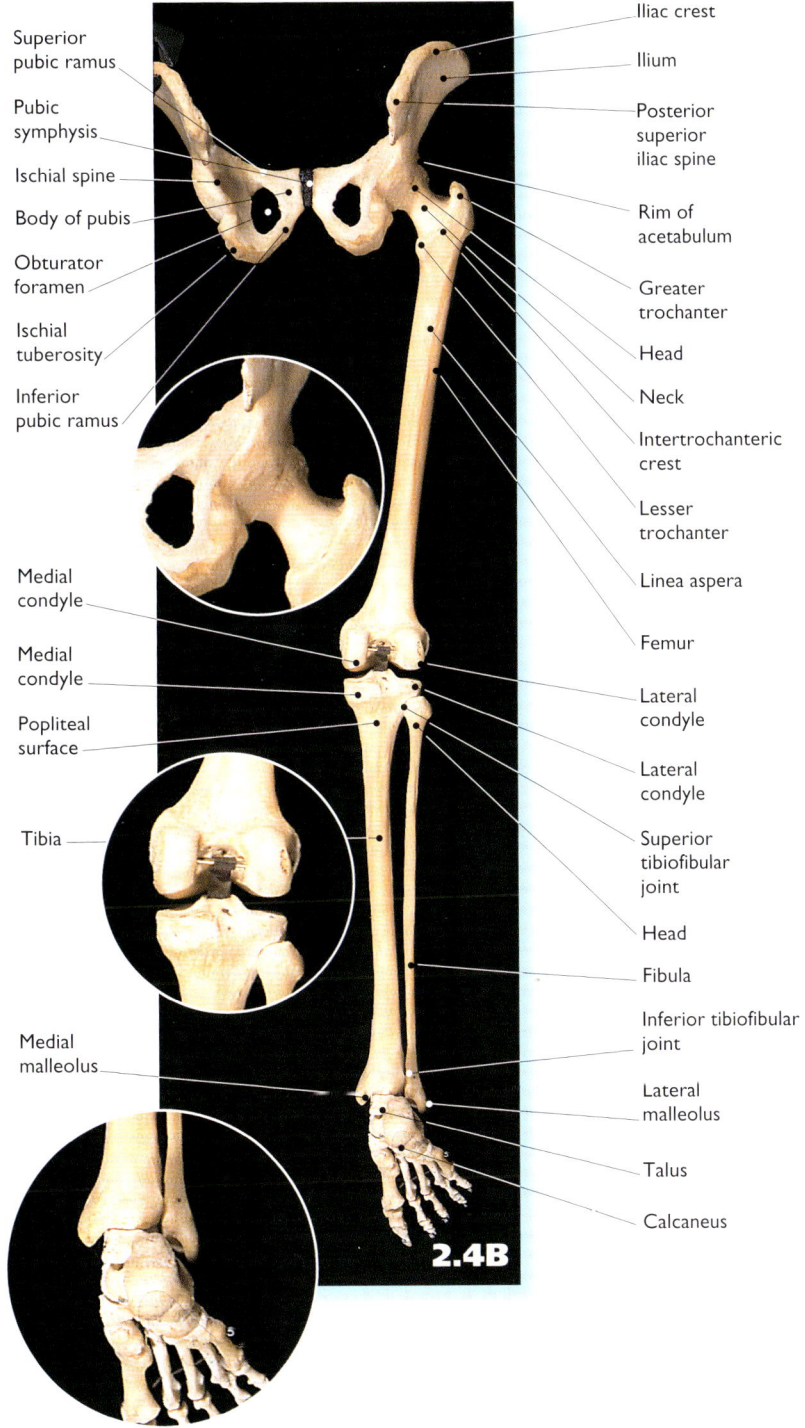

2.4B

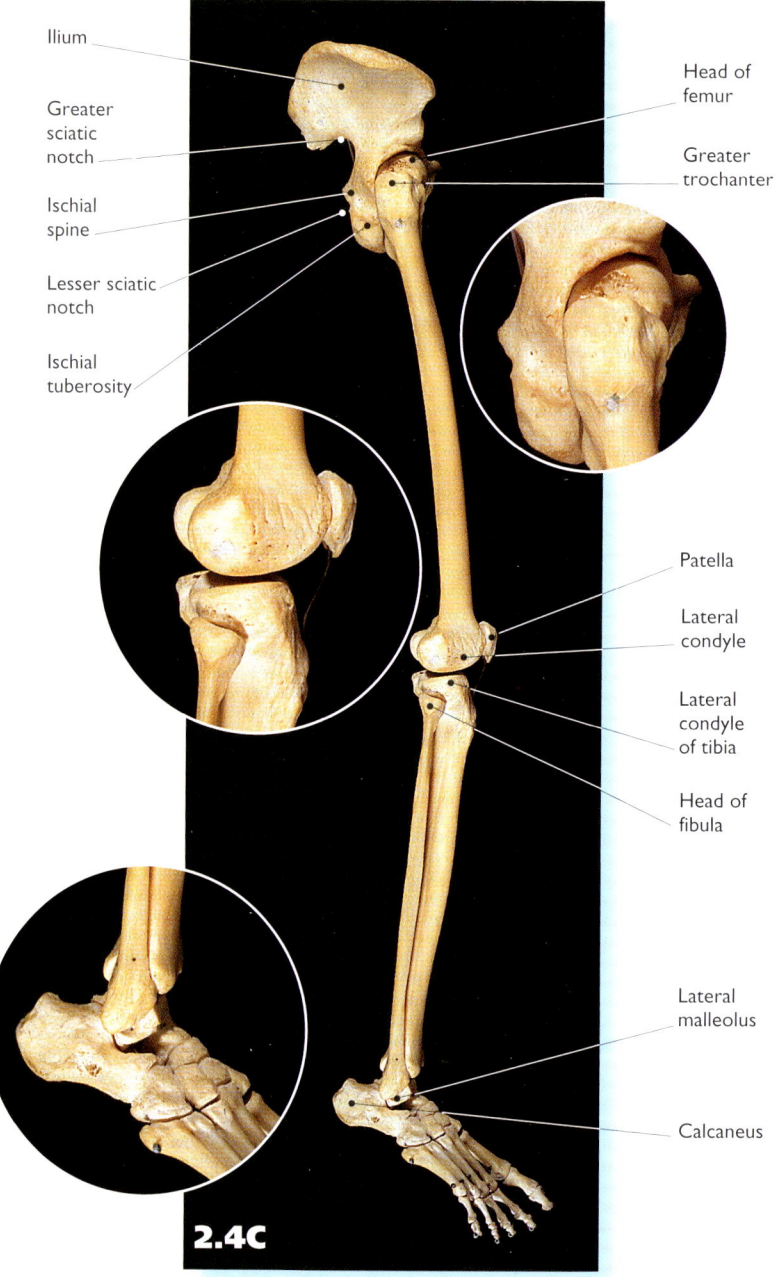

which are converted into the greater and lesser sciatic foramina by the rather small and transversely placed sacrospinous ligament and by the larger and tough, almost vertical, sacrotuberous ligament. The sacrum (with the coccyx at its lower end) and the two hip bones form the bony pelvis.

Femur – bone of the thigh, with the ball-shaped head at the upper end for the hip joint; it is joined to the shaft by the neck at an angle of about 125°. The greater trochanter is the large prominence at the upper junction of the shaft and neck; the lesser trochanter is the smaller cone-shaped projection at the lower part of the neck and adjacent shaft, facing medially and backwards. The expanded lower end has medial and lateral epicondyles at each side and curved medial and lateral condyles for the knee joint. The epiphysis at the lower end should begin to ossify in the ninth fetal month – a fact of possible medicolegal significance as an indication of maturity.

Patella – kneecap, of which the posterior surface is smooth with facets for articulating with the condyles of the femur, and the lower end is rather pointed compared with the upper end.

Tibia – medial and main bone of the leg, of which the large upper end has flat medial and lateral condyles for the knee joint, with the tibial tuberosity in the centre of the front of the shaft below the condyles. The medial surface of the shaft is flat and subcutaneous and commonly called the shin. The smaller lower end has the medial malleolus on its medial side and an articular surface for the ankle joint.

Fibula – lateral and non-weight-bearing bone of the leg, with the slightly expanded upper end, the head, having an *oblique* articular facet on its upper surface for the superior tibiofibular joint. The thin shaft has a rather flattened lower end, the lateral malleolus, with a *vertical* articular facet on its medial surface for the ankle joint.

Tarsal bones – bones of the hind part of the foot. The talus and calcaneus are the most important of the seven tarsal bones. The talus, with a convex upper surface, lies below the tibia and is gripped between the two malleoli to form the ankle joint. The rounded head of the talus faces forwards to articulate with the navicular bone and the calcaneus, and there is a concave articular facet on the under surface for another joint with the calcaneus. The calcaneus is the largest foot bone, forming the heel, with facets on the upper surface for joints with the talus; it is the only tarsal bone with an epiphysis (on the posterior surface). The projection on the medial side is the sustentaculum tali, which forms part of the support for the talus. The navicular bone is in front of the talus on the medial side, with the three cuneiform bones in front of the navicular bone. On the lateral side, the cuboid bone is in front of the calcaneus.

Metatarsal bones and phalanges – like the corresponding metacarpal bones and phalanges in the hand, each metatarsal bone and phalanx has a shaft with a base at the proximal end and a head at the distal end, to make tarsometatarsal, metatarsophalangeal, and interphalangeal joints. The most important is the metatarsophalangeal joint of the great toe.

Arches of the foot – medial and lateral, longitudinal and transverse. Because of the orientation of the calcaneus, which does not lie flat, but is angled upwards, and of the shapes of other bones, the foot has an arched form. The medial longitudinal arch is composed of the calcaneus, talus,

Summary

- The **backbone** of the body is the spine or vertebral column. Its component vertebrae are held together by various small joints and ligaments, including the intervertebral discs which act like shock absorbers between the bodies of individual vertebrae.

- The **skull** sits on top of the cervical part of the spine, with one of its largest bones, the mandible, making the temporomandibular or jaw joint on each side.

- The thoracic part of the spine with ribs and cartilages, and the sternum at the front, form the **thorax**.

- The lumbar part of the spine forms the **central part of the abdomen**, with the two hip bones forming the **bony pelvis**.

- The **main bones of the upper limb** are the humerus, radius and ulna, with the clavicle and scapula forming the pectoral girdle.

- The most important of the small **wrist bones** is the scaphoid bone (the one most frequently fractured).

- The **main bones of the lower limb** are the femur, tibia and fibula, with the hip bone (fused ilium, ischium and pubis) forming the pelvic girdle.

- The largest **foot bone** is the calcaneus or heel bone.

navicular, the three cuneiforms, and the three medial metatarsals (with the two sesamoid bones under the head of the first metatarsal); the lateral longitudinal arch is formed by the calcaneus, the cuboid, and the two lateral metatarsals. The transverse arch (really a half arch in each foot) is made up by the cuneiforms, the cuboid, and the bases of the metatarsals.

Part 3

Head, neck and vertebral column

The head and neck are the most intricate parts of the body, with many major nerves and blood vessels in close proximity to one another. Apart from housing such vital structures as the eye, ear and brain, the head contains the beginning of the alimentary and respiratory tracts, with the pharynx extending into the neck and the larynx (voicebox) branching off the lower pharynx.

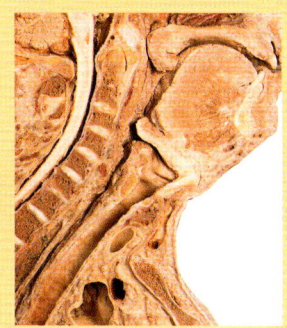

On the under surface of the brain is the pituitary gland, one of the major components of the endocrine system. From the brainstem at the lower part of the brain, and from the spinal cord (which is continuous with the brainstem) within the vertebral column, emerge the cranial and spinal nerves that are responsible for all kinds of motor and sensory activities.

This chapter includes the brain, lying within the cranial cavity of the skull, and the spinal cord, which extends through the cervical and thoracic parts of the vertebral column to the level of L1 vertebra. (See p. 20 for external features of the skull.)

Cranial cavity

In life the cranial cavity is lined by the dura mater (3.1), the outermost and toughest of the three membranes or meninges that cover the brain (p. 49). In places the dura forms partitions that help to keep the brain in place: the falx cerebri, between the two cerebral hemispheres, and the tentorium cerebelli, forming a roof for the posterior cranial fossa, but with a large central gap for the brainstem to pass through. The dura also forms the venous sinuses of the skull (see below).

Anterior cranial fossa – front part of the interior of the skull base (3.2, 3.3) which, on either side, forms the roofs of the orbits and, centrally, the roof of nose. The inferior surfaces of the frontal lobes of the brain lie in this fossa. Adjacent to the midline, where the crista galli projects upwards at the front, the cribriform plates of the ethmoid bone are pierced by the filaments of the olfactory nerve, which run into the olfactory bulb on the under surface of the frontal lobes.

Fractures may cause loss of smell due to rupture of olfactory nerve filaments.

Middle cranial fossa – middle part of the base, butterfly-shaped, with a central part containing the pituitary fossa (with the pituitary gland) and the optic canals. On each side is a lateral part where the temporal lobe of the brain lies, with the cavernous venous sinus adjacent to the pituitary fossa; the internal carotid artery emerges from the roof of the fossa and divides into the anterior and middle cerebral arteries. More laterally, there are grooves for the middle meningeal vessels (liable to be injured at the pterion, p. 20) and the superior orbital fissure, foramen rotundum, foramen ovale, and foramen spinosum.

The pituitary fossa is a key landmark in lateral radiographs of the head.

Fractures may cause haemorrhage from middle meningeal vessels with pressure on the motor area of the cerebral cortex, and, if involving the roof of the temporomandibular joint cavity, leakage of cerebrospinal fluid from the external acoustic meatus.

Pituitary gland – properly called the hypophysis cerebri (3.4), this is a major organ of the endocrine system, and is itself under the control of the hypothalamus (p. 44). It is connected to the floor of the third ventricle by the pituitary stalk, and consists mainly of posterior and anterior parts. The hormones of the posterior pituitary – antidiuretic hormone, which influences urine production by the kidneys, and oxytocin, which stimulates uterine contraction and milk ejection from the breasts – are produced by hypothalamic neurosecretory cells whose fibres store the secretion and run down the pituitary stalk. Although the anterior pituitary is also connected to the stalk, other hypothalamic cells produce controlling factors which pass into a network of very small veins that surround the stalk – the hypophyseal portal system (like a very miniature portal system of the liver, p. 134) – and so reach the anterior pituitary to deliver the stimuli for hormone production by its own cells. The main anterior pituitary hormones are growth hormones and those that control the thyroid and adrenal glands, ovaries, testes, and breasts.

Tumours of the pituitary growing upwards and backwards may press on the optic chiasma causing visual defects.

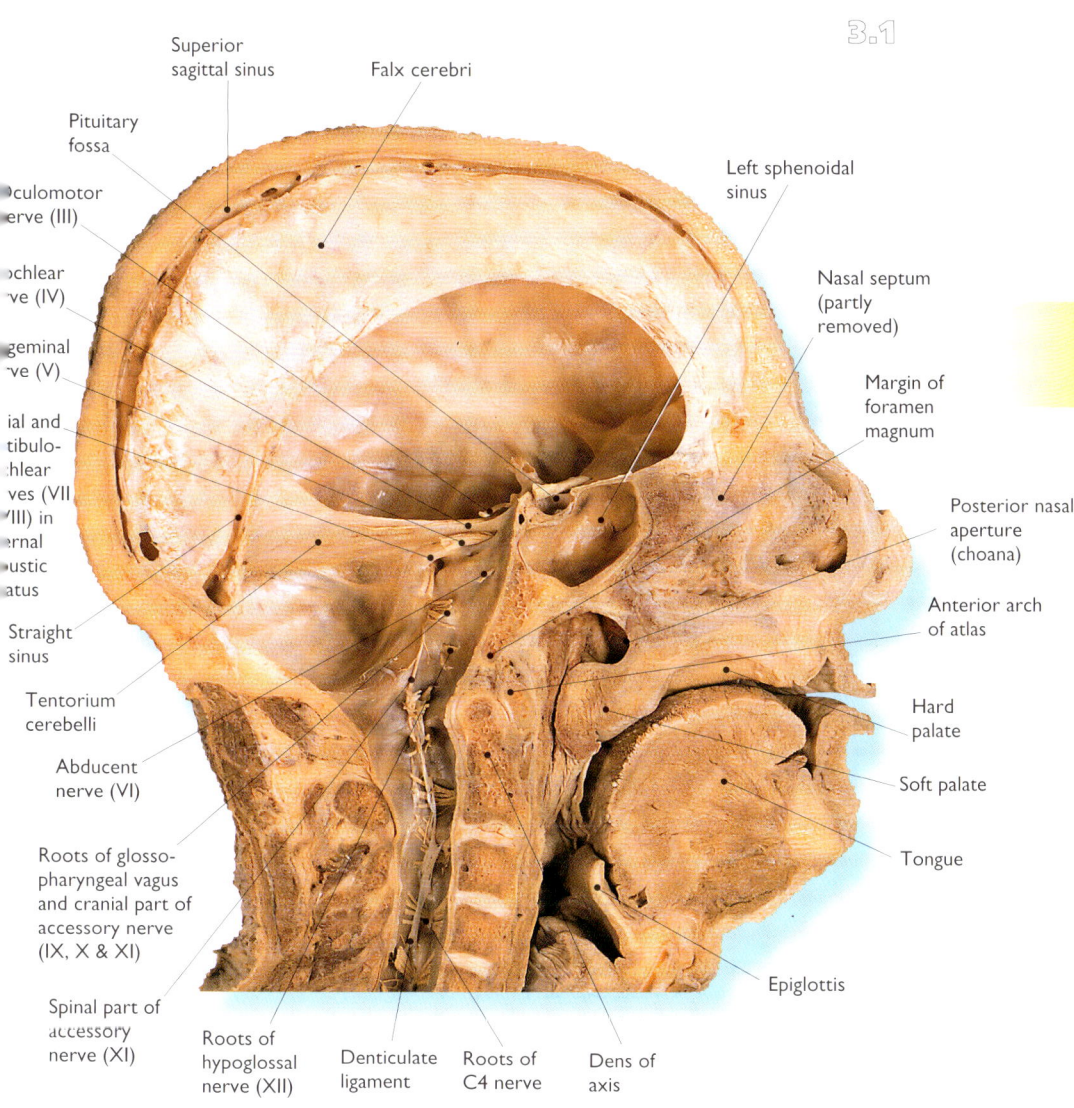

3.1. Left half of the head and cranial cavity (median sagittal section), with the dura mater intact, after removal of the brain and spinal cord (compare with **3.4**)

Human Anatomy

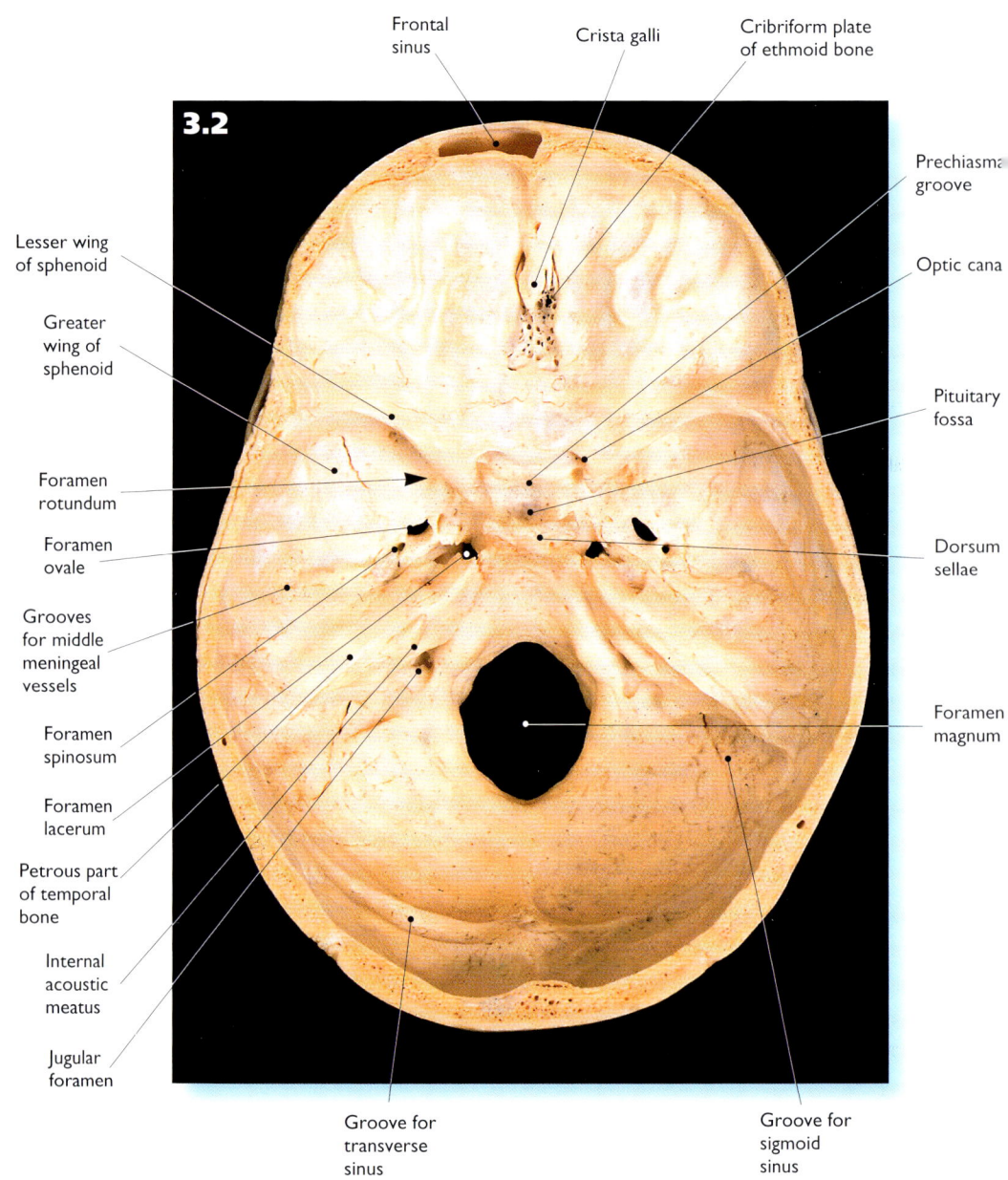

3.2. Internal surface of the base of the skull

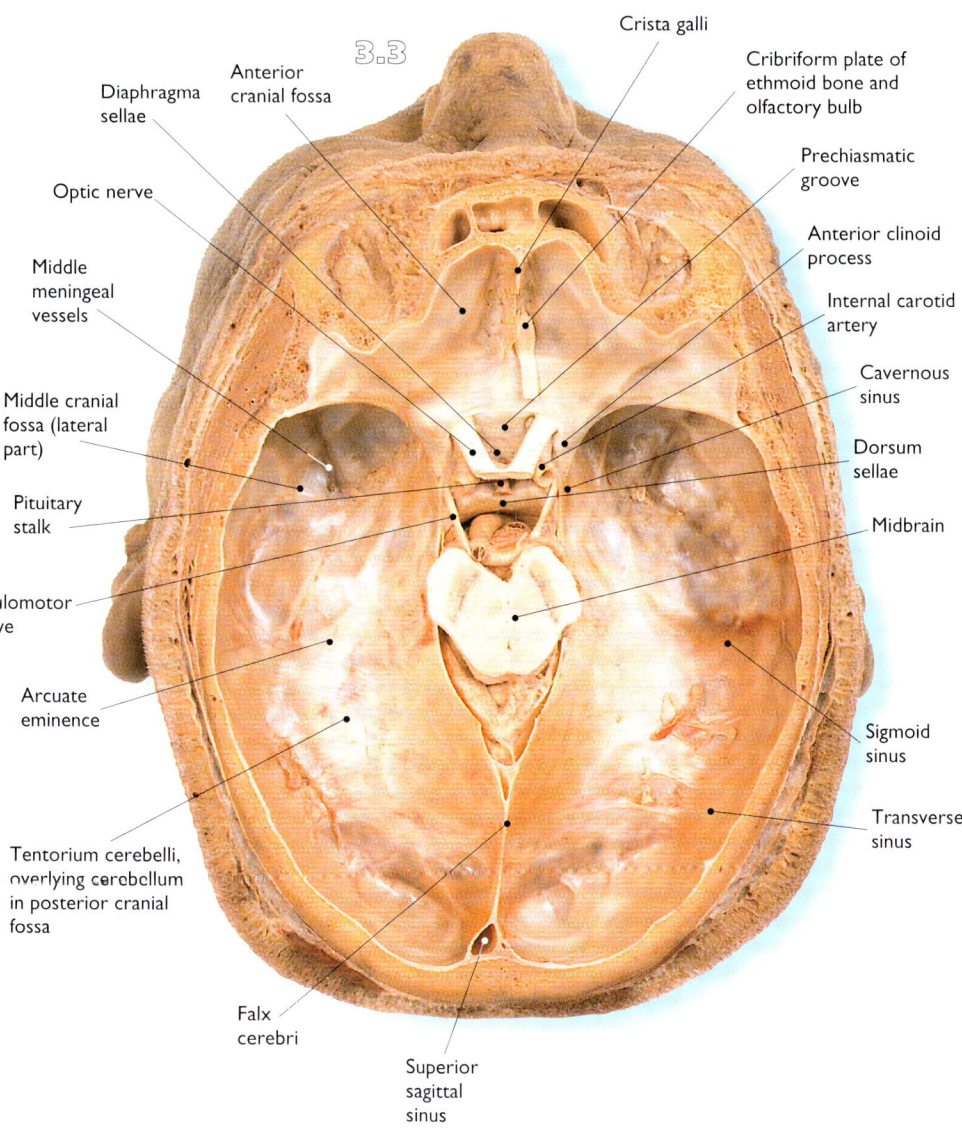

3.3. Cranial fossae, after removal of the brain by cutting through the midbrain part of the brainstem

Posterior cranial fossa – posterior part of the base, containing the foramen magnum and lodging the brainstem and cerebellum, and some large venous sinuses. The petrous part of the temporal bone makes a ridge that separates the middle from the posterior fossa and contains the internal acoustic meatus. At the back and sides of the posterior fossa are grooves for the transverse and sigmoid sinuses. The hypoglossal canal is above the occipital condyle.

Venous sinuses – veins within the skull formed by splitting of the dura mater (**3.1**, **3.3**). The superior sagittal sinus runs back below the midline of the cranial vault, to turn to the right and become the right transverse sinus, which in turn runs down as the sigmoid sinus to the jugular foramen and emerges as the internal jugular vein. The straight sinus receives the great cerebral vein and runs back in the junction of the falx cerebri and tentorium cerebelli, turning to the left as the left transverse sinus, which continues as the left sigmoid sinus and left internal jugular vein. The paired cavernous sinuses lie on either side of the pituitary gland and body of the sphenoid bone. Passing through each cavernous sinus are the internal carotid artery, the three nerves of the extra-ocular muscles (oculomotor, trochlear, and abducent nerves), and the ophthalmic and maxillary branches of the trigeminal nerve.

 These sinuses are important because blood can drain into them from the orbits and face, providing a possible route for infection to reach the inside of the skull.

Other sinuses include the superior petrosal sinus, which runs back from the cavernous sinus, along the top of the petrous part of the temporal bone, to join the transverse sinus, and the inferior petrosal sinus, which also runs back from the cavernous sinus, but at a lower level, in the groove between the petrous temporal and occipital bones, and passes through the jugular foramen to become the highest tributary of the internal jugular vein.

Pituitary fossa – usually indents one or both sphenoidal air sinuses (**3.4**).

Nasal septum – formed by the vomer and the ethmoid bone, but the front part is of cartilage (**3.4A**) and so not present in the bony skull.

Petrous part of temporal bone – commonly called the petrous temporal, it forms the prominent ridge (**3.3**) that is the boundary between the middle and posterior cranial fossae. It contains the internal acoustic meatus.

Hypoglossal canal – lies above the occipital condyle.

Mandibular foramen – in the medial surface of the ramus of the mandible and guarded in front by the spike-like lingula.

Mylohyoid line – oblique ridge on the medial surface of the body of the mandible, for attachment of the mylohyoid muscle, with the groove for the mylohyoid nerve running below it from the mandibular foramen.

Skull foramina

Only the most important skull foramina are listed here, with the principal structures that pass through them (see **2.1C, 3.2**).

Optic canal – optic nerve and ophthalmic artery.

Superior orbital fissure – oculomotor, trochlear, and abducent nerves, and lacrimal, frontal, and nasociliary branches of ophthalmic nerve.

Foramen rotundum – maxillary nerve.

Foramen ovale – mandibular nerve.

Foramen spinosum – middle meningeal vessels.

Foramen lacerum – internal carotid artery, entering at the back and emerging from upper the part.

Carotid canal – internal carotid artery, entering the back of the foramen lacerum.

Internal acoustic meatus – facial and vestibulocochlear nerves.

Jugular foramen – sigmoid sinus (emerging as internal jugular vein), and glossopharyngeal, vagus, and accessory nerves.

Hypoglossal canal – hypoglossal nerve.

Stylomastoid foramen – facial nerve.

Foramen magnum – medulla oblongata, vertebral arteries, and spinal parts of accessory nerves.

Head and neck in sagittal section

Much useful anatomy can be learned from a sagittal section in or very near the midline (**3.4, 3.5**), and the features listed below should be especially noted.

Nose – is at approximately the same level as the cerebellum at the back.

Hard palate – is at approximately the same level as the foramen magnum.

Posterior nasal aperture (choana) – opens into the nasopharynx (nasal part of the pharynx), which has the pharyngeal tonsil (adenoids) on the posterior wall.

Mouth – with the tongue in its floor, opens into the oropharynx (oral part of the pharynx), between the soft palate and epiglottis.

Inlet of the larynx – below the epiglottis, opens into the laryngopharynx (laryngeal part of the pharynx).

Hyoid bone – is at the level of the C3 vertebra.

Thyroid cartilage – is at the level of the C4 and C5 vertebrae.

Cricoid cartilage – is at the level of the C6 vertebra.

Vocal folds (vocal cords) – are at a level midway between the laryngeal prominence (Adam's apple) and the lower border of the thyroid cartilage.

Frontal lobe of the brain – rests on the floor of the anterior cranial fossa.

Human Anatomy

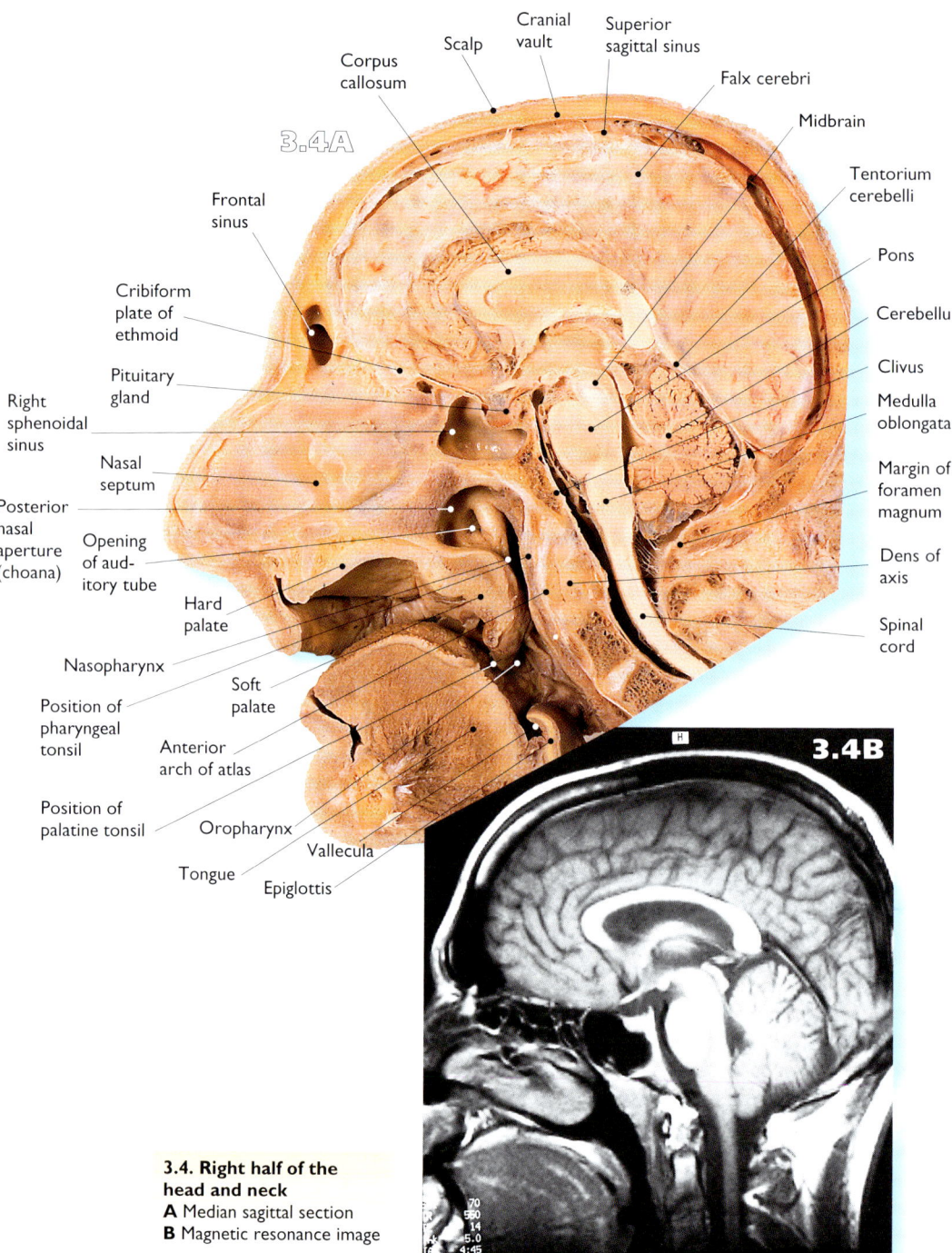

3.4. Right half of the head and neck
A Median sagittal section
B Magnetic resonance image

Head, neck and vertebral column

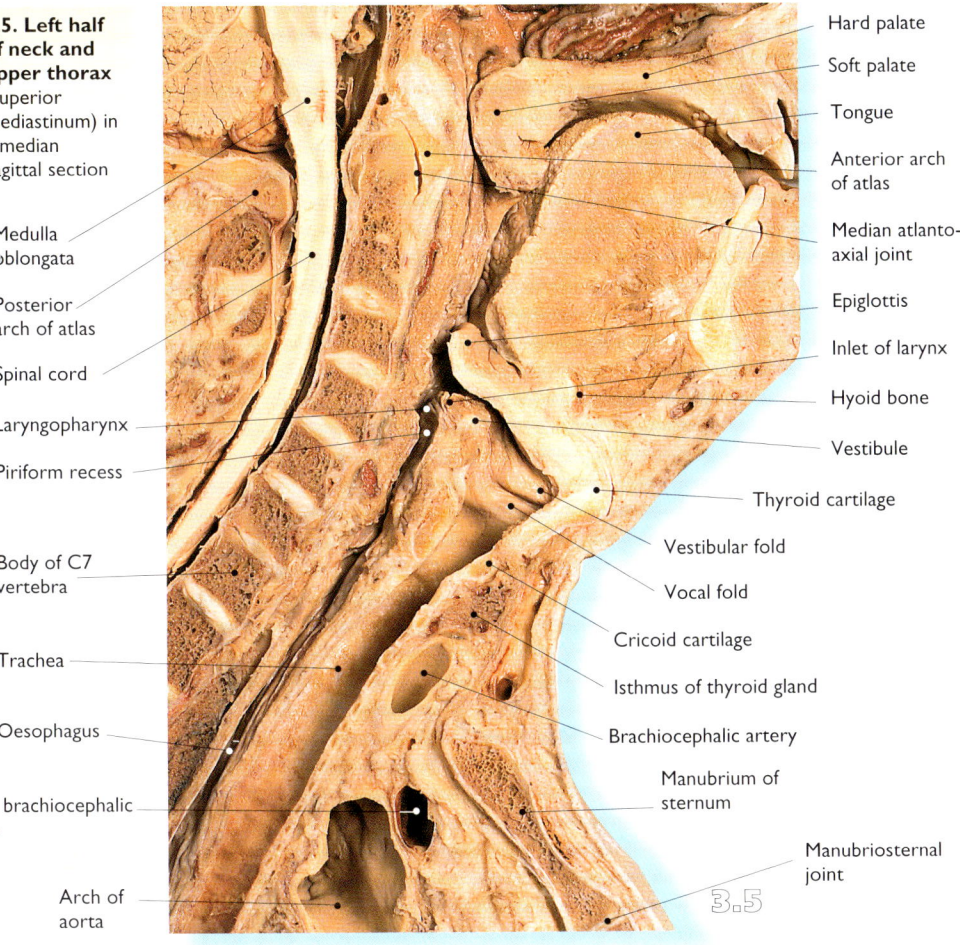

5. Left half of neck and upper thorax (superior mediastinum) in median sagittal section

- Medulla oblongata
- Posterior arch of atlas
- Spinal cord
- Laryngopharynx
- Piriform recess
- Body of C7 vertebra
- Trachea
- Oesophagus
- brachiocephalic
- Arch of aorta
- Hard palate
- Soft palate
- Tongue
- Anterior arch of atlas
- Median atlanto-axial joint
- Epiglottis
- Inlet of larynx
- Hyoid bone
- Vestibule
- Thyroid cartilage
- Vestibular fold
- Vocal fold
- Cricoid cartilage
- Isthmus of thyroid gland
- Brachiocephalic artery
- Manubrium of sternum
- Manubriosternal joint

Falx cerebri – part of the dura mater (p. 36), lies between the cerebral hemispheres; here (3.4) the left hemisphere has been removed to show the surface of the falx, which covers most of the medial surface of the right hemisphere.

Tentorium cerebelli – another part of the dura mater, this separates the lower back parts of the cerebral hemispheres from the cerebellum and forms the roof of the posterior cranial fossa.

Midbrain – upper part of the brainstem (p. 47), passing through the central gap in the tentorium cerebelli.

Pons – middle part of the brainstem, in front of the clivus of the skull.

Medulla oblongata – lower end of the brainstem, passing through the foramen magnum to become the spinal cord at the level of the atlas (C1 vertebra).

Brain, spinal cord and nerves

Brain

The brain (**3.6, 3.7**), consisting of the cerebrum, brainstem, and cerebellum, is the part of the central nervous system that lies within the skull. The functions of certain areas are clearly defined; among the most important are those that control the movements of skeletal muscles (voluntary movement) and those at which various kinds of sensory impressions reach consciousness. Other parts are concerned with the body's own internal control mechanisms (often closely associated with the endocrine system), and with such functions as memory, thought, emotion, and all the vast gamut of behaviour. Attention is focused here only on neurons concerned with major motor and sensory activities.

Gray matter – predominantly nerve cell bodies, concentrated in the cortex on the surface of the cerebral and cerebellar hemispheres (*see* below) and in subcortical groups or nuclei (**3.8**). In each cerebral hemisphere these include the caudate and lentiform nuclei (collectively called the corpus striatum), which, with some other groups, form the basal nuclei, still often called by their old name, basal ganglia, and mainly concerned with helping to coordinate muscular activity. One of the largest and most important cellular masses is the thalamus, the main relay station for conscious sensations on the way to the cerebral cortex. The thalamus forms a slight bulge in the lateral wall of the third ventricle (*see* below), and the region just below this is the hypothalamus, which contains the neurosecretory cells that control the pituitary gland.

White matter – predominantly nerve fibres, concentrated below the cortex and forming communicating networks. Some fibres form well-recognized tracts with specific functions; many have come from or go to the spinal cord, e.g. the main motor tracts, as well as tracts for the different types of sensation and special senses.

Cerebrum – forebrain, with a central part and two cerebral hemispheres, whose surface is thrown into folds or gyri (singular, gyrus), with intervening grooves or sulci (singular, sulcus) (**3.6**). The main connection between the hemispheres is the corpus callosum, a bundle of 200 million nerve fibres, best seen when the brain is bisected longitudinally (**3.7**).

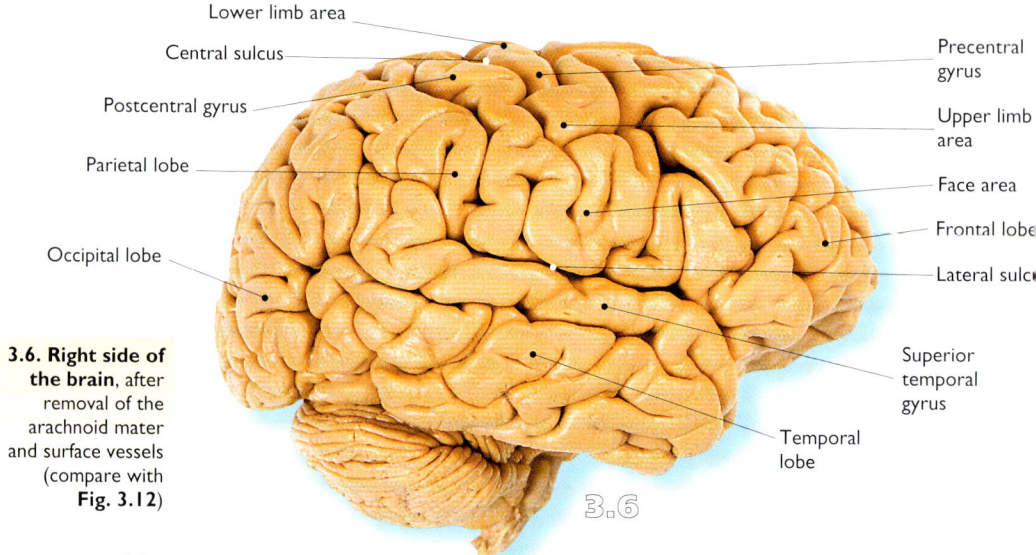

3.6. Right side of the brain, after removal of the arachnoid mater and surface vessels (compare with **Fig. 3.12**)

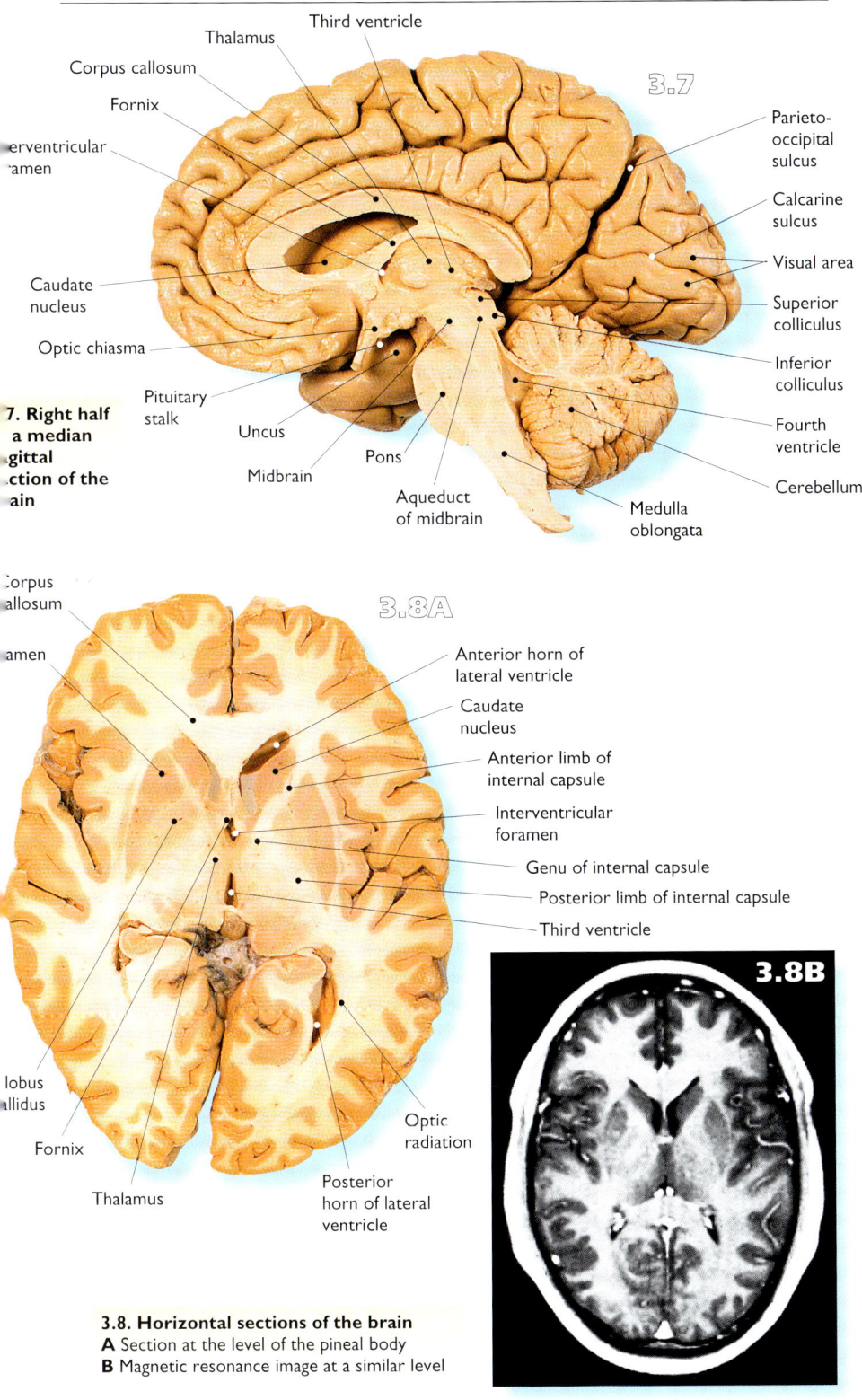

3.7. Right half of a median sagittal section of the brain

3.8. Horizontal sections of the brain
A Section at the level of the pineal body
B Magnetic resonance image at a similar level

Central sulcus – one of the key features of the whole brain, it separates the frontal and parietal lobes (thus separating motor and sensory areas – *see* below), running down the lateral surface from near the middle of the upper margin towards the lateral sulcus (but not continuing directly into it – an identifying feature) (**3.6**).

Precentral gyrus – in front of the central sulcus, at the back of the frontal lobe. It is the *main motor area of cortex* and contains nerve cells responsible for controlling skeletal muscles via connections with the motor nuclei of cranial nerves and anterior horn cells of the spinal cord, with coordinating connections through basal nuclei, thalamus, and cerebellum. The parts of the body are represented 'upside down' in the motor cortex: the lower limb is controlled from the uppermost part (supplied by the anterior cerebral artery), the upper limb in the middle, and the face, larynx, etc., in the lower part (all supplied by the middle cerebral artery). The precise regions concerned with highly important functions, such as finger, thumb, and lip movements, occupy comparatively large areas of cortex.

> Vascular damage to, or pressure on, the motor cortex and the fibres leading from it causes **spastic paralysis**.

Postcentral gyrus – behind the central sulcus, at the front of the parietal lobe. It is the *main sensory area of cortex*, where sensations, such as touch, reach consciousness. There is a similar upside down representation of body parts to that in the motor cortex.

Lateral sulcus – prominent longitudinal sulcus on the lateral surface, separating frontal and temporal lobes. Some cortex of the (usually) left frontal lobe near the front end of the sulcus is the main speech area (Broca's area).

Superior temporal gyrus – in the temporal lobe below the lateral sulcus, it contains the auditory area of cortex, which is for the conscious appreciation of sound.

Calcarine sulcus – on the medial surface of the occipital lobe (**3.7**). The adjacent cortex is the visual area (supplied by the posterior cerebral artery), where visual impulses reach consciousness.

> Thrombosis of the posterior cerebral artery may cause **visual defects**.

Internal capsule – area of white matter between the thalamus and caudate and lentiform nuclei (**3.8, 3.9**). In horizontal sections of the hemisphere it appears rather like a capital L on its side, with an anterior limb, genu, and posterior limb. *It is one of the supremely important areas of the whole brain and, indeed, of the whole body*: through the genu run corticonuclear fibres from the cerebral cortex to the motor nuclei of cranial nerves, and through the posterior limb run corticospinal fibres from the cortex to the anterior horn cells of the spinal cord. Damage to these internal capsule fibres by haemorrhage or thrombosis of the striate arteries (p. 50) results in a 'stroke', with paralysis of the *opposite* side of the body (hemiplegia), because in the medulla of the brainstem most fibres cross over to the opposite side to form the corticospinal tracts (*see* below). Other internal capsule fibres include those that run from the thalamus to sensory areas of the cortex (thalamocortical fibres).

> **Vascular damage** of the internal capsule is the commonest cause of spastic paralysis.

Cerebellum – connected by the superior, middle, and inferior cerebellar peduncles to the midbrain, pons, and medulla, respectively. Through them

Head, neck and vertebral column

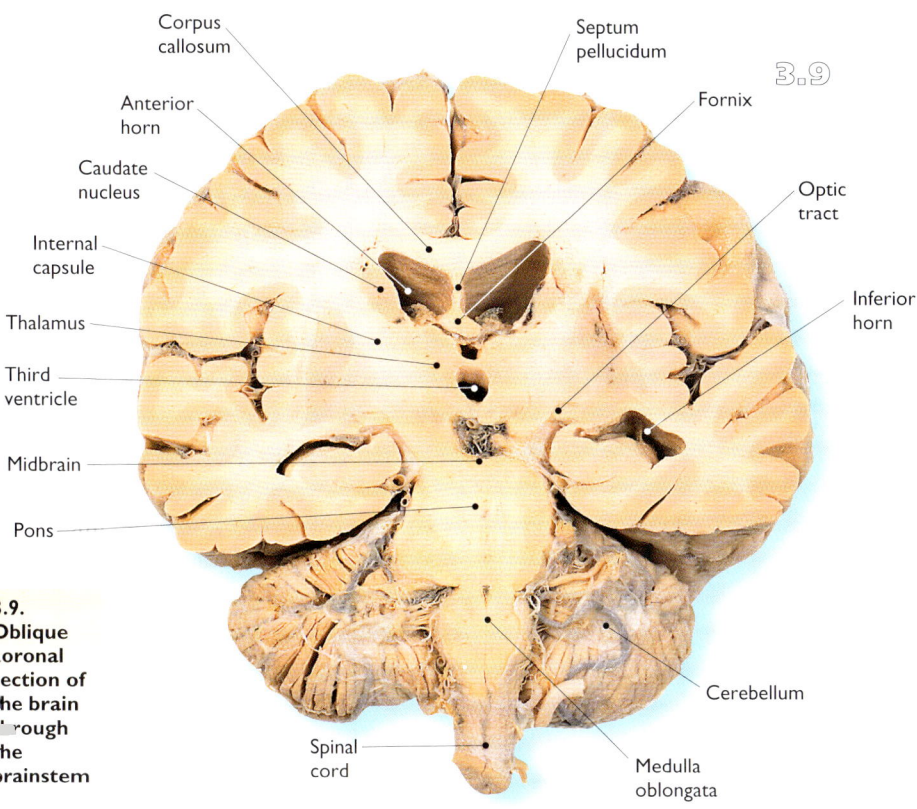

3.9. Oblique coronal section of the brain through the brainstem

it has multiple connections with the rest of the brain and spinal cord. Concerned with muscular coordination, it does not *initiate* movements (that depends on the cerebral cortex), but it helps movements to be carried out in a smooth and controlled manner. The cerebellum has nothing to do with conscious sensation.

Cerebellar disease causes jerky and uncoordinated movements (but not paralysis), tremors and speech defects.

Brainstem – hangs down from the central part of the cerebrum (3.7, 3.10, 3.11) and consists from above downwards of the midbrain, pons, and medulla oblongata (pons, medulla, and cerebellum are sometimes called the hindbrain). In the brainstem are groups of nerve cells (cranial nerve *nuclei*) which either give rise to the motor (efferent) fibres of cranial nerves (p. 50) or receive sensory (afferent) fibres from cranial nerve *ganglia*, situated on the nerves outside the brainstem and corresponding to the posterior root ganglia of spinal nerves (p. 56). Among the fibres that pass through the brainstem to and from other parts of the brain and spinal cord are the motor fibres from the cerebral cortex. They become grouped together to form a bulge, the pyramid, on either side of the midline of the medulla; here, most of the fibres cross to the opposite side (motor decussation or decussation of the pyramids) to form the lateral corticospinal tract that continues into the spinal cord (p. 55).

Respiratory and cardiac centres – certain cell groups in the medulla that are associated with the glossopharyngeal and vagus nerves, they control breathing and heart rate. Death occurs when such control ceases irreversibly; tests carried out to establish whether death has, indeed, occurred are tests of function of different parts of the brainstem, assessed by activity (or rather the lack of activity) in certain cranial nerves and their interconnections within the brainstem.

Ventricles of the brain – cavities within various parts of the brain (3.7–3.9) that contain cerebrospinal fluid (CSF). Each cerebral hemisphere has a lateral ventricle (which includes anterior, posterior and inferior horns) which communicates through an interventricular foramen with a narrow central cavity, the third ventricle, which in turn leads back through the aqueduct of the midbrain to the fourth ventricle, at the back of the brainstem with a tent-like bulge towards the cerebellum.

Tests for brainstem death are necessary to determine whether organs can be removed for transplantation.

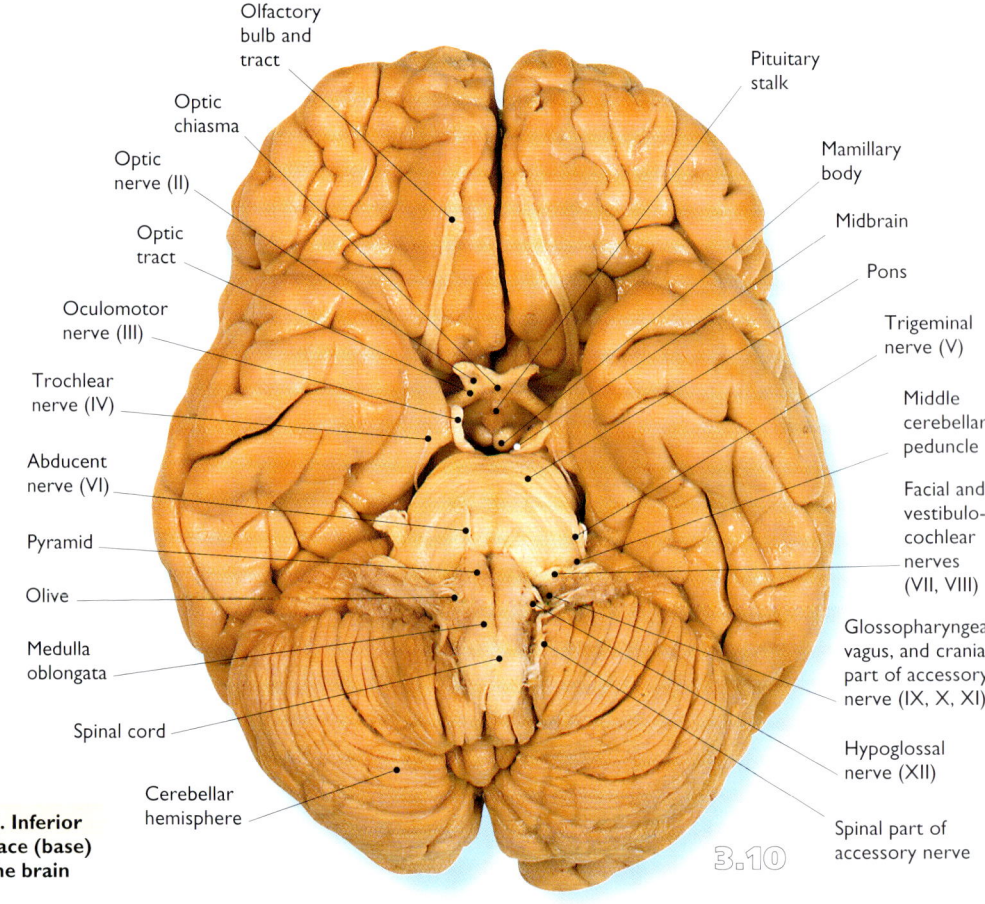

3.10. Inferior surface (base) of the brain

Head, neck and vertebral column

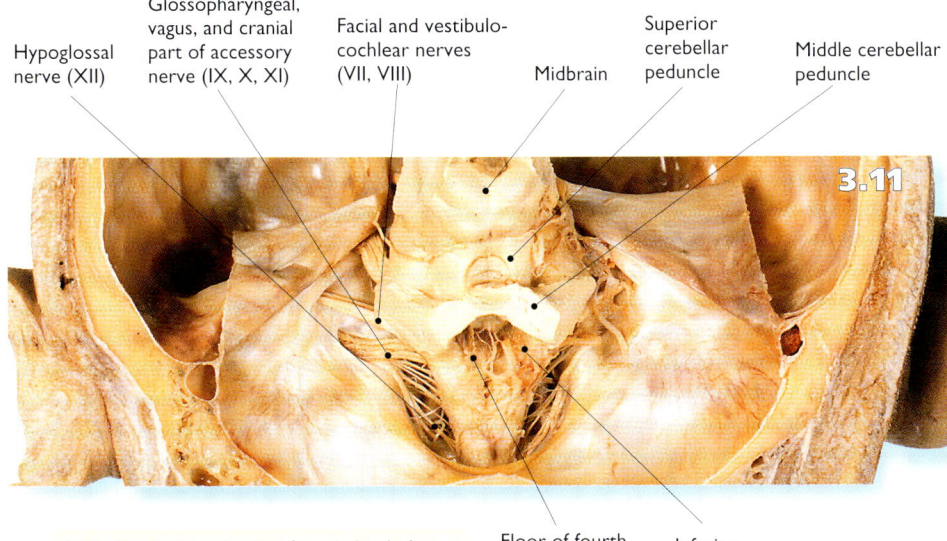

3.11. Brainstem *in situ*, from behind after removal of the cerebrum and cerebellum

Cerebrospinal fluid – total volume about 130 ml, it acts as a protective waterbath to support the brain and spinal cord, and also as a medium for exchange of materials to and from nervous tissue. It is constantly secreted from specialized blood capillaries, the choroid plexuses, within parts of the lateral, third, and fourth ventricles. From each lateral ventricle, CSF passes through the interventricular foramen into the third ventricle, and then through the aqueduct of the midbrain into the fourth ventricle. From the back of the fourth ventricle below the cerebellum, CSF escapes from the ventricular system into the subarachnoid space (*see text below*) through three small apertures in the arachnoid – one median and two lateral. Since it is continuously secreted, CSF must be constantly absorbed; this occurs into the bloodstream through arachnoid granulations that project into the superior sagittal sinus at the top of the cranial cavity.

Obstruction to the outflow of CSF results in **hydrocephalus** (enlargement of the ventricular system).

Meninges – membranes that enclose the brain and spinal cord. The outermost, the dura mater (**3.1**), is described on p. 36. Lying in contact with the inside of the dura is the arachnoid mater (**3.12**), a much thinner membrane with thin spidery processes that connect it to the even thinner pia mater, which is part-and-parcel of the brain surface. In life, the subarachnoid space between the arachnoid and pia is filled with CSF. When the brain is removed from the skull, the arachnoid (not the dura) should come with it, although it may be torn in places (e.g. when cutting through cranial nerves and brainstem). These same three meninges continue through the foramen magnum to surround the spinal cord within the vertebral canal.

Blood supply of the brain – by the vertebral and internal carotid arteries, whose branches form the arterial circle

49

(of Willis) on the base of the brain (**3.13**). The vertebral artery (from the subclavian, running up through the foramina in the upper six cervical vertebrae) enters the skull through the foramen magnum and unites with its fellow to form the single midline basilar artery, which lies on the ventral surface of the pons. It divides into the two posterior cerebral arteries – each is joined by the posterior communicating artery to the internal carotid as that vessel divides into the middle cerebral artery (which runs laterally in the lateral sulcus to emerge on the lateral surface of the cerebral cortex) and the anterior cerebral artery (which is united to its fellow by the very short anterior communicating artery and runs on to the medial surface of the cerebral hemisphere). Apart from cortical, brainstem, and cerebellar branches, there are very small but highly important striate branches of the anterior and middle cerebral arteries which penetrate the brain substance to supply the internal capsule (p. 46).

> Anterior and middle cerebral vascular lesions cause **paralysis**; posterior cerebral lesions cause **visual defects**.

Various cerebral veins, which usually do not accompany arteries, drain into adjacent venous sinuses. Like veins of the heart, they are singularly unaffected by disease.

Cranial nerves

The cranial nerves (**3.10**, **3.11**) can be referred to by their names or numbers (by long tradition in Roman figures, or as first, second, third, etc.).

> The cranial nerves most commonly damaged are I, II, III, VI and VII (the commonest of all).

I Olfactory – the nerve for smell (olfaction), it is formed by about 20 nerve filaments

> Tearing of all nerve filaments of one side gives complete **anosmia** (loss of smell) on that side.

which pierce the roof of the nose (cribriform plate of the ethmoid bone) to enter the olfactory bulb of the brain in the anterior cranial fossa. From the bulb fibres pass directly to the cerebral cortex (of the uncus of the temporal lobe) without synapse in the thalamus – an afferent pathway unique to olfaction, since all other senses involve the thalamus on their way to the cortex.

II Optic – the nerve for vision, it is formed by fibres from the retina of the eye and passes back through the optic canal to the optic chiasma (see Visual pathway, p. 72).

> A complete lesion of one optic nerve causes complete blindness in that eye.

III Oculomotor – the motor nerve to four of the six muscles that move the eye (medial, superior and inferior rectus, and inferior oblique), and to the levator muscle of the upper eyelid. It also carries parasympathetic fibres via the ciliary ganglion to constrict the pupil for light reflexes and accommodation (adjusting the shape of the lens and pupil for near vision, p. 72). It leaves the brainstem near the midline of the midbrain and runs through the cavernous sinus to enter the orbit through the superior orbital fissure.

> Paralysis of each of the three 'eye nerves' (III, IV and VI) gives squint (strabismus) and double vision (diplopia), and the eye takes up a characteristic position for each nerve affected.

IV Trochlear – the smallest cranial nerve and the only one to emerge from the dorsal surface of the brainstem (from the midbrain behind the inferior colliculus). It is the motor nerve to the superior oblique muscle of the eye, and runs through the cavernous sinus to enter the orbit through the superior orbital fissure.

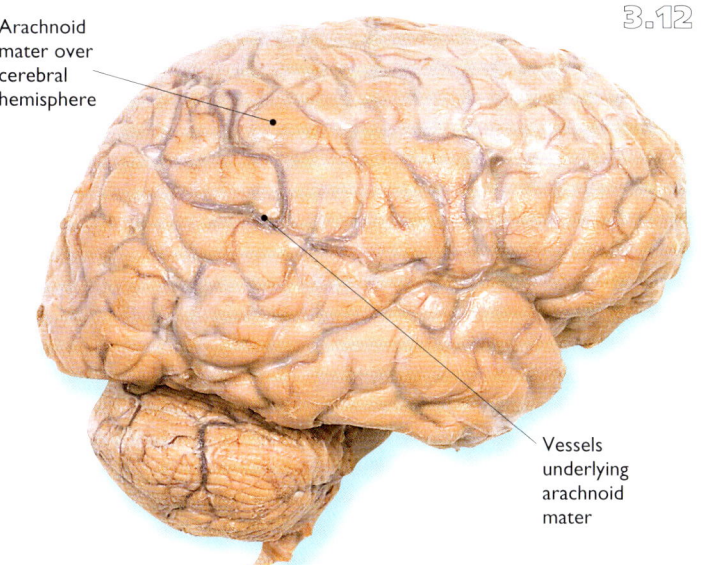

3.12. Right side of the brain, as removed from the skull with the arachnoid mater intact

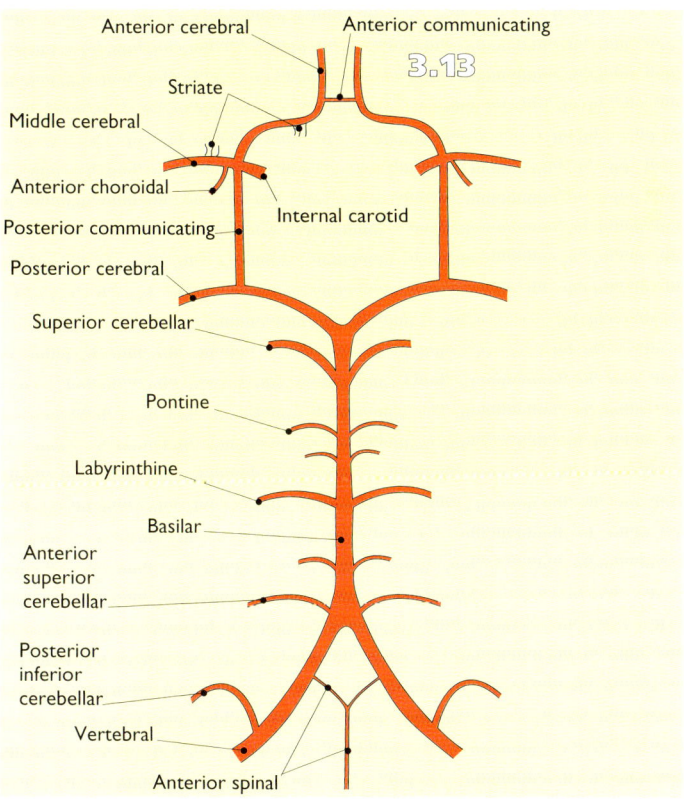

Fig. 3.13. Arterial circle at the base of the brain. The vessels 'fit on' to **Fig. 3.10**, with the basilar artery lying over the pons and the anterior cerebral arteries lying deep to the optic nerves

V Trigeminal – the largest cranial nerve, it supplies through its three branches – the ophthalmic, maxillary, and mandibular nerves – sensory fibres for many structures in the head, including much of the skin of the face and scalp, and the mucous membranes of the nose, mouth, palate, and pharynx, the teeth, the conjunctiva, and (most important of all) the cornea of the eye. Motor fibres for the muscles of mastication run in the mandibular nerve. The main nerve leaves the brainstem at the junction of the pons and middle cerebellar peduncle, and passes over the apex of the petrous part of the temporal bone to enter the trigeminal cave of dura mater (Meckel's cave), where the trigeminal ganglion (with afferent cell bodies) is situated. The three branches diverge from the ganglion: the ophthalmic nerve passes through the cavernous sinus and enters the orbit through the superior orbital fissure; the maxillary nerve also passes through the sinus and then through the foramen rotundum; and the mandibular nerve runs downwards through the foramen ovale.

VI Abducent – the motor nerve to the lateral rectus muscle of the eye. It leaves the brainstem at the junction of the pons and the pyramid of the medulla, and passes through the cavernous sinus to enter the orbit through the superior orbital fissure.

VII Facial – the motor nerve for the muscles of the face (but not the skin, which is the trigeminal nerve), with some fibres for the special sensation of taste from the anterior part of the tongue, and parasympathetic secretomotor fibres for the submandibular and sublingual glands (via the submandibular ganglion) and for the lacrimal gland (via the pterygopalatine ganglion) by fibres distributed via branches of the trigeminal nerve. The facial nerve leaves the brainstem at the junction of the pons and medulla to enter the internal acoustic meatus and run through the temporal bone, lying medial to and then behind the middle ear, before emerging through the stylomastoid foramen.

VIII Vestibulocochlear – really two nerves in one that supply the inner ear: the vestibular part is concerned with balance (equilibrium) and the cochlear part with hearing. The combined nerve leaves the brainstem with the facial nerve at the junction of the pons and medulla to enter the internal acoustic meatus.

IX Glossopharyngeal – a mixed nerve that supplies only one small muscle of the pharynx (stylopharyngeus), sensory fibres to the palate and tongue (including taste from the posterior part), and highly important sensory fibres to monitor blood pressure and blood carbon dioxide levels from special receptors associated with the carotid arteries. Also parasympathetic secretomotor fibres for the parotid gland (via the otic ganglion by fibres which join the auriculotemporal nerve, from the mandibular branch of the trigeminal nerve). The nerve rootlets that form the glossopharyngeal, vagus, and cranial part of the accessory nerves leave the side of the brainstem lateral to the olive of the medulla and pass through the jugular foramen.

X Vagus – a mixed nerve with wide distribution not only in head and neck, but also (uniquely for a cranial nerve) in the thorax and abdomen (vagus means wandering). It supplies muscles of the palate, pharynx, oesophagus and larynx, the heart, smooth muscle of the bronchi, much

Facial nerve paralysis causes drooping of the mouth on the affected side, with uncontrolled dribbling of saliva, inability to close the eye and wrinkle the forehead, and inability to blow or whistle properly.

of the alimentary tract (most importantly, the stomach and its glands), and afferent fibres from all these structures. For its cranial course, see Glossopharyngeal nerve above.

XI Accessory – in two parts: the cranial part, which joins the vagus to provide the skeletal muscle supplies of the palate, pharynx, oesophagus, and larynx; and the spinal part (what is usually meant by the term accessory nerve) whose cells of origin are in the upper cervical segments of the spinal cord, and which supply the sternocleidomastoid and trapezius muscles. The cranial part leaves the brainstem as described for the glossopharyngeal nerve; the rootlets of the spinal part leave the cervical part of the spinal cord behind the denticulate ligament and unite to run up through the foramen magnum and join the cranial part before leaving through the jugular foramen.

> Operations on the neck (e.g., to remove lymph nodes) may damage the **accessory nerve**, causing paralysis of trapezius and inability to shrug the shoulder.

XII Hypoglossal – motor nerve to muscles of the tongue. It leaves the brainstem by two roots between the pyramid and olive of the medulla, and the roots unite as they pass through the hypoglossal canal.

Spinal cord

The spinal cord, continuous with the medulla of the brainstem (**3.5**), is the part of the CNS that lies within the vertebral canal. It extends from the C1 vertebra to the L1 vertebra (in the adult; in the newborn it reaches the L3 vertebra, but the vertebral column grows at a greater rate than does the cord). The spinal nerves (see below) emerge from the side of the cord; the part of the cord that gives attachment to a pair of spinal nerves is referred to as a segment of the cord. Like the brain, the cord is surrounded by the same three meninges, but unlike the brain the gray matter is concentrated centrally, with no 'cortex'.

Meninges – dura mater, continuous with that inside the skull, lines the vertebral canal down as far as the second

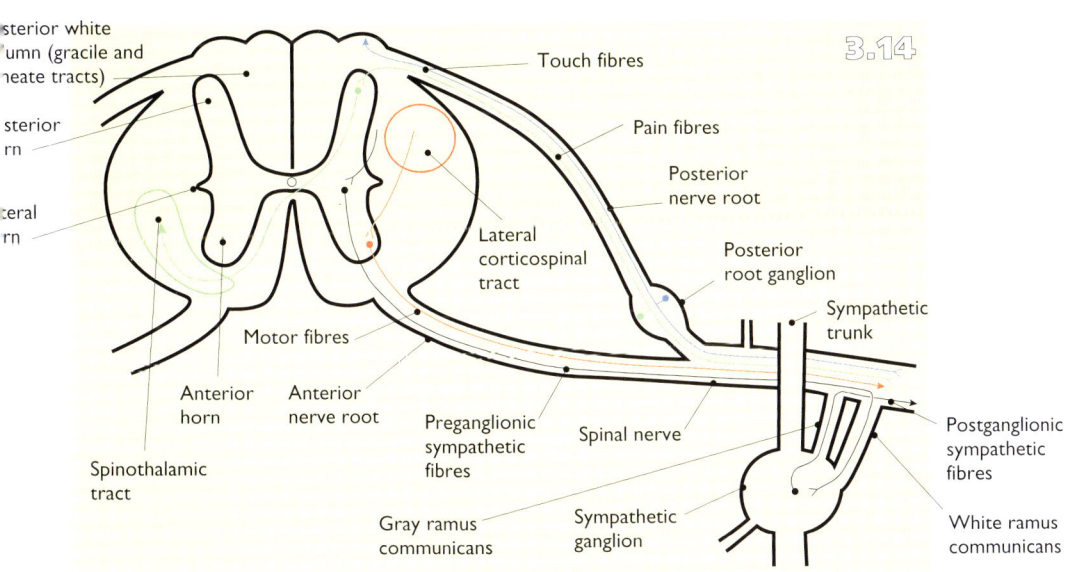

3.14. Major tracts of the spinal cord and fibre components of the spinal nerves

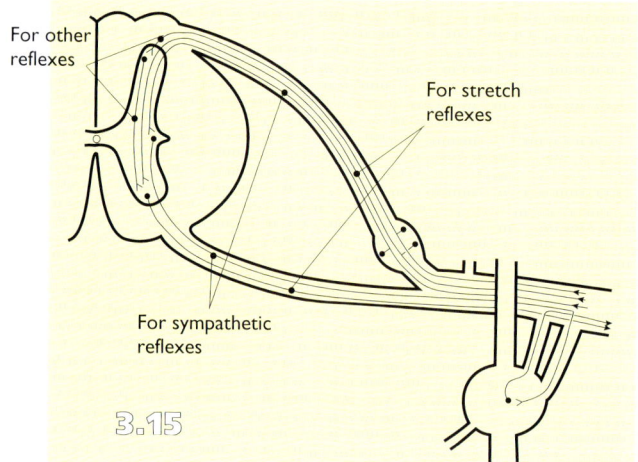

3.15. Reflex pathways in the cord. The stretch reflexes (tendon jerks) depend on direct synaptic connections between afferent and efferent fibres, but for others there are intervening neurons

piece of the sacrum. Inside it is the arachnoid mater and the subarachnoid space with CSF; pia mater adheres to the surface of the cord and the emerging nerve roots. Specimens of CSF can be obtained by lumbar puncture – passing a needle into the subarachnoid space through the midline of the back, usually between the spines of L3 and L4 vertebrae (level with the highest points of the iliac crests). The spinal cord, having ended at the L1 level, is not in danger of being damaged by the needle, and the nerve roots that form the lower spinal nerves (*see* below) are simply displaced, not penetrated.

Gray matter – nerve cell bodies that are concentrated in the cord's central part (which on cross-section is H-shaped); the extremities of the H are the horns of gray matter (**3.14**). Some posterior horn cells are concerned with transmission of pain and temperature sensations, while anterior horn cells give rise to motor fibres that supply skeletal muscles. All segments of the cord have anterior and posterior horns, but a more limited number of segments have smaller lateral horns, whose cells are part of the ANS: from segments T1 down to L2 they are sympathetic, and in segments S2–S4 they are parasympathetic.

Between and around the cells and fibres mentioned above, there are masses of interneurons. Some take part in spinal reflexes – the neuronal circuits within the spinal cord concerned with such involuntary activities as the sudden withdrawal on touching something hot. However, the stretch reflexes, commonly called tendon jerks (such as the knee jerk that occurs on tapping the patellar tendon with the knee partly flexed, the biceps jerk in the arm, and the Achilles' tendon jerk in the leg) do not involve interneurons; there is a direct synaptic connection between the afferent fibres from the muscle that has been stretched momentarily (by tapping the tendon) and the motor nerve cells and their fibres that produce the momentary muscle contraction or 'jerk' of the appropriate joint (**3.15**).

White matter – nerve fibres that are arranged around the periphery of the cord and referred to as columns of white matter (**3.14**). The posterior white columns are entirely occupied by the (ascending) gracile and cuneate tracts, which form the main pathway for touch and associated sensations. The lateral and anterior white columns contain various ascending and descending tracts, of which the most important are the (descending) corticospinal and other associated motor tracts, the (ascending) spinothalamic tracts for pain and temperature, and the (ascending) spinocerebellar tracts that assist in muscular coordination.

Gracile and cuneate tracts – from cell bodies in the posterior root ganglia (*see* below) of all the spinal nerves of the same side; the gracile tract is composed of fibres from sacral, lumbar, and lower thoracic nerves, and the cuneate tract from upper thoracic and cervical nerves. Fibres run up in the posterior white column (3.14) to end in the medulla by synapsing with cells of the gracile and cuneate nuclei, whence fibres that form the medial lemniscus cross to the opposite side of the brainstem to pass to the thalamus, where there are further synapses with cells whose fibres pass to the appropriate sensory areas of the cerebral cortex. The tracts form the *main pathway* for touch, proprioception, vibration sense, and the sensation of fullness of the bladder and rectum.

> Damage to the gracile and cuneate tracts of one side causes **loss of touch sensation** on the same side of the body.

Lateral and anterior spinothalamic tracts – formed by fibres from posterior horn cells of the *opposite* side, i.e. they are crossed tracts (3.14). These posterior horn cells are in synaptic connection with incoming fibres from posterior root ganglion cells of their own side. The tracts run up in the anterior part of the lateral white column and in the anterior white column. In the brainstem many fibres end by synapsing with cell groups there, which in turn send their fibres to the thalamus, while other fibres pass directly to the thalamus. From the thalamus, fibres pass to the appropriate areas of the cerebral cortex. These tracts are the *main pathway* for pain and temperature sensations.

Note that the pathway for touch (which crosses over in the medulla of the brainstem) is different from that for pain and temperature (which crosses in the spinal cord). Thus, disease or injury of the posterior columns may interrupt the transmission of touch sensation while leaving pain and temperature sensation intact ('dissociated sensation'), and vice versa. Note also that each pathway has essentially three groups of neurons: the first with cell bodies in posterior root ganglia, the second with cell bodies in the medulla (touch) or posterior horns (pain and temperature), and the third with cell bodies in the thalamus.

Anterior and posterior spinocerebellar tracts – from posterior horn cells, which give rise to crossed and uncrossed fibres that run at the periphery of the lateral white column to the cerebellum. They assist with muscular coordination and have nothing to do with conscious sensation.

Lateral corticospinal tract – this is the *supremely important motor tract*; it is the downward continuation of the crossed fibres from the motor decussation in the medulla and occupies the posterior part of the lateral white column (3.14). The fibres end by synapsing (usually via interneurons) with the anterior horn cells whose axons supply skeletal muscles. The smaller anterior corticospinal tract, which contains uncrossed fibres, runs in the anterior white column, near the median fissure, but the fibres eventually cross to anterior horn cells of the opposite side.

> Damage to spinothalamic tracts of one side causes **loss of pain and temperature sensations** on the opposite side of the body.

> Damage to corticospinal tracts of one side causes **spastic paralysis** of muscles on the opposite side of the body.

Extrapyramidal tracts – collective name for several tracts (e.g. vestibulospinal and reticulospinal, often intermingled with corticospinal fibres) derived from various cell groups in the brainstem. Their fibres synapse with the same anterior horn cells as corticospinal fibres, but are called extrapyramidal because (unlike corticospinal fibres) they do not run through the pyramid of the medulla. Anterior horn cells are thus subject to many influences from both cortical and subcortical cell groups.

Upper and lower motor neurons – corticospinal (and corticonuclear) and extrapyramidal fibres constitute the upper motor neurons. Anterior horn cells with their fibres running to skeletal muscles constitute the lower motor neurons. Typical causes of damage to upper motor neurons are birth injury to the brain (cerebral palsy, the spastic child), vascular damage to the internal capsule (stroke, *see* above), or spinal cord injury that damages the tracts. Polio (anterior poliomyelitis, a virus infection of anterior horn cells) or a cut peripheral nerve are examples of lower motor neuron damage.

> Damage to upper motor neurons leads to **spastic paralysis**, with increased stretch reflexes; damage to lower motor neurons leads to **flaccid paralysis** with reduced or absent reflexes.

Blood supply of the spinal cord – by (single) anterior and (paired) posterior spinal arteries, derived at the upper end from the vertebral arteries and forming longitudinal trunks which are supplemented at various, but variable, segmental levels by small radicular arteries that run along the spinal nerve roots. There are corresponding veins.

Spinal nerves

There are 31 pairs of spinal nerves – eight cervical (C), twelve thoracic (T), five lumbar (L), five sacral (S), and one coccygeal (Co). Each one of each pair is attached to its own side of its own segment of the cord by a posterior (dorsal) and an anterior (ventral) root (**3.14**), each root being formed by bundles of nerve fibres. Thus, the fourth cervical nerves (C4 nerves) are attached to the fourth cervical segment (C4 segment).

> Posterior nerve roots contain **afferent** (sensory) nerve fibres; anterior nerve roots contain **efferent** (motor) nerve fibres.

The sites of the cell bodies that give origin to the fibres in each nerve root are different. The posterior root contains afferent (sensory) fibres, whose cell bodies are in the posterior root ganglion, which is the slight swelling on the posterior

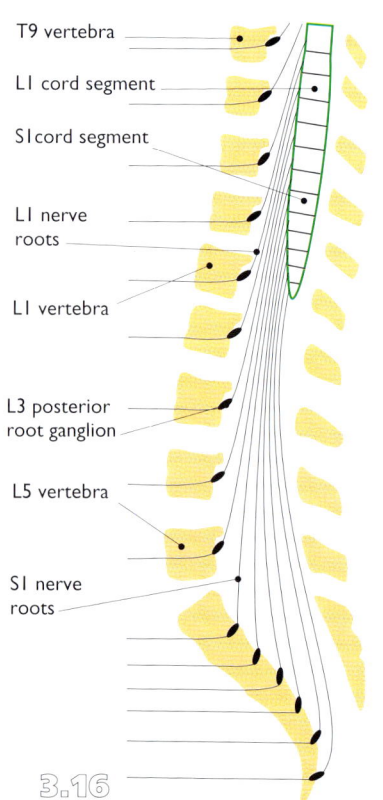

3.16. Lower end of the spinal cord and cauda equina (only posterior nerve roots are shown)

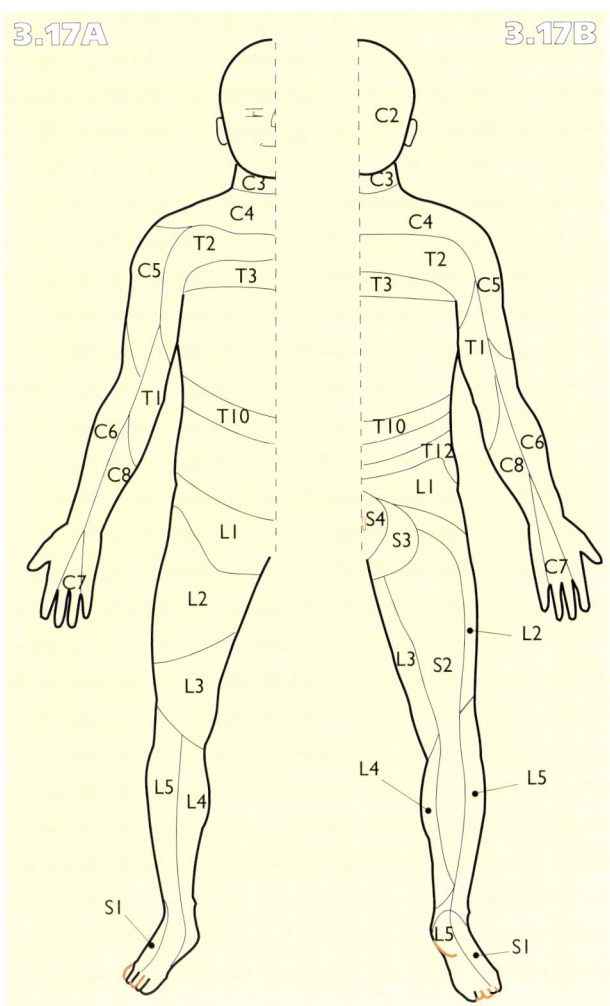

3.17. Dermatomes of the body
A Front
B Back
All repeated

nerve root situated in the intervertebral foramen, just before the two roots unite to form the spinal nerve itself. The anterior root contains efferent (motor) fibres, whose cells of origin are in the anterior horns of the spinal cord (lower motor neurons – see above), for the supply of skeletal muscle fibres or, in the lateral horns, as the source of preganglionic autonomic fibres (p. 15). The lateral horn cells in segments T1 down to L2 are sympathetic and those in segments S2–S4 are parasympathetic. A typical spinal nerve thus contains motor, sensory, and autonomic fibres.

The different lengths of the spinal cord and vertebral column mean that nerve roots must become longer and longer in order to reach their own intervertebral foramina. Thus, below L1 vertebra (where the cord ends) there is a sheaf of nerve roots, the cauda equina ('horse's tail', **3.16**). It follows that injury to the lumbar part of the vertebral column can only damage nerve roots (i.e. lower motor neurons), with flaccid paralysis of the muscles supplied; it cannot cause spastic paralysis (p. 56), because the upper motor neurons in the spinal cord are not involved.

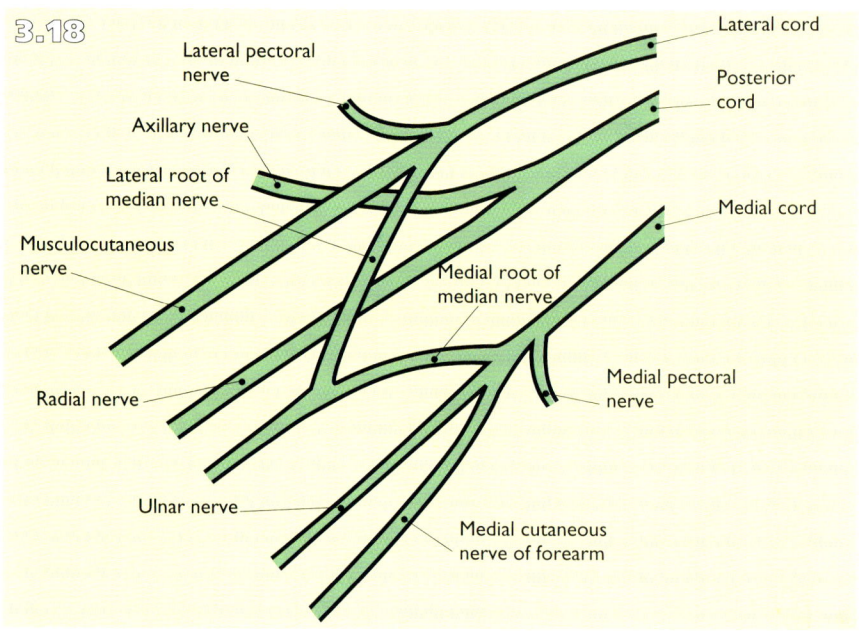

3.18. Cords of the right brachial plexus and their main branches
(the roots, trunks and divisions are not shown)

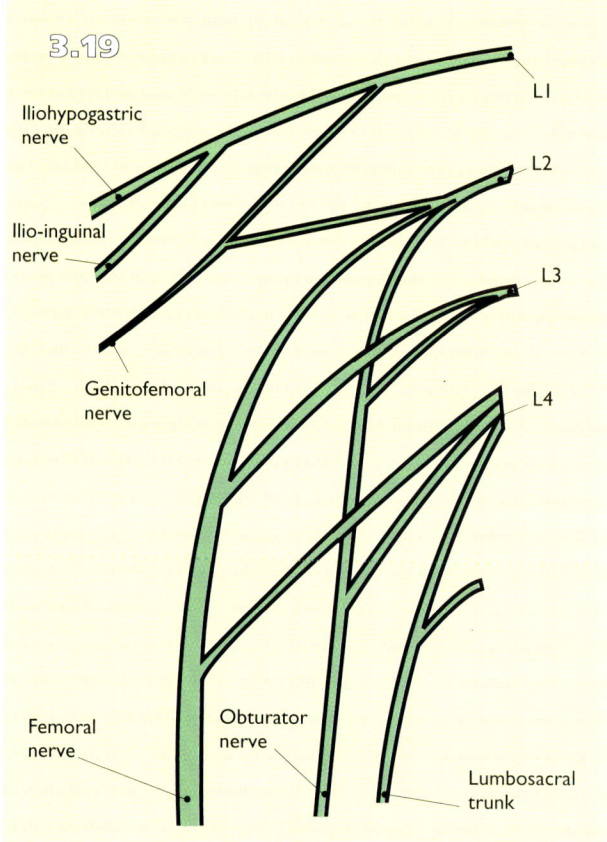

3.19. Right lumbar plexus and principal branches

Head, neck and vertebral column

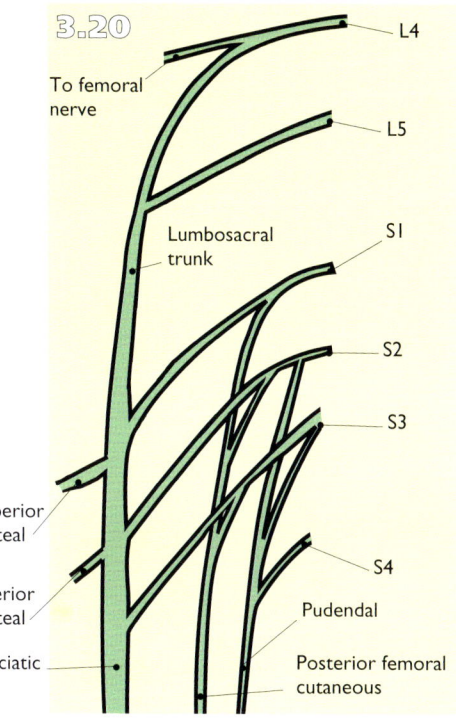

3.20. Sacral plexus and principal branches

Each spinal nerve emerges from its own intervertebral foramen and immediately divides into two branches (rami), which both contain motor and sensory fibres. The posterior ramus is the smaller and supplies muscles and skin of the back near the midline. The anterior ramus is larger and more important, and is what is commonly meant by the term spinal nerve; some rami join their fellows as the roots of the great nerve plexuses – cervical, brachial, lumbar, and sacral. The last three provide the innervation of the limbs. Because of the way nerves unite and divide in plexuses, any given nerve may contain fibres from more than one spinal nerve. Knowledge of the distribution of dermatomes (the areas of skin supplied by any one nerve, 3.17) is often useful clinically (e.g. in determining the level of a spinal cord injury) and also assists in understanding the phenomenon of referred pain. Thus, irritation of part of the diaphragm, supplied through the phrenic nerve mainly by the C4 nerve, may give rise to pain that appears to come from above the shoulder, which is the area of skin supplied by the C4 nerve.

Cervical plexus – roots from C1–C4 anterior rami, it gives small motor branches to deep neck muscles and forms some cutaneous nerves for the neck and head, but by far the most important branch is the phrenic nerve, which supplies its own half of the diaphragm (p. 112).

Brachial plexus – roots from C5–T1 anterior rami (**3.18**), it forms the nerves of the upper limb to supply muscles and skin. The parts of the plexus are the roots, trunks, divisions and cords, in that order. The roots unite to form upper (C5 and 6), middle (C7) and lower (C8 and T1) trunks. Each trunk gives rise to anterior and posterior divisions. The three posterior divisions unite to form the posterior cord, while the anterior divisions form the lateral and medial cords; it is these cords which give rise to the largest branches of the plexus (**3.18**).

Lumbar plexus – roots from L1–L5 anterior rami (**3.19**), it supplies the lowest part of the anterior abdominal wall and muscles of the anterior and medial parts of the thigh. The largest branches are the femoral and obturator nerves and the lumbosacral trunk, which is the contribution that the lumbar plexus makes to the sacral plexus.

Sacral plexus – roots from L4–S3 anterior rami (**3.20**), it supplies the rest of the lower limb and structures of the pelvis and perineum. The largest branches are the sciatic, posterior femoral cutaneous, pudendal, and superior and inferior gluteal nerves.

Human Anatomy

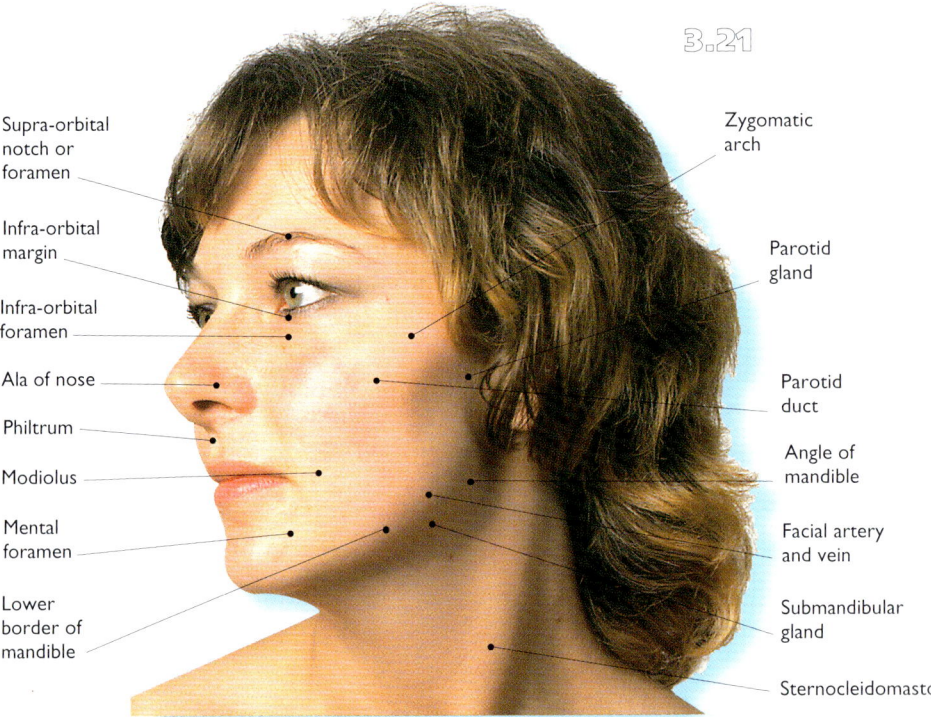

3.21. Surface features of the left side of the face (see also 3.35)

Segmental supply of muscles – although most muscles are supplied by nerves whose motor fibres come from more than one spinal cord segment, there is usually one segment that predominates. The following list indicates which segments of the cord supply certain key muscles, and which are involved in the stretch reflexes (the 'jerks' that occur when tapping tendons, such as the patellar tendon to induce the knee jerk):

C4 – diaphragm
C5 – deltoid
C6 – biceps (and biceps jerk)
C7 – triceps (and triceps jerk)
C8 – wrist flexors and extensors
T1 – small muscles of the hand
L2 – psoas major
L3 – quadriceps femoris (and knee jerk)
L4 – tibialis anterior and posterior
L5 – peroneus longus and brevis
S1 – gastrocnemius (and ankle jerk)
S2 – small muscles of the foot

Face and scalp

The face (**3.21, 3.22**), the front part of the head, extends between both ears and from the hairline (or where the hairline ought to be) to the chin. The scalp covers the vault of the skull and includes the forehead (common to face and scalp). The obvious features of the face are the openings of the eyes, ears, nose, and mouth, while towards the back, below and in front of the ear, is the parotid gland. Most of the facial muscles, commonly called as a group 'muscles of facial expression', pass from various parts of the facial skeleton to skin and often blend with one another; hence, they are unlike most muscles, which pass from bone to bone. The most important are the three mentioned below – orbicularis oculi, orbicularis oris, and buccinator. The whole group is supplied by the facial nerve and must not be confused

Head, neck and vertebral column

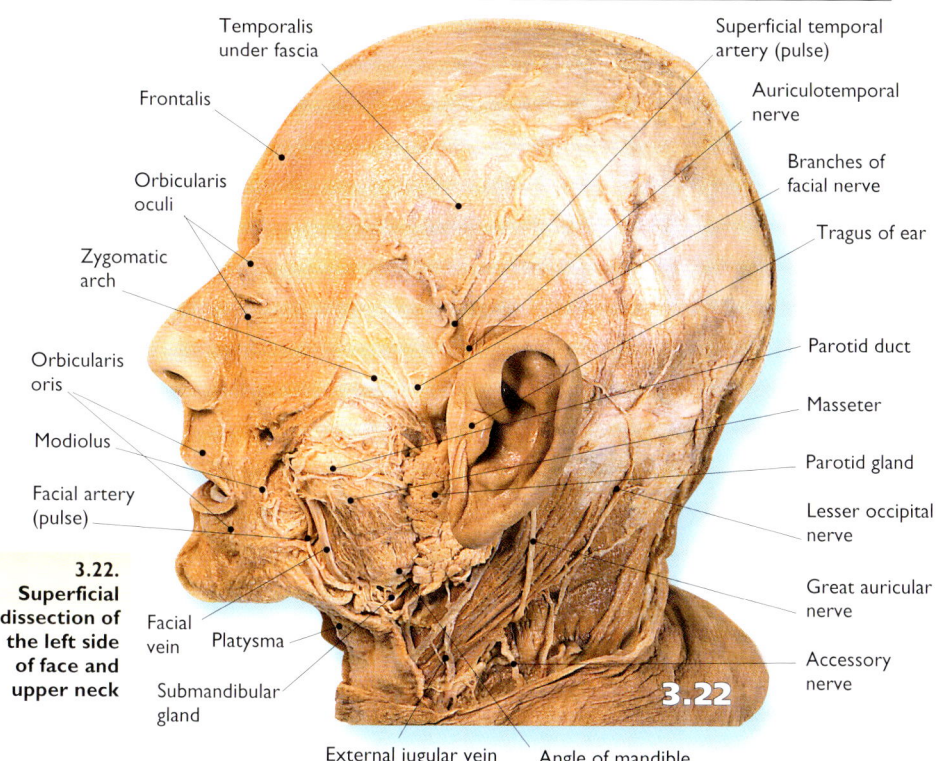

3.22. Superficial dissection of the left side of face and upper neck

with the group called 'muscles of mastication', which moves the lower jaw – the temporalis, masseter, and the lateral and medial pterygoids; these are supplied by the mandibular branch of the trigeminal nerve.

> **Bell's palsy** (of uncertain cause) is the commonest type of facial nerve paralysis (p. 52).

Scalp – the main components are hairy skin, thin muscles at the front and back (frontalis, which has no bony attachment, and occipitalis, attached to the back of the occipital bone), and a tough connective tissue layer (galea aponeurotica) that connects the two muscles, which are both supplied by the facial nerve and are collectively called occipitofrontalis. Only some very loose tissue connects the muscles and aponeurosis to the cranial vault, hence the scalp can move on the bone, and there is a plane of cleavage here where the scalp can be dragged off the bone. The main arterial supplies are the supra-orbital, superficial temporal, and occipital arteries (*see below*).

> **Wounds of the scalp** bleed profusely because the dense connective tissue surrounding the vessels prevents the cut edges from contracting.

Cutaneous nerves of face and scalp – largely from the three branches of the trigeminal nerve: the ophthalmic nerve supplies skin above the level of the eye and on the front of the nose, and extends far back over the vault of the skull; the maxillary nerve supplies the triangular area between the ear, eye, and corner of the mouth (including the upper lip); and the mandibular nerve supplies the skin over the mandible (including the lower lip),

> Branches of the maxillary nerve provide the **sensory supply** for the upper lip, and of the mandibular nerve for the lower lip.

continuing up into a strip in front of the ear. The only facial skin *not* supplied by the trigeminal nerve is that over the angle of the mandible, which is supplied by the great auricular nerve (cervical plexus). Branches from C2 and C3 nerves supply the back of the scalp (the C1 nerve does not supply any skin).

Orbicularis oculi – encircles the eye, running through both lids, and is responsible for 'screwing up' and closing the eye. The upper eyelid has its own muscle, levator palpebrae superioris, for opening the eye, which is supplied by the oculomotor nerve (p. 70); note, therefore, that facial nerve paralysis (p. 52) does not lead to ptosis (drooping) of the upper lid.

Orbicularis oris – encircles the opening of the mouth, to form the muscle of the lips along with several other muscles that blend with it.

Buccinator – attached to the bone of maxilla and mandible opposite the three molar teeth, it blends at the front with muscles round the mouth and at the back with the superior constrictor of the pharynx. It is important for blowing and for keeping food between the teeth, although it must not be classified as a muscle of mastication (it does not move the jaw), and it is supplied, like other facial muscles, by the facial nerve.

Parotid gland – the largest salivary gland, it is at the side of the face and overlaps the masseter muscle below and in front of the ear and the sternocleidomastoid behind; it extends inwards behind the ramus of the mandible towards the styloid process and lies within a tough connective tissue capsule. Embedded within the gland, from superficial to deep, are the facial nerve, retromandibular vein, and the end of the external carotid artery and its terminal branches (superficial temporal and maxillary). Also embedded are some lymph nodes and secretory nerve fibres from the auriculotemporal nerve via the (parasympathetic) otic ganglion, situated on the medial side of the mandibular nerve just below the foramen ovale.

Mumps, a virus infection, causes painful swelling of the gland.

Parotid duct – runs forwards from the anterior border of the gland and lies along the middle third of a line drawn from the tragus of the ear to the midpoint of the philtrum (the rectangular area above the middle of the upper lip). The duct pierces the buccinator obliquely and opens into the mouth opposite the second upper molar tooth.

Facial nerve – after emerging from the stylomastoid foramen and running through the parotid gland, branches fan out from the front of the parotid gland to supply the facial muscles. Note that this nerve *does not supply facial skin* (although it does supply a very small area of the tympanic membrane and external acoustic meatus).

Facial artery and vein – the artery moves from the neck on to the face 3 cm in front of the angle of the mandible at the anterior border of masseter, where the facial pulse can be felt. The artery runs up beneath facial muscles towards the inner canthus (angle) of the eye; it is a tortuous vessel, in contrast to the facial vein which is straight, lies just behind it, and runs into the upper neck to drain into the internal jugular vein.

The **pulse** is felt where the artery crosses the mandible 3 cm in front of the angle of the mandible.

Supra-orbital artery – emerges from the orbit through the supra-orbital notch or foramen to enter the scalp.

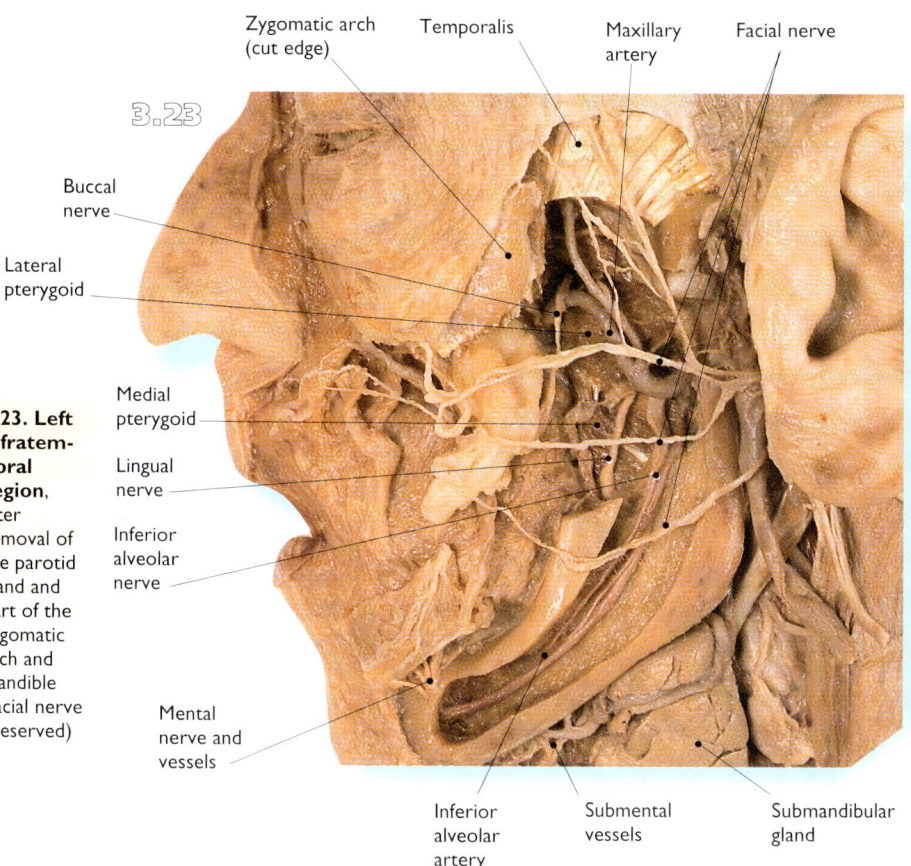

3.23. Left infratemporal region, after removal of the parotid gland and part of the zygomatic arch and mandible (facial nerve preserved)

Superficial temporal artery – a terminal branch of the external carotid within the parotid gland, it passes outwards behind the temporomandibular joint and then turns up in front of the tragus of the ear.

*The superficial temporal **pulse** is felt in front of the tragus of the ear.*

Occipital artery – arising from the external carotid in the neck opposite the facial artery (which passes upwards and *forwards*), it runs upwards and *backwards* to the scalp as one of its main supplies.

Lymph nodes and lymphatics – there are a few lymph nodes in the parotid gland and behind the ear, but there are no nodes within the scalp (only lymphatic channels). All lymph from the head drains to cervical nodes.

Temporalis – from the side of the skull it passes deep to the zygomatic arch and becomes attached to the coronoid process of the mandible and the front of the ramus, almost as far down as the last molar tooth.

Masseter – from the zygomatic arch it runs downwards to the outer side of the ramus of the mandible.

Lateral pterygoid – from the *lateral side of the lateral pterygoid plate* and adjacent part of the base of the skull, its fibres run *backwards* to become attached to the neck of the mandible, the capsule of the temporomandibular joint, and the interarticular disc.

Medial pterygoid – mainly from the *medial side of the lateral pterygoid plate* (not the medial pterygoid plate), it runs *downwards and backwards* to the inner side of the angle of the mandible.

Temporomandibular joint – lies between the mandibular fossa and articular tubercle of the squamous part of the temporal bone and the head of the mandible. Inside the capsule there is a fibrocartilaginous interarticular disc that divides the joint cavity into two. If you lay a fingertip just in front of the tragus of the ear and open your mouth wide, you can feel that the head of the mandible has moved downwards and forwards. The lateral pterygoid muscle is responsible for this movement, pulling the head of the mandible out of its notch on the disc below the mandibular fossa on to the articular tubercle in front of the fossa, and allowing the chin to drop down. The *lowest* fibres of temporalis are responsible for restoring the normal position: they pull the coronoid process backwards because at their origin they lie *horizontally* before hooking down over the root of the zygomatic arch. In less-wide opening, the head of the mandible simply rotates slightly, without being pulled out of its fossa. Accessory muscles of mastication (in the floor of the mouth and attached to the hyoid bone, such as the mylohyoid and geniohyoid) assist the opening. The other three mastication muscles (temporalis, masseter, and the medial pterygoid) all help to *close* the mouth. The pterygoids also produce the side-to-side movements of chewing.

In **dislocation of the jaw** the head of the mandible gets 'stuck' on the articular eminence and must be manually helped back into the fossa.

Inferior alveolar nerve – from the mandibular nerve just below the foramen ovale, it emerges between the two pterygoid muscles and runs down to enter the mandibular foramen with the companion vessels behind it (**3.23**). It supplies all the lower teeth, the skin of the chin, and mucous membrane of the lower lip. It gives off the nerve to the mylohyoid just before entering the foramen.

For **dental anaesthesia** see p. 66.

Lingual nerve – from the same origin as the inferior alveolar, it also emerges between the two pterygoids, but 1 cm in front. It runs down and forwards to enter the mouth by passing under the lower border of the superior constrictor of the pharynx. It lies against the periosteum of the mandible (or on the origin of mylohyoid) just below and behind the third molar tooth, and enters the tongue to supply sensory fibres to the anterior part; it does not supply tongue *muscles,* which are innervated by the hypoglossal nerve (p.65). When high up under the lateral pterygoid, the chorda tympani branch of the facial nerve joins the lingual nerve to provide taste fibres for the anterior part of the tongue and secretory fibres for the submandibular and sublingual glands via the (parasympathetic) submandibular ganglion, which is attached to the lingual nerve at the side of the tongue.

Buccal nerve – another mandibular nerve branch, it emerges through the lateral pterygoid and runs down over the buccinator to below the parotid duct; it supplies cheek skin as well as mucous membrane on the inside of buccinator. In dissections of the infratemporal region (as in **3.23**), note the three mandibular nerve branches running downwards: buccal, lingual, and inferior alveolar, in that order from front to back, with the last two coming out between the two pterygoid muscles.

Auriculotemporal nerve – also from the mandibular, it has two roots which embrace the middle meningeal artery; the nerve then runs upwards, in front of the ear, with the superficial temporal vessels (**3.22, 3.23**) to supply face and scalp skin and secretory nerve fibres to the parotid gland (*see* above).

Posterior superior alveolar nerve – from the maxillary nerve to give two or more branches that run down the posterior wall of the maxilla and pierce the bone to supply the posterior upper teeth.

Maxillary artery – runs through or between the pterygoid muscles to pass through the pterygomaxillary fissure and enter the nose, where it is called the sphenopalatine, the main vessel of the nasal cavity (p. 68). Among the many branches are the middle meningeal artery (p. 36), which passes vertically *upwards* to the foramen spinosum, and the inferior alveolar artery, which runs *downwards* behind its companion nerve to enter the mandibular foramen.

Mouth

The mouth is the start of the alimentary tract, with lips at the front (containing the orbicularis oris), cheeks at the sides (containing the buccinator), the palate in the roof, and the oropharyngeal isthmus at the back (the opening into the oral part of the pharynx – see Palate, below). The vestibule of the mouth is the space that separates the lips and cheeks from the teeth and gingivae (gums); the parotid duct opens into it opposite the second upper molar tooth, with numerous small mucous glands in the lips and cheeks. The mouth cavity is the part internal to the teeth and gums, with the hard and soft palates as its upper boundary and the tongue in its floor, formed by the pair of mylohyoid muscles with the smaller geniohyoids lying above them. The ducts of the submandibular and sublingual glands open into the cavity at the sides below the tongue.

Sublingual gland – almond-shaped salivary gland that lies against the body of the mandible and makes a bulge in the mucous membrane over the floor of the mouth. Secretory fibres for this and the submandibular gland (in the neck, p. 80) come from the lingual nerve via the (parasympathetic) submandibular ganglion.

Tongue – a mass of skeletal muscle on each side of a midline fibrous septum, covered by a mucous membrane roughened by papillae and containing mainly mucous glands, with lymphoid follicles (lingual tonsil) at the back. There are also special nerve endings for taste (taste buds), found mainly towards the sides and back of the mucous membrane. The largest tongue muscle is the genioglossus, with bony attachments to the mandible and hyoid bone. All the tongue muscles are supplied by the hypoglossal nerve of their own side (**3.37A**). The mucous membrane of the front part is supplied by the lingual nerve for ordinary sensations, like touch and temperature, but with fibres from the facial nerve's chorda tympani branch (which joins the lingual nerve below the foramen ovale) for the taste buds of this part. The back In the rare **hypoglossal nerve paralysis**, the protruded tongue deviates towards the side of the lesion, because of the unopposed action of the muscles of the opposite side.

part is supplied by the glossopharyngeal nerve for both ordinary sensations and taste, with a small part of the front of the vallecula (p. 84) being supplied by the internal laryngeal branch of the vagus.

Gingivae – commonly called the gums, these are attached to the alveolar margins of the jaws and surround the necks of the teeth; they consist of dense fibrous tissue covered with mucous membrane.

Teeth – composed of a special mineralized tissue, dentine, with a central pulp cavity that contains vessels and nerves. Each tooth has an upper part or crown covered by enamel (the hardest of all tissues), a neck surrounded by the gum, and a root covered by cementum and anchored in the tooth socket by fibrous tissue, the periodontal ligament (periodontium).

Adult, or permanent, dentition consists of 32 teeth, eight in each half of each jaw, numbered and named from the midline laterally (listed here with approximate date of eruption in years): 1, central incisor (7 yr); 2, lateral incisor (8 yr); 3, canine (11 yr); 4, first premolar (9 yr); 5, second premolar (10 yr); 6, first molar (6 yr); 7, second molar (12 yr); and 8, third molar (18 yr or in later years of maturity, hence often called the 'wisdom tooth'). The deciduous dentition of the child ('milk teeth') consists of 20 teeth, five in each half jaw, lettered and named from the midline laterally (listed here with approximate date of eruption in months): A, central incisor (6 m); B, lateral incisor (8 m); C, canine (18 m); D, first molar (12 m); and E, second molar (24 m). Note that the deciduous molars are replaced by the permanent premolars, since the permanent molars have no precursors in the deciduous dentition.

To work on the teeth of the lower jaw dentists commonly need to produce inferior alveolar and lingual nerve block by injecting anaesthetic solution through the inside of the cheek, so that it percolates round the nerves where they are labelled in 3.23 and diffuses into them (the needle must not penetrate the nerves themselves). The teeth of the upper jaw can be anaesthetized by local injection into the mucous membrane that overlies the appropriate part of the jaw, because the bone of the maxilla is less dense and more pervious than that of the mandible, so allowing the anaesthetic to penetrate into the bone and reach the roots of the teeth where the nerves enter them.

> Local injection can anaesthetise upper teeth, but anaesthesia of lower teeth requires **nerve block**, due to differing bone densities in the upper and lower jaws.

Palate – consists of the horizontal, bony hard palate (**2.3**), formed by parts of the maxillae and palatine bones and covered by a tough mucous membrane (mucoperiosteum), and of the muscular soft palate (**3.24**), which hangs down from the back of the hard palate (like a mobile curtain) to separate the front part of the nasopharynx from the oropharynx. One pair of its muscles (the palatoglossus) runs to the side of the tongue to form the palatoglossal arch, which is the dividing line between the mouth and oropharynx; the tonsils (p. 87) lie just behind this arch. A similar pair (the palatopharyngeus) run into the pharynx (p. 85), while two other pairs, the tensor veli palatini (tensor palati) and levator veli palatini (levator palati) pass into the palate from above and raise it during swallowing, so helping to close off the nasopharynx and direct food and drink downwards. The lower border of the soft palate is not straight, but has a central downwards projection, the uvula, with its own pair of tiny muscles. All the muscles are supplied by pharyngeal branches of the vagus (p. 82), except for the tensor which is supplied by a branch from the nerve to the medial pterygoid muscle (mandibular nerve).

> Saying 'Ah' with the mouth open raises the soft palate and enables more of the **posterior pharyngeal wall** to be seen.

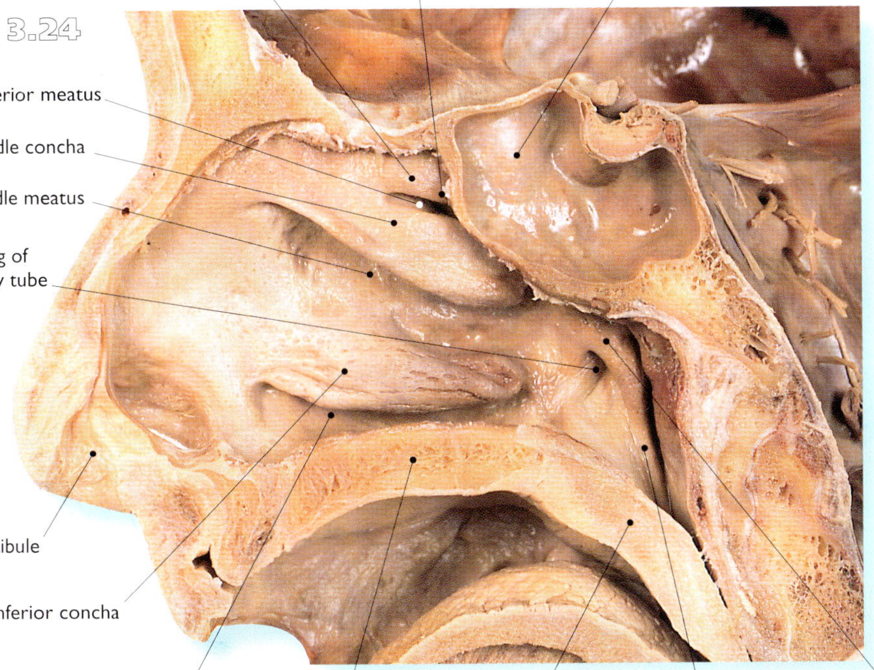

Head, neck and vertebral column

Superior concha · Spheno-ethmoidal recess · Sphenoidal sinus

Superior meatus
Middle concha
Middle meatus
Opening of auditory tube

Vestibule

Inferior concha

Inferior meatus · Hard palate · Soft palate · Salpingopharyngeal fold · Tubal elevation

3.24. Lateral wall of the right half of the nasal cavity

Nose and paranasal sinuses

The nose, which is the start of the respiratory tract and the organ of olfaction (smell), consists of the external nose and the nasal cavity. Draining into the cavity are the four pairs of paranasal air sinuses, named from the bones in which they lie; they are of uncertain function, but they add some resonance to the voice and by their shapes they may help to orientate the orbits so that the eyes can provide binocular vision.

External nose – the part that sticks out on the face. It is bony only in its upper part (the pair of nasal bones); the rest is cartilaginous. The openings are the nostrils (external nares).

Nasal septum – divides the nasal cavity into right and left halves. It is formed by the vomer at the back and part of the ethmoid bone centrally, with the rest being cartilaginous (see 3.4A). It is

---
Conditions such as the **common cold** and **hay fever** cause increased secretion and swelling of the mucous membrane, hence obstruction to the flow of air.

The lower anterior part of the septum is the common site for **nose-bleed** (epistaxis).

67

rarely exactly in the midline, so that a 'deviated septum' is a normal occurrence without significance. Only if it is grossly deviated may it cause problems by obstructing one or more of the sinus openings.

Nasal cavity – on either side of the nasal septum (**3.24**), the roof of each half is only 1–2 mm wide, although the floor (the upper surface of the hard palate) is more than 1 cm wide. The lateral wall is the most complicated feature; its skeleton is made up of parts of the maxilla, the palatine and ethmoid bones, and the inferior nasal concha (the superior and middle nasal conchae are part of the ethmoid bone).

Superior, middle, and inferior nasal conchae – form scroll-like projections from the lateral wall (**3.24**), these are still sometimes called by their old names, the turbinate bones. They increase the surface area of the nasal mucous membrane and so help to warm inspired air. Immediately behind the *superior* concha is the spheno-ethmoidal recess, into which drain the sphenoidal sinus and posterior ethmoidal air cells. Behind the *middle* concha is the sphenopalatine foramen, through which the spheno-palatine artery enters the nose. About 1 cm behind the *inferior* concha is the opening of the auditory tube (in the nasopharynx).

Superior meatus – the space under the superior concha, into which drain the posterior ethmoidal air cells.

Middle meatus – under the middle concha, it features a swelling, the ethmoidal bulla (due to ethmoidal air cells), at the upper boundary of a curved groove, the semilunar hiatus, into which drain anterior and middle ethmoidal air cells, the maxillary sinus, and the frontonasal duct (from the frontal sinus).

Inferior meatus – under the inferior concha, into which drains the nasolacrimal duct.

Blood supply – mainly by the sphenopalatine artery (the end of the maxillary), with anastomoses with the anterior ethmoidal (internal carotid) and facial (external carotid) branches, in particular on the lower anterior part of the septum. There are corresponding veins.

Nerve supply – most of the nasal cavity (including the sinuses) is lined by respiratory mucous membrane (stratified, with cilia), with sensory supplies by branches of the ophthalmic and maxillary nerves (trigeminal). Only a small area of the roof, the uppermost part of the septum and over the superior concha, is olfactory, with receptors for smell supplied by filaments of the olfactory nerve which run through the foramina in the cribriform plate of the ethmoid bone to enter the olfactory bulb on the under surface of the frontal lobe of the brain. Nasal glands receive secretory fibres from the (parasympathetic) pterygopalatine ganglion (the 'ganglion of hay fever'), which is attached to the maxillary nerve just below the base of the skull, behind the foramen rotundum.

Frontal sinus – in the frontal bone above the orbit (**3.3**), draining into the middle meatus via the frontonasal duct.

Ethmoidal sinus – in the ethmoid bone on the medial wall of the orbit and lateral wall of the nose, and made up of a number of ethmoidal air cells which drain into the middle meatus (including the semilunar hiatus) or the superior meatus.

Sphenoidal sinus – in the body of the sphenoid bone (**3.24**); the adjacent pair do not communicate with one another, they may vary greatly in size, and one or both may be indented by the pituitary fossa. Each drains into the spheno-ethmoidal recess behind the superior concha.

Maxillary sinus – in the body of the maxilla (and sometimes known by its old name, the maxillary antrum), it drains into the semilunar hiatus of the middle meatus, through an opening that is high up on its medial wall, not near its floor, so that efficient drainage depends on the epithelial cilia (microscopic hairs), which beat to direct mucous secretion and debris towards the opening.

> Infection may spread from the nose or throat to any of the sinuses, but especially the maxillary, leading to **sinusitis**.

Eye and lacrimal apparatus

The eye (eyeball), the organ of vision, is almost a complete sphere, about 25 mm (1 inch) in diameter, lodged in the front half of the orbit (orbital cavity) of the skull, and protected by the eyelids. The eye consists of three layers – the sclera, choroid, and retina (from outside inwards); the retina contains the light receptors. At the front the sclera is replaced by, and continuous with, the transparent cornea, which admits light into the eye. At the back, the optic nerve occupies the posterior half of the orbit, with most of the extra-ocular muscles that move the eye and other nerves and vessels all embedded in the orbital fat. The lacrimal apparatus includes the lacrimal gland, which secretes tears, and the duct systems that dispose of these tears.

Eyelids – each contains part of the orbicularis oculi muscle (p. 62), which closes the eye, and a plaque of dense fibrous tissue, the tarsal plate, which strengthens the protective capacity of the lid. The upper lid has an extra muscle to elevate it, the levator palpebrae superioris (3.25), unusual in that it contains some smooth muscle fibres as well as skeletal fibres. The gap between the lids when the eye is open is the palpebral fissure. The edges of the lids contain the eyelashes and the tarsal (Meibomian) glands, which are modified sebaceous glands.

> The **facial nerve** (VII) closes the eye (orbicularis oculi) but the **oculomotor nerve** (III) opens it.

Sclera – the 'white of the eye', the tough, fibrous outer layer (3.26), to which are attached the extra-ocular muscles. The visible surface of the sclera is covered by a thin transparent membrane, the conjunctiva, which is continuous with the outer epithelial covering of the cornea and which also lines the inner surface of the eyelids.

> 'Something in the eye' like a speck of dust readily irritates the conjunctiva, giving **conjunctivitis** with enlarged and easily seen blood vessels.

Cornea – the transparent bulge at the front of the eye, continuous with the sclera at the sclerocorneal junction (limbus), and through which the iris and pupil can be seen.

> Foreign bodies that damage the cornea may lead to **loss of transparency** with the formation of opacities and so interfere with vision.

Choroid – the thin and pigmented vascular layer that lies internal to the sclera. The front part of the choroid is the ciliary body, which contains smooth muscle. From it is suspended the lens (whose shape can be altered by ciliary muscle to focus – accommodation); the part of the ciliary body in front of the lens forms the pigmented iris, which gives the eye its colour and whose central opening is the pupil.

Part of the ciliary muscle forms the sphincter pupillae, for constricting the pupil, and there are a few radial dilator pupillae fibres behind the sphincter fibres. The choroid, ciliary body, and iris are sometimes collectively known as the uveal tract (from the Latin for grape, having the colour of a black grape).

The area between the cornea and the iris is the anterior chamber, and that between the iris and the lens is the posterior chamber. Both chambers are continuous with one another through the pupil and contain a fluid, the aqueous humour, which is derived from ciliary blood vessels and continuously circulates from the posterior chamber into the anterior chamber. Here it is absorbed into a small channel, the canal of Schlemm (sinus venosus sclerae), at the iridocorneal angle, from where it drains away into ciliary veins.

Interference with the drainage of aqueous humour leads to an increase in intra-ocular pressure (**glaucoma**), which can eventually cause blindness due to retinal degeneration.

Retina – the innermost layer, it contains the rods and cones, which are the light receptors. At the posterior pole of the eye is a particularly sensitive part of the retina, the macula lutea, where the clarity and sharpness of vision (visual acuity) are greatest. A little to the medial (nasal) side of the macula is the optic disc, devoid of rods and cones and therefore a blind spot, where nerve fibres leave the retina to pass back into the optic nerve. From the optic disc branches of the central artery of the retina fan out and corresponding veins converge on to it. These vessels and the surface of the retina can be observed through an ophthalmoscope, a procedure commonly called examining the fundus of the eye.

Macular degeneration is the common cause of loss of central vision in the elderly.

Detachment of the retina or retinal haemorrhage causes blind spots over the affected area.

All the region internal to the retina (and behind the lens and ciliary body) is filled with a clear, gelatinous fluid, the vitreous body (vitreous humour); this has no connection with the aqueous humour; it helps to maintain the globular shape of the eye.

Extra-ocular muscles – four rectus muscles (superior and inferior, medial and lateral) and two oblique muscles (superior and inferior) (3.25, 3.27). All except the inferior oblique arise from the back of the orbit and run forwards; the inferior oblique arises from the front, near the nasolacrimal canal, and runs backwards and laterally. These muscles are attached to the sclera in such a way that the muscles responsible for turning the eye *inwards* are the medial, superior, and inferior recti, and those for turning it *outwards* are the lateral rectus and the superior and inferior obliques. Turning the eye *upwards* depends on the superior rectus and inferior oblique, and *downwards* on the inferior rectus and superior oblique.

Motor nerve supplies – lateral rectus by the abducent nerve, superior oblique by the trochlear nerve, and the other four by the oculomotor nerve, which also supplies the skeletal fibres of the levator of the upper lid (the smooth muscle part receives sympathetic fibres).

The ciliary muscle and sphincter pupillae are supplied by parasympathetic fibres of the oculomotor nerve via the short ciliary branches of the ciliary ganglion, which lies on the lateral side of the optic nerve near the back of the orbit. Sympathetic fibres which enter the orbit with the ophthalmic artery cause dilatation of the pupil.

Head, neck and vertebral column

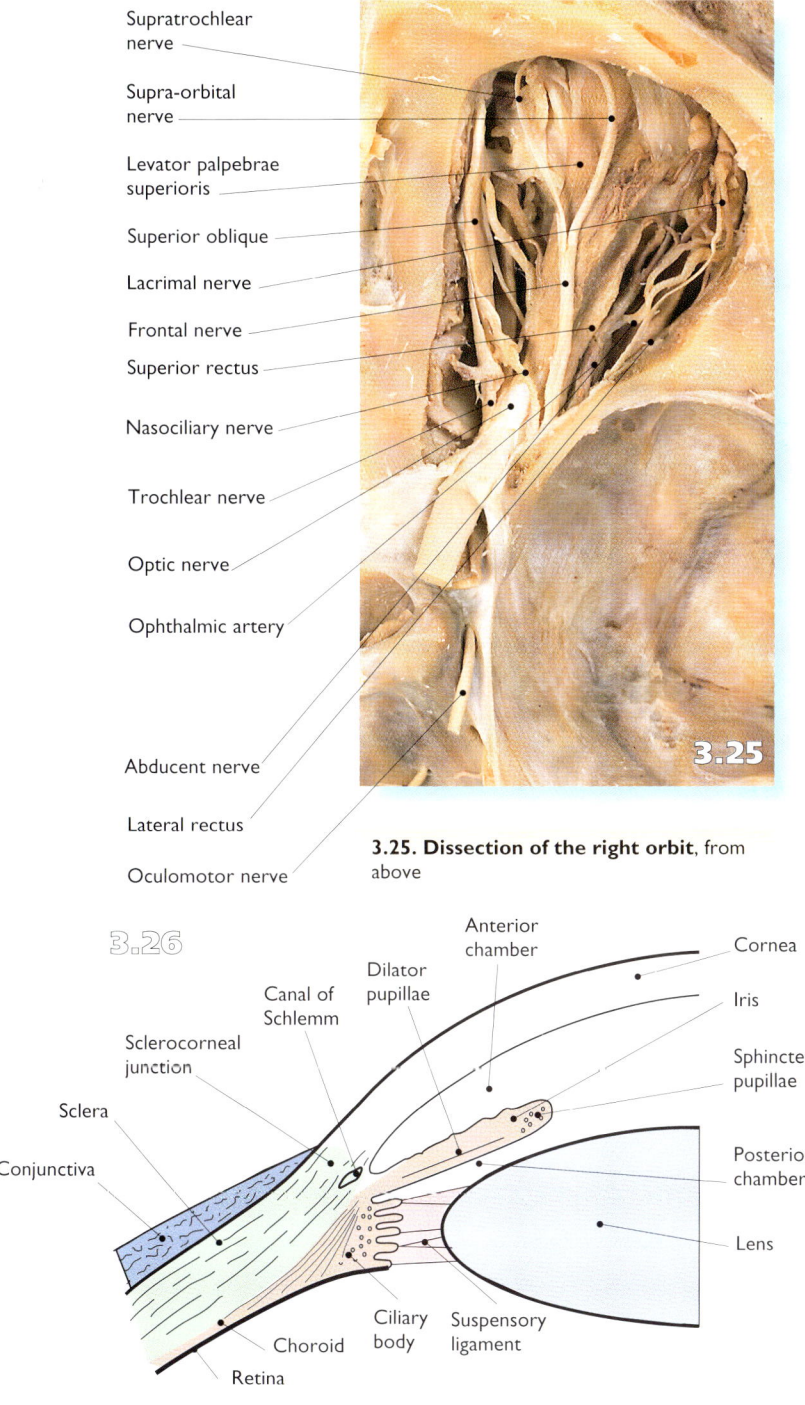

3.25. Dissection of the right orbit, from above

3.26. A section through the eye in the region of the sclerocorneal junction

71

Sensory nerve supplies – the cornea, the most important part of the surface of the whole body, is supplied by the long and short ciliary nerves, which arise respectively from the ophthalmic branch of the trigeminal nerve and from the oculomotor nerve via the (parasympathetic) ciliary ganglion. They provide the afferent fibres for the corneal reflex; there are connections in the brainstem with neurons of the facial nerve that supply the orbicularis oculi, thus causing the protective closure of the eye.

> After the use of **local anaesthetic** drops (e.g. to remove a foreign body), the eye must be carefully protected since the corneal reflex is lost until the anaesthetic effect has worn off.

Visual pathway – light impulses that fall on the rods and cones pass back in the optic nerve to the optic chiasma (**3.28**), on the under surface of the brain in front of the pituitary gland. At the chiasma, fibres from the nasal (medial) side of both retinas cross over, so that the optic tracts which run back from the chiasma contain fibres from the *temporal side* of the retina of one eye and from the *nasal side* of the retina of the *opposite* eye. Each optic tract runs back round the side of the brainstem to reach a group of cells on the under surface of the thalamus, the lateral geniculate body, where the retinal fibres end by synapsing with cells whose fibres form the optic radiation, which passes to the visual area of the cerebral cortex, mostly on the medial surface of the occipital lobe.

> The **extent of visual loss** following damage (e.g. by haemorrhage or tumours) to the visual pathway enables the site of the damage to be identified.

Light reflexes – the general light reflex (e.g. blinking and turning away from a sudden bright light) involves connections in the brainstem and spinal cord so that the head and perhaps other parts of the body can respond.

The pupillary light reflexes depend on connections between retinal fibres in the optic nerve and certain neurons of the oculomotor nucleus; because of fibre cross-overs in the optic chiasma and between the oculomotor nuclei of both sides, shining a light into one eye causes constriction of the pupils of both eyes. The final pathway is via the (parasympathetic) ciliary ganglion, which lies near the back of the orbit on the lateral side of the optic nerve.

> **Examination of the pupils** in both conscious and unconscious patients is an important part of clinical examination.

The accommodation–convergence reflex, sometimes called the near reflex, which enables the lens to focus for near vision and the eyes to converge slightly, as for reading, involves certain areas of the cerebral cortex as well as of the brainstem.

Lacrimal apparatus – concerned with the secretion and disposal of tears, which keep the visible part of the eye and the conjunctiva moist.

Lacrimal gland – in the upper outer corner of the orbit (**3.29**), with about a dozen small ducts constantly discharging a small amount of secretion on to the surface of the eye. At the medial end of each eyelid is a tiny opening (lacrimal punctum) into a lacrimal canaliculus, which leads into the lacrimal sac situated in the lacrimal groove at the front of the orbit.

> **Blinking** helps to spread secretion over the cornea and conjunctiva.

The sac continues down as the nasolacrimal duct, which opens into the inferior meatus of the nose (hence the 'snuffly nose' when crying, although excess tears escape on to the face). The secretory nerve supply involves branches of the facial, maxillary, and ophthalmic nerves and the (parasympathetic) pterygopalatine ganglion (p. 15).

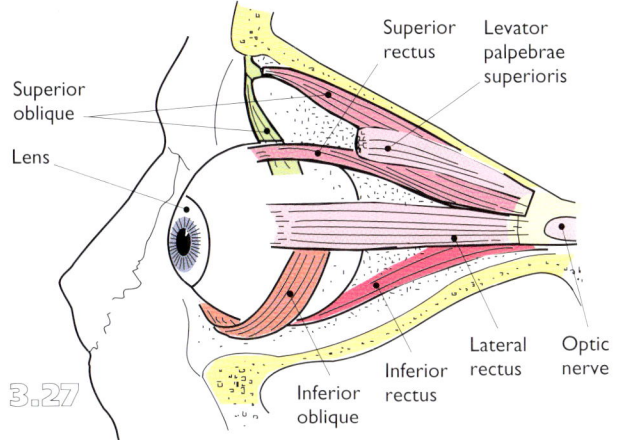

Fig. 3.27. Extra-ocular muscles of the left eye (the lateral rectus obscures the view of the medial rectus)

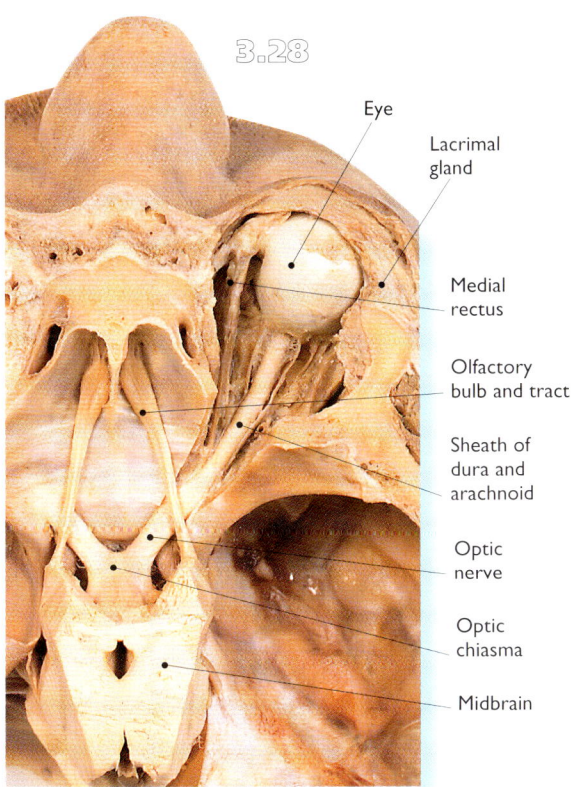

3.28. Right orbit and optic nerve, in a horizontal section of the head

Human Anatomy

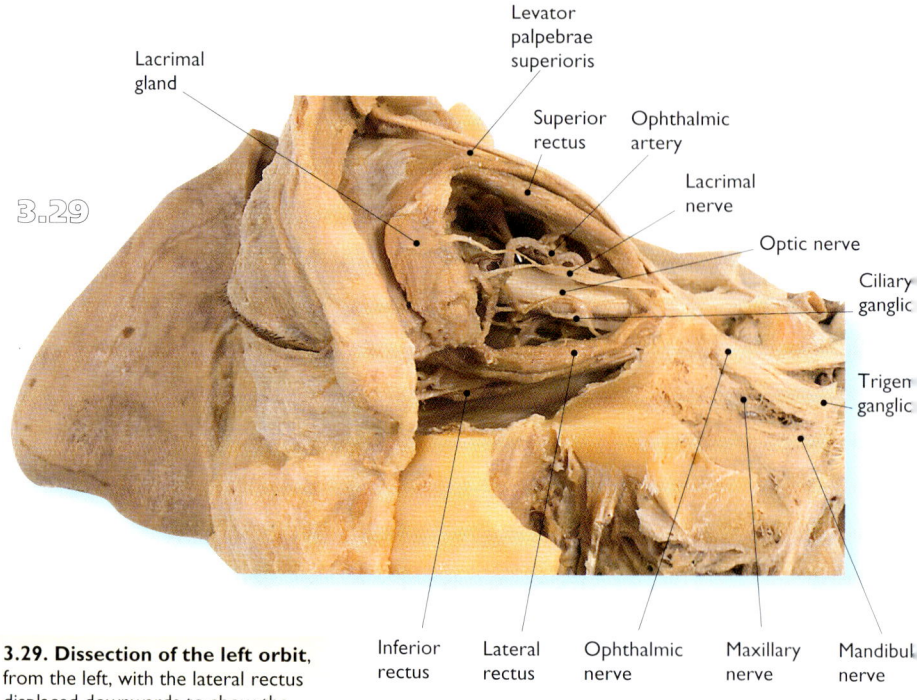

3.29. Dissection of the left orbit, from the left, with the lateral rectus displaced downwards to show the ciliary ganglion

Ear

The ear, the organ of hearing and balance, has three parts, named the external, middle, and internal ear. All three are concerned with hearing, but only the internal ear with balance.

External ear – consists of the auricle (pinna), which projects from the side of the head, and the external acoustic meatus (earhole). The auricle and the outer part of the meatus have a cartilaginous framework, but the deeper part of the meatus is part of the temporal bone. Special glands in the skin lining the meatus secrete wax (cerumen), whose purpose is to trap particles before they reach the eardrum (see below).

 The commonest cause of **deafness** is excess wax which prevents the tympanic membrane from vibrating. Infections of meatal skin are very painful, because the skin adheres very tightly to the underlying cartilage and bone.

Middle ear – a small cavity within the temporal bone, separated from the external acoustic meatus by the tympanic membrane (eardrum, 3.30, 3.31). The cavity is bridged by three tiny bones, the auditory ossicles (malleus, incus, and stapes, meaning hammer, anvil, and stirrup, named from their shapes). It communicates at the front with the nasopharynx (p. 84) by the very narrow (1 mm or less) auditory tube (Eustachian tube). This is formed partly by the temporal bone, and partly by cartilage which can be moved slightly by small muscles attached to it, in particular the tensor palati (tensor veli palatini); this increases the diameter of the tube and

Infections of the middle ear (**otitis media**) may cause rupture of the tympanic membrane ('perforation of the eardrum'), and may also invade the mastoid air cells (mastoiditis).

Head, neck and vertebral column

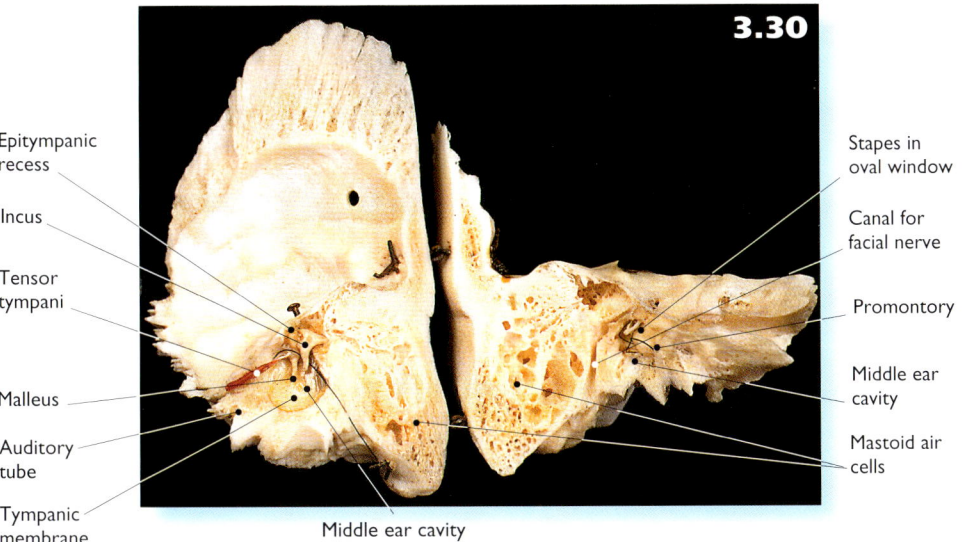

Fig. 3.30. Bisected right temporal bone, to show the middle ear cavity. The fine threads over the promontory represent the tympanic plexus (glossopharyngeal nerve) which supplies the mucous membrane lining the middle ear cavity

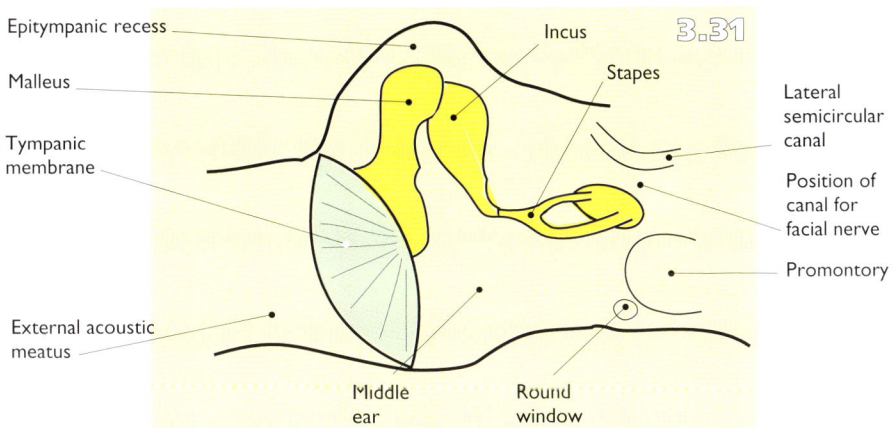

Fig. 3.31. The right middle ear

helps to equalize the air pressure between the nose and middle ear cavity. At the back, the cavity communicates with the sponge-like mastoid air cells which invade the mastoid process.

Internal ear – a complicated structure within the temporal bone that is concerned with hearing and balance. As explained below, it has bony and membranous parts (**3.32, 3.33**); to avoid confusion it is essential to remember what makes up these various parts and, in particular, to distinguish between those called *canals* (which are bony) and those called *ducts* (which are membranous).

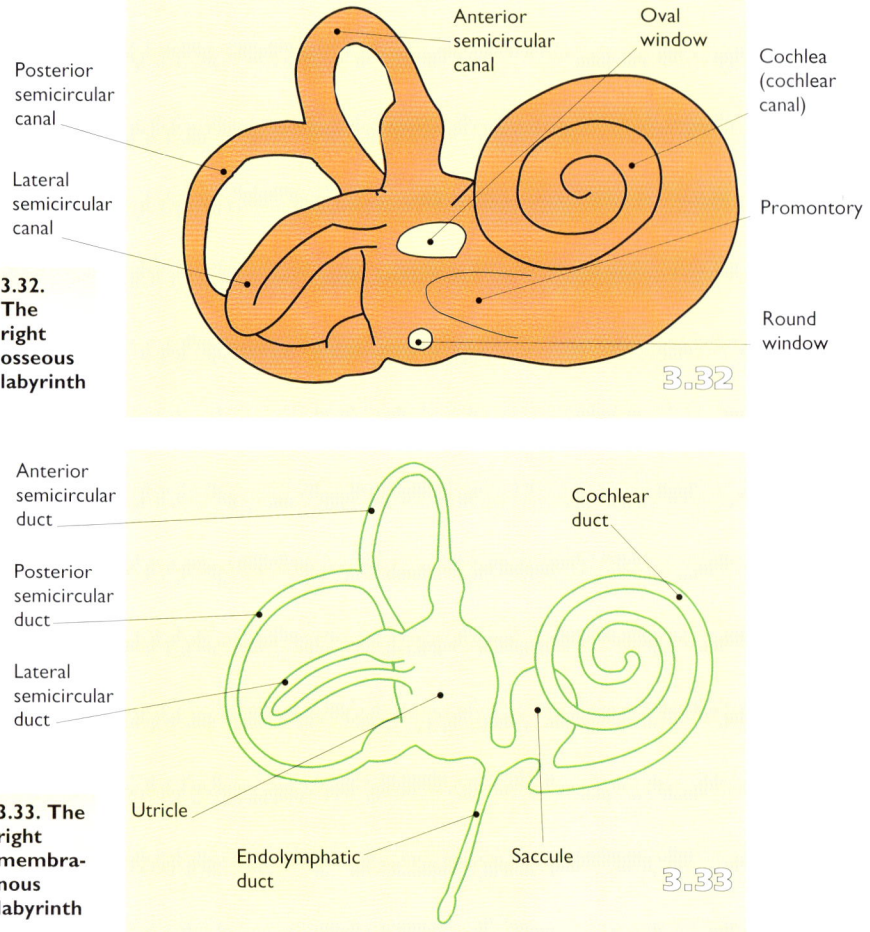

3.32. The right osseous labyrinth

3.33. The right membranous labyrinth

The irregular-shaped space within the temporal bone comprising the internal ear is the osseous (bony) labyrinth. From front to back its parts are the cochlear canal (cochlea), the vestibule, and the semicircular canals.

These bony spaces are occupied by a similarly shaped, thin fibrous sac, the membranous labyrinth. From front to back its parts are the cochlear duct (which occupies the bony cochlear canal), the utricle and saccule (which occupy the bony vestibule), and the semicircular ducts (which occupy the bony semicircular canals).

All the parts of the membranous labyrinth are filled with a fluid, the endolymph; outside the membranous labyrinth is another fluid, the perilymph, which separates the membranous labyrinth from the surrounding bony labyrinth. The two fluids do not communicate with one another.

Hearing – sound waves that cause the tympanic membrane to vibrate are conducted across the middle ear cavity by the malleus, incus, and stapes. The movement of the stapes, which fills a small opening (the oval window) in the cochlear canal, causes movement of the perilymph, which in turn causes movement of the endolymph within

> A common cause of **conductive deafness** in the elderly is otosclerosis, where the stapes becomes fixed and cannot transmit vibrations to the inner ear.

the cochlear duct. This, in its turn, stimulates the specialized auditory cells of the cochlear duct to send impulses into the brain by the cochlear nerve – the auditory part of the vestibulocochlear (eighth cranial) nerve. By various brainstem connections, the impulses are conveyed to the auditory area of the cerebral cortex.

Note that the stimulation of the special nerve receptors for hearing is by a rather indirect pathway: first, by vibration of the tympanic membrane, then through the chain of auditory ossicles, then to the perilymph, then to the endolymph, and only then to the nerve receptors. It follows that disturbance of any part of this pathway could lead to impairment of hearing – deafness. Of the two types of deafness, conductive deafness is due to impairment of the conduction of vibrations in the external or middle ear (e.g. by wax in the external ear affecting the tympanic membrane or by middle ear disease preventing movement of the ossicles); sensorineural deafness is due to conditions that affect the internal ear or eighth nerve.

Balance – the vestibular nerve, the balance part of the vestibulocochlear nerve, supplies special nerve receptors in the utricle, saccule, and semicircular ducts that are stimulated by the movement of endolymph within these parts of the membranous labyrinth (which constitute the vestibular system). The body can make adjustments to its position according to these vestibular stimuli. In susceptible people, certain types of movement (as in travel by car, ship or plane) cause disturbances of vestibular function which stimulate the vomiting centre in the brainstem - motion sickness. It is usually sudden changes in position of the head that cause the movement of endolymph, and hence the feeling of giddiness.

Neck and vertebral column

The skeleton of the neck is the cervical part of the vertebral column, and the thoracic and lumbar parts of the vertebral column (p. 21) form the back of the thorax and abdomen, respectively (**2.2B**). Significant muscles at the front and side of the neck are mentioned below. At the back of the neck and at the back of the thoracic and lumbar regions, there is on each side of the midline a large longitudinal muscle mass, the erector spinae (its old name was sacrospinalis).

Erector spinae – extends from the sacrum to the skull and forms the bulge beside the line of vertebral spines (**3.34, 6.4**). It consists of large numbers of muscle bundles of varying lengths, with multiple attachments to vertebral spines, laminae, and transverse processes and to the adjacent parts of ribs. It is the great extensor muscle of the vertebral column, and is one of the few muscles to be supplied segmentally by the *posterior rami* of spinal nerves.

Sternocleidomastoid – prominent landmark (**3.21, 3.35**) running obliquely upwards from the manubrium of the sternum and adjacent part

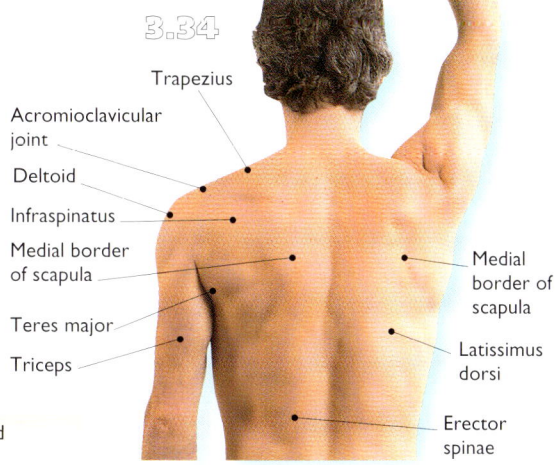

3.34. Surface features of the trunk, from behind

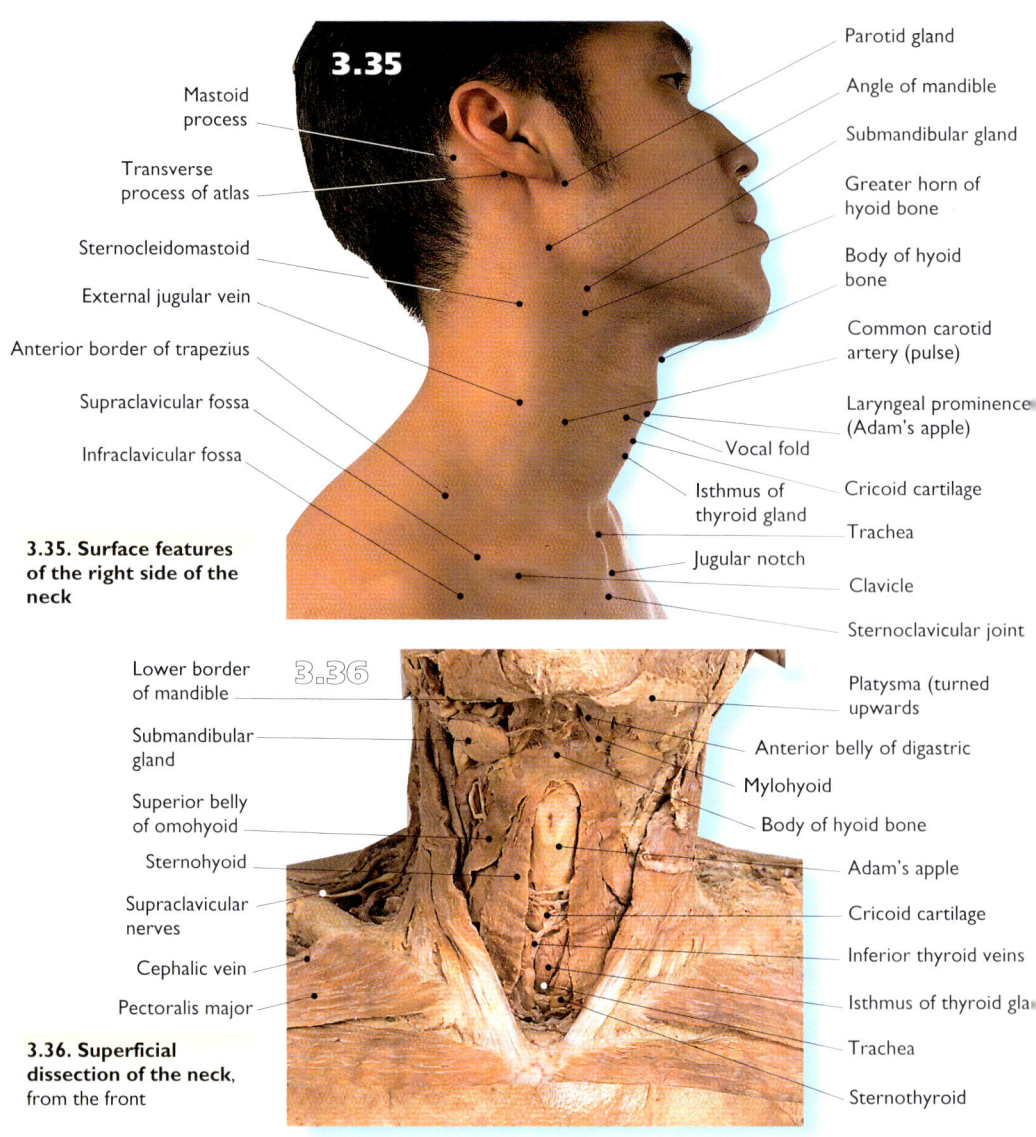

3.35. Surface features of the right side of the neck

3.36. Superficial dissection of the neck, from the front

of the clavicle to the mastoid process of the temporal bone. The part of the neck in front of it up to the midline is the anterior triangle; the part behind it, as far as trapezius, is the posterior triangle. The muscle overlies much of the carotid vessels and the internal jugular vein (**3.36**, **3.37A**). Acting singly, it tilts the face upwards and to the opposite side; acting with its opposite fellow, the pair protrude the neck (as in peering over someone's shoulder). They are supplied by the spinal part of the accessory nerve.

Cervical plexus – cutaneous branches fan out from behind sternocleidomastoid: great auricular and lesser occipital nerves upwards, transverse cervical nerve forwards (**3.22**), and branches of the supraclavicular nerve downwards (**3.36**). By far the most important branch is the phrenic nerve (*see* below).

Hyoid bone – the body and greater horns are palpable below the mandible (3.35, 3.36), on a level with the C3 vertebra. It is connected to the thyroid cartilage by the thyrohyoid membrane, which is pierced by the internal laryngeal nerve (from the superior laryngeal branch of the vagus) and the superior laryngeal artery (from the superior thyroid).

Laryngeal prominence (Adam's apple) – in the middle of the front of the neck (3.35, 3.36), and more obvious in males than in females because the two laminae (plates) of the thyroid cartilage that form it (at the level of C4 and C5 vertebrae, as part of the larynx – p. 83) join at a more acute angle in adolescent and adult males.

> The whole larynx and hence the Adam's apple move upwards during **swallowing**.

At the back of each lamina are upward and downward projections, the superior and inferior horns; the lower make the cricothyroid joints with the cricoid cartilage. The vocal folds within the larynx lie at a level midway between the laryngeal prominence and the lower border of the thyroid cartilage.

Cricoid cartilage – shaped like a signet ring, with a narrow anterior arch and a broad posterior lamina, both of which give attachment to the cricothyroid membrane of the larynx. The arch is felt about 5 cm above the jugular notch of the manubrium of the sternum, at the level of the C6 vertebra, immediately in front of the junction of pharynx and oesophagus. From the cricoid cartilage the trachea continues downwards *and backwards*, disappearing into the thorax behind the jugular notch.

> **Backward pressure** on the cricoid cartilage can prevent the upward passage of vomit into the pharynx.

Common carotid artery – source of the carotid pulse (3.35), *vitally important in indicating circulation to the brain*. Arising on the left from the arch of the aorta and on the right from the brachiocephalic trunk, each artery divides into internal and external carotid arteries at about the level of the upper border of the thyroid cartilage (C4 vertebra) (3.37).

> The **carotid pulse** is felt by pressing backwards in the angle between sternocleidomastoid and the thyroid cartilage (larynx).

Internal carotid artery – enters the skull through the carotid canal, to run through the cavernous sinus and divide into the anterior and middle cerebral arteries, which are major components of the arterial circle at the base of the brain (3.3, 3.13).

External carotid artery – instantly identified from the common or internal carotids because it has numerous branches (3.37B); the other two have no branches in the neck. The external carotid ends by entering the parotid gland and dividing into the superficial temporal and maxillary arteries (3.22, 3.23).

External jugular vein – prominent vessel that runs down across sternocleidomastoid and disappears behind the clavicle to join the subclavian vein (5.6).

Scalenus anterior – small prevertebral muscle (3.37A, 5.3) that runs from the transverse processes of C3–C6 vertebrae to the scalene tubercle of the first rib. It is an important landmark in the lower neck: the phrenic nerve passes vertically downwards in front of it and the roots of the brachial plexus emerge behind it.

Phrenic nerve – from C3, C4, and C5 (mainly C4) roots of the cervical plexus, it passes obliquely downwards over the scalenus anterior (3.37A, 5.3) to enter the thorax as *the only motor* *nerve to its own half of the diaphragm* (p. 112).

Brachial plexus – the roots, trunks, divisions, and cords (p. 59) are each in a distinct position in the neck or axilla. The roots are in the neck between two of the prevertebral muscles (scalenus anterior and scalenus medius). The trunks (upper, middle, and lower) are low down in the posterior triangle of the neck; the upper trunk gives rise to the suprascapular nerve (**3.37A, 5.3**), which supplies the supraspinatus and infraspinatus muscles of the shoulder. The divisions, which have no branches, lie behind the clavicle and form the lateral, medial, and posterior cords in the axilla (p. 95).

Cervical lymph nodes – superficial nodes, which lie mainly along the external jugular vein, below the mandible, and behind the ear, and deep nodes along the internal jugular vein, including jugulodigastric (tonsillar) nodes below the angle of the mandible. Head and neck structures drain to these nodes, which in turn pass lymph to the right lymphatic duct or thoracic duct (on the left).

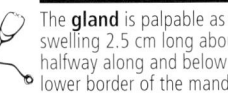

Palpation for cervical lymph nodes is an essential part of clinical examination.

Submandibular gland – salivary gland lying in the angle between the inner surface of the body of the mandible and the outer surface of mylohyoid (**3.36, 3.37A**), with a small deep part that hooks deeply around the posterior border of that muscle. The submandibular duct, 2 cm long, runs forwards on the hyoglossus muscle at the lower part of the side of the tongue, above the lingual artery and with the lingual nerve (with the submandibular ganglion attached

The **gland** is palpable as a slight swelling 2.5 cm long about halfway along and below the lower border of the mandible.

to it) hooking under the duct. The duct opens into the floor of the mouth beside the frenulum of the tongue.

Internal jugular vein – main vein of the head and neck, continuous with the sigmoid sinus in the skull through the jugular foramen (**5.6**). It runs down on the lateral side of the internal and common carotid arteries (**3.37A**) to join the subclavian vein behind the sternoclavicular joint and form the brachiocephalic vein. It receives the inferior petrosal sinus and the pharyngeal, lingual, facial, and superior and middle thyroid veins, in that order from above downwards. On the left, the thoracic duct (p. 115) joins the left side of the angle between the internal jugular and subclavian veins.

Right lymphatic duct – a short vessel formed by channels that drain the right side of the head and neck, right upper limb, and right side of the thorax, it joins the right side of the angle between the internal jugular and subclavian veins (similar to the thoracic duct on the left side).

Glossopharyngeal nerve – the smallest of the last four cranial nerves, it only supplies one muscle (the stylopharyngeus). It gives sensory fibres to the back of the tongue and part of the pharynx, and has a highly important carotid branch, only found with meticulous dissection, that runs down to the start of the internal carotid artery to supply specialized receptors in its wall and surrounding tissue. It conveys, to centres in the brainstem, information on blood pressure and the carbon dioxide content of the blood, and thus takes part in the reflex control of the heart rate.

Vagus nerve – runs straight down between the internal jugular vein and the internal and common carotid

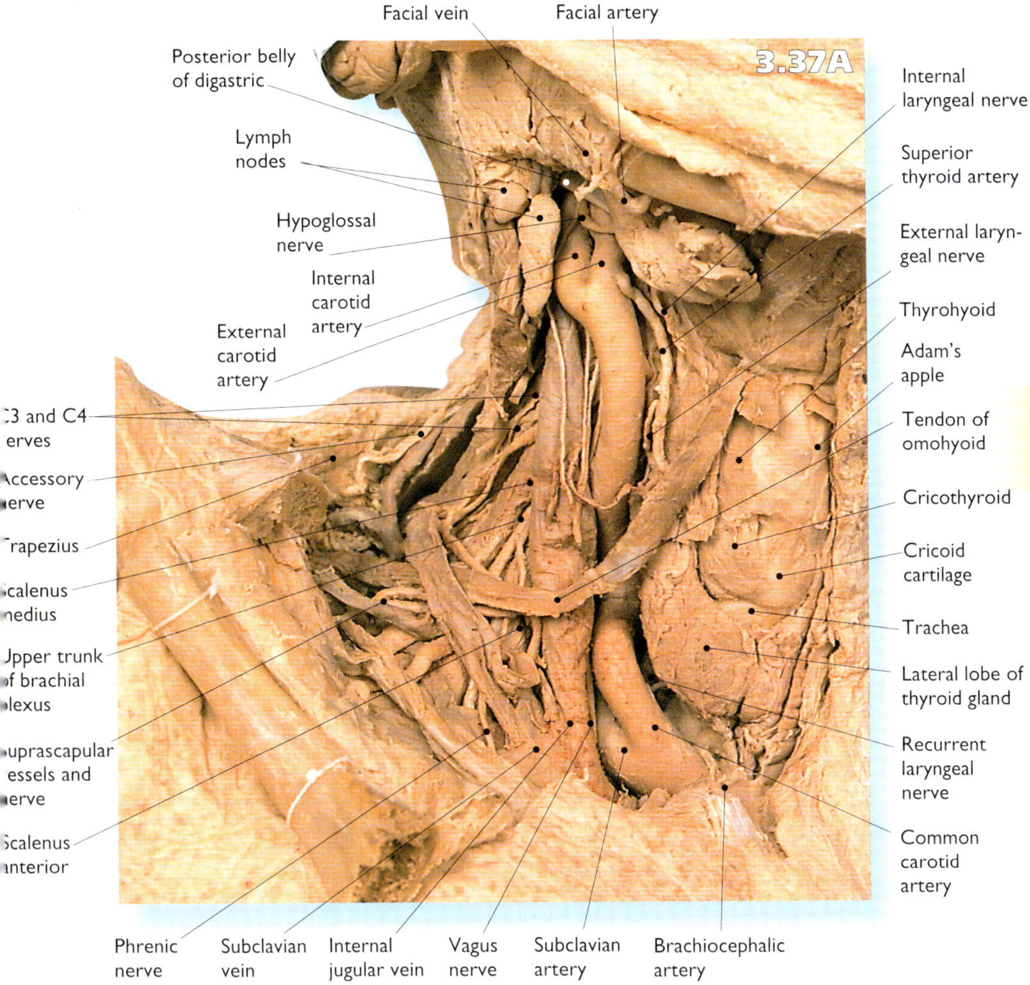

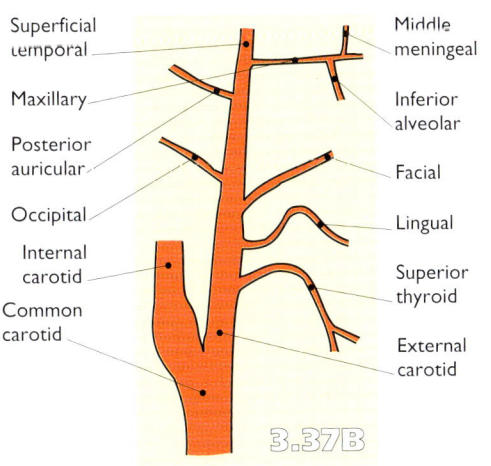

3.37. Great vessels and nerves of the right side of the neck. A Dissection from the front and the right, after removal of the sternocleidomastoid and with part of the clavicle turned down. **B** The carotid arteries and branches

arteries (3.37A) to enter the thorax. Among its branches in the neck are the pharyngeal branches and the superior laryngeal nerve, which divides into the internal laryngeal nerve (sensory to the larynx below the vocal folds), which passes downwards and forwards just below the greater horn of the hyoid bone to enter the larynx through the thyrohyoid membrane (3.37A, 3.39), and the external laryngeal nerve (motor to the cricothyroid, the only laryngeal muscle visible on the outside of the larynx), which runs down behind the superior thyroid artery (3.37A). There are also cervical cardiac branches that run down to the cardiac plexus (as well as thoracic cardiac branches).

Recurrent laryngeal nerve –from the vagus, but arising in the lowest part of the neck on the right (hooking under the right subclavian artery) and from within the thorax on the left (hooking under the arch of the aorta, 5.4). It runs up in the groove between trachea and oesophagus, and enters the pharynx and larynx (3.38), passing behind the cricothyroid joint and supplying all the laryngeal muscles (except the cricothyroid, supplied by the external laryngeal nerve) and the mucous membrane below the vocal folds.

> The **recurrent laryngeal nerves** are among the most important in the body, since by their supply of the vocal fold muscles they control the size of the airway.

Accessory nerve (spinal part) – runs down and backwards through the sternocleidomastoid to the trapezius, which it enters about 5 cm above the clavicle (3.37A). The nerve supplies both muscles.

Hypoglossal nerve – curls forwards just above the tip of the greater horn of the hyoid bone (3.37A) to run into the tongue and supply its muscles.

Sympathetic trunk – lies behind the internal or common carotid arteries (but outside the carotid sheath), giving off from its three ganglia various branches to blood vessels and other cervical structures, and also cardiac branches.

Vertebral artery – arising from the subclavian artery, it enters the foramen in the transverse process of the C6 vertebra and runs up through the same foramen in the succeeding vertebrae, eventually emerging from that of the atlas and then curling over the posterior arch of the atlas to enter the skull through the foramen magnum and unite with its fellow to form the basilar artery (3.13).

Thyroid and parathyroid glands

Thyroid gland – consists of a small central isthmus in front of tracheal rings 2–4, and on each side a lateral lobe, overlapped by the thin infrahyoid ('strap') muscles and sternocleidomastoid, and lying in front of the common carotid artery, hugging the sides of the lower larynx and upper trachea (3.36, 3.37A, 5.3). The upper pole extends up to near the top of the lamina of the thyroid cartilage, and the lower pole down to tracheal rings 5 or 6. Being attached by connective tissue to the larynx, the gland *moves with swallowing*. It usually has two arteries and three veins. The superior thyroid artery comes down from

> The gland is usually only visible or palpable when enlarged (then called a **goitre**).

> The gland is best **palpated** with the examiner behind the patient, so that both hands can be brought forwards to feel the sides and front of the neck.

Head, neck and vertebral column

the start of the external carotid to the upper pole, and the inferior thyroid artery, from the thyrocervical trunk, arches up behind the lower pole. The recurrent laryngeal nerve (see above) may be in front of or behind this artery. Super-ior and middle thyroid veins drain to the internal jugular, and one or more inferior thyroid veins enter the left brachiocephalic vein by running straight down in front of the trachea (where they may be a hazard in tracheotomy). The gland's iodine-containing secretion, thyroxine, is a general metabolic stimulant.

> The nerve is the most important structure related to the thyroid gland because it may be injured during **thyroid surgery**.

Parathyroid glands – usually two on each side, these are very small pea-like structures lying in contact with or even within the lower part of the back of the lateral lobe of the thyroid gland. All are supplied by the inferior thyroid arteries. The endocrine secretion, calcitonin, helps to control blood calcium.

Larynx

The larynx (voice box) has a framework of cartilages and membranes (3.38–3.41). The rather pyramidal-shaped arytenoid cartilages, with a vocal and a muscular process at their bases, sit on top of the (posterior) lamina of the cricoid cartilage to make the crico-arytenoid joints, and the inferior horns of the thyroid cartilage make the cricothyroid joints with the

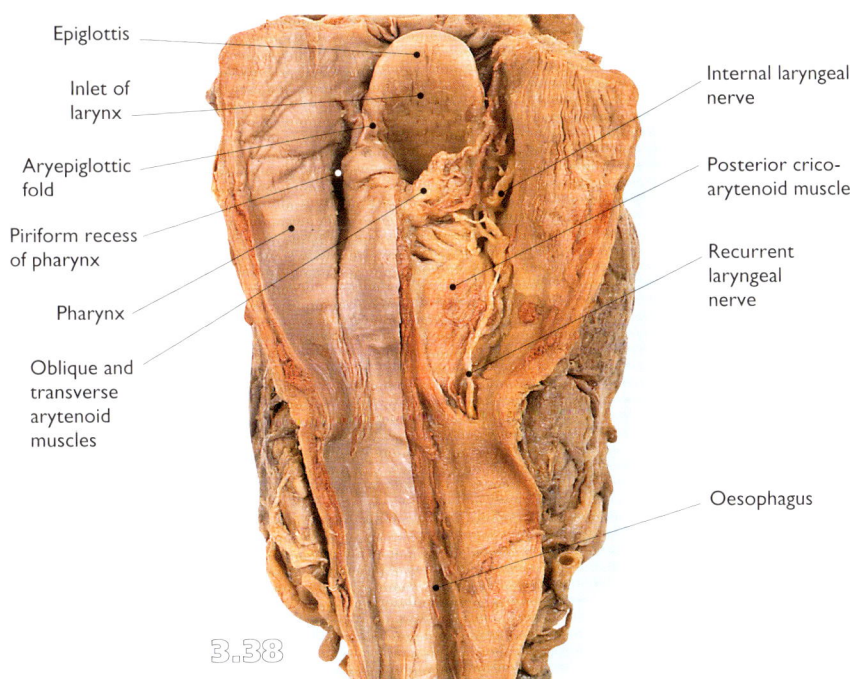

3.38. Larynx, pharynx, and oesophagus, from behind. The pharynx and oesophagus have been incised in the midline and turned forwards; the mucous membrane has been dissected away on the right side

83

sides of the cricoid cartilage. The epiglottic cartilage, covered by mucous membrane to form the epiglottis, is at the front of the laryngeal inlet from the pharynx. The aryepiglottic folds of mucous membrane and muscle form the lateral boundaries of the inlet, with the arytenoid cartilages and interarytenoid muscles at the back. The cavity of the larynx between the inlet and vocal folds (*see* below) is the vestibule of the larynx. At the cricoid cartilage (level of the C6 vertebra) the larynx becomes continuous with the trachea. Because of the attachment of some pharyngeal muscles (*see* below) to the larynx, the larynx moves upwards when swallowing.

Cricothyroid membrane – the most important of the membranes of the larynx. Attached all round the upper margin of the ring-like cricoid cartilage, it stretches up (like the lower part of a round tent) to be attached at the front to the midline junction of the thyroid laminae, midway between the laryngeal prominence and the lower borders of the laminae, and at the back to the vocal processes of the arytenoid cartilages (**3.40**). These attachments alter the round shape to a V-shape, with the apex at the front. This upper free margin of the membrane is covered by mucous membrane and forms, on each side, the anterior 60% of the vocal fold or vocal cord; the posterior 40% is the vocal process of the arytenoid cartilage (**3.41**). The up-rush of air past the folds causes them to vibrate, hence the production of sounds. Slight rotation movements at the crico-arytenoid joints, but more importantly gliding movements up and down the sloping sides of the cricoid lamina (moving the arytenoids farther apart or closer together), alter the size of the rima of the glottis (the gap between the folds through which the air passes, **3.41**) and so help to modify the sounds produced. The vestibular folds lie just above the vocal folds; they are separate structures that do not move like the vocal folds, so they are often called the false vocal folds.

Posterior crico-arytenoid muscle – runs from the back of the cricoid lamina to the muscular process of the arytenoid cartilage. It is the *only muscle that can abduct the vocal fold*, i.e. increase the size of the rima of the glottis.

> The **most important muscle of the larynx**, because it increases the size of the airway.

The other intrinsic muscles either adjust the tension in the vocal folds, adduct them, or alter the shape of the laryngeal inlet.

Nerve supply – the motor nerve supply of laryngeal muscles is the recurrent laryngeal nerve, except for the cricothyroid (supplied by the external laryngeal nerve). The sensory supply of the mucous membrane below the vocal folds is also by the recurrent laryngeal nerve, but above the folds is by the internal laryngeal nerve (so its all from the vagus, but by different branches).

Pharynx

The pharynx is a muscular tube that extends from the base of the skull to the C6 vertebra, where it becomes the oesophagus (*see* **3.4A, 3.5**). The nasal part (nasopharynx) is part of the respiratory tract, and has the opening of the auditory tube (p. 74) in the lateral wall and the pharyngeal tonsil in the posterior wall. The oral and laryngeal parts (oropharynx and laryngopharynx) are common to the respiratory and alimentary tracts. The oropharynx has the (palatine) tonsils just behind the palatoglossal

> 'Sore throats' (**pharyngitis**) and infection of the tonsils (**tonsillitis**) are common causes of enlarged and painful cervical lymph nodes.

folds (junction with the mouth) and in front of the palatopharyngeal folds, with the valleculae at the base of the

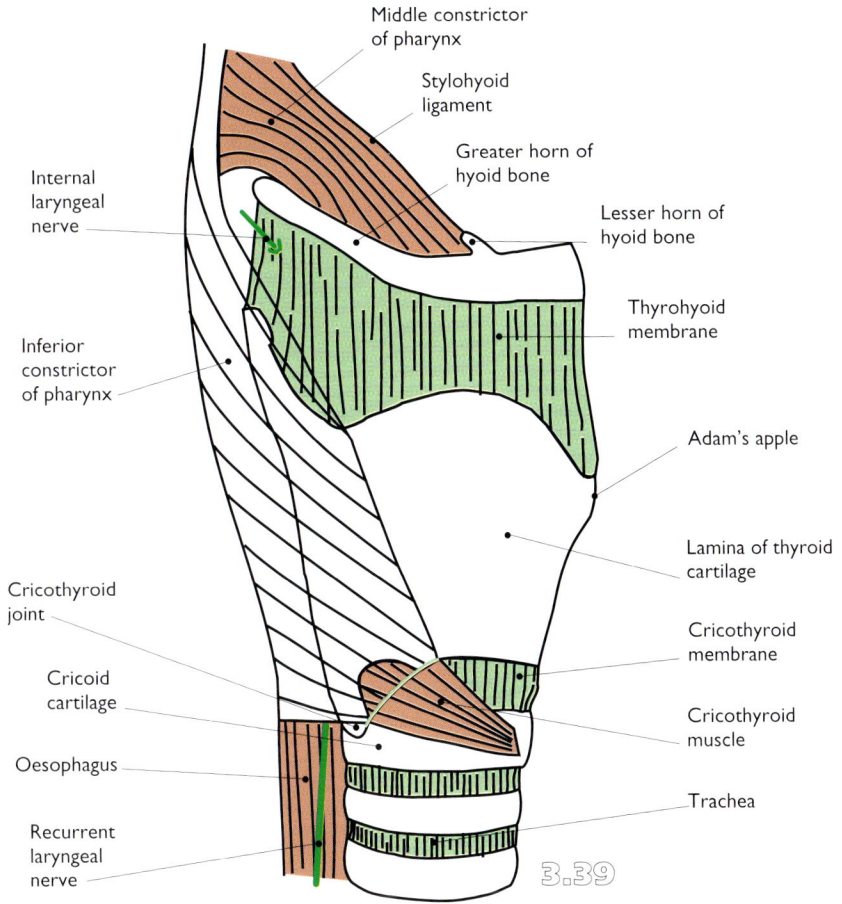

3.39. The right side of the external surface of the larynx

tongue in front of the epiglottis. The laryngopharynx has the larynx with the laryngeal inlet projecting backwards into it, with the piriform recess at each side.

Muscles – mainly the three pairs of constrictor muscles, arranged like three tumblers stacked one inside the other, but with large gaps at the front – openings into the nose, mouth, and larynx. The inferior constrictor arises from the side of the cricoid and thyroid cartilages, the middle constrictor from the horns of the hyoid bone (3.39), and the superior constrictor comes from the inside of the mandible, pterygomandibular raphe, and medial pterygoid plate. Their fibres run backwards and upwards to converge at the back on to the midline pharyngeal raphe, which is attached to the pharyngeal tubercle of the base of the skull.

Three other pairs of small muscles run down from above to blend with the constrictors – the stylopharyngeus (from the styloid process), palatopharyngeus (from the soft palate), and salpingopharyngeus (from the cartilaginous part of the auditory tube). These, but more importantly the inferior constrictors, raise the larynx during swallowing; the sternothyroid, the elasticity of the trachea, and the

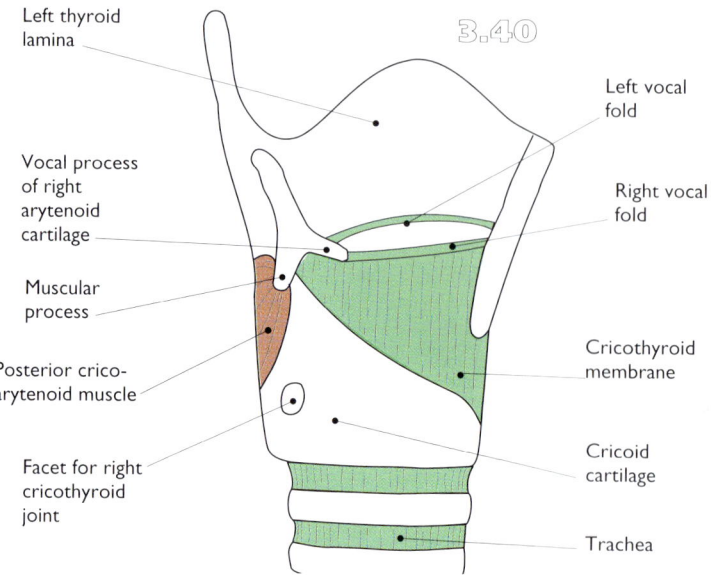

3.40. The vocal folds of the larynx, from the right, with the right lamina of the thyroid cartilage removed. The left arytenoid cartilage is obscured by the right one

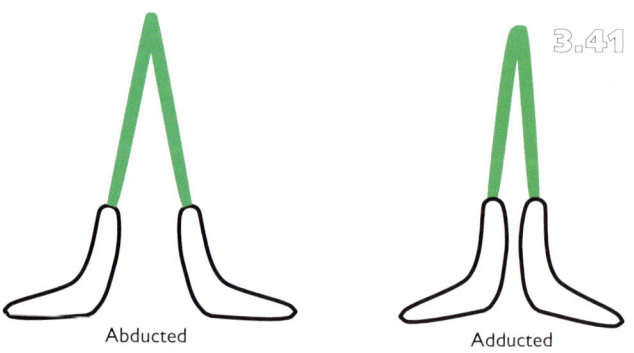

3.41. The vocal folds in abducted and adducted positions

upper attachment of the oesophagus to the back of the cricoid cartilage pull it down.

Nerve supply – mainly from the pharyngeal plexus, found on the back of the middle constrictor, and formed by pharyngeal branches of the vagus (which provide motor and sensory fibres) and glossopharyngeal nerves (which provide sensory fibres only, although the stylopharyngeus has its motor supply from a separate glossopharyngeal branch). The sensory supply to the mucosa of the nasopharynx (like the back of the nose) is mostly by the maxillary branches of the trigeminal nerves.

In swallowing (deglutition), the tongue is raised (a voluntary action) towards the hard palate and forces the food bolus into the oral part of the pharynx, while the soft palate is raised to block off the nasopharynx. The rest of the swallowing process is involuntary; sequential contraction of the pharyngeal constrictors carries on into the oesophagus and so throughout its whole length.

Tonsils – masses of lymphoid tissue (properly called the palatine tonsils) which lie in the oropharynx between the palatoglossal and palatopharyngeal arches (once collectively known as 'the pillars of the fauces'). The mucous membrane on the pharyngeal surface contains numerous downgrowths or crypts which may become the site of infection, especially in the young. With the pharyngeal tonsil at the back of the nasopharynx and the lingual tonsil in the base of the tongue, there is thus a protective ring of lymphoid tissue at the start of the alimentary and respiratory tracts.

Summary

- Injury to the side of the head may rupture the **middle meningeal artery**, causing a dangerous build-up of pressure on the cerebral cortex.

- The most important tracts within the brain and spinal cord are the **corticospinal** (motor), **gracile** and **cuneate** (touch), and **spinothalamic** (pain).

- Arterial disease (haemorrhage and thrombosis) affecting the internal capsule is the common cause of **stroke** (hemiplegia).

- The **visual pathway** includes the retina, optic nerve, optic chiasma, optic tract, lateral geniculate body, optic radiation and the calcarine area of the cerebral cortex.

- The **cornea** is supplied by ciliary branches of the ophthalmic branch of the trigeminal nerve.

- The **muscles of the face** are supplied by the facial nerve, but facial skin is supplied by the ophthalmic, maxillary, and mandibular branches of the trigeminal nerve.

- The **muscles of mastication** are supplied by the mandibular branch of the trigeminal nerve.

- The **hyoid bone** lies at the level of C3 vertebra, the **thyroid cartilage** at C4 and C5 vertebrae, and the **cricoid cartilage** opposite C6 vertebra.

- The **carotid pulse** is felt in the angle between sternocleidomastoid and the thyroid cartilage, the **facial pulse** 2.5 cm in front of the angle of the mandible, and the **superficial temporal pulse** in front of the tragus of the ear.

- The **isthmus of the thyroid gland** lies in front of the second to fourth rings of the trachea, with the lateral lobes extending between the levels of C5 to T1 vertebrae. The gland is not obvious to the naked eye, unless enlarged.

- The most commonly palpable **cervical lymph nodes** are those in the angle between the mandible and sternocleidomastoid, and between sternocleidomastoid and the clavicle.

- The most important muscle of the larynx is the **posterior cricoarytenoid** – the only one that can abduct the vocal fold.

Part 4

Upper limb

The upper limb accounts for 5% of the body weight. The movements of the clavicle and scapula, humerus, radius and ulna have one collective purpose - to put the hand into the desired position for whatever it is required to do. Since the limb is essentially suspended from the trunk of the body by muscles only and not by a large joint, it has great freedom of movement. The shoulder joint, kept out to the side of the trunk by the clavicle, is the most mobile of all body joints.

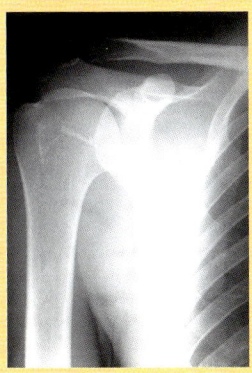

The power and the range of upper limb activity are enormous, extending from the the relatively crude movements of wielding a hammer to the most delicate brush strokes of the artist or the steady manipulations of the neurosurgeon. The coordination of motor and sensory activities in the hand is matched only by those of the eye. The twisting movements of the forearm that turn over the hand and the unique rotatory movement at the base of the thumb, allowing it to be carried towards the palm of the hand to give a firm grip, have given a degree of manual dexterity that has contributed to the human species becoming the world's most dominant animal.

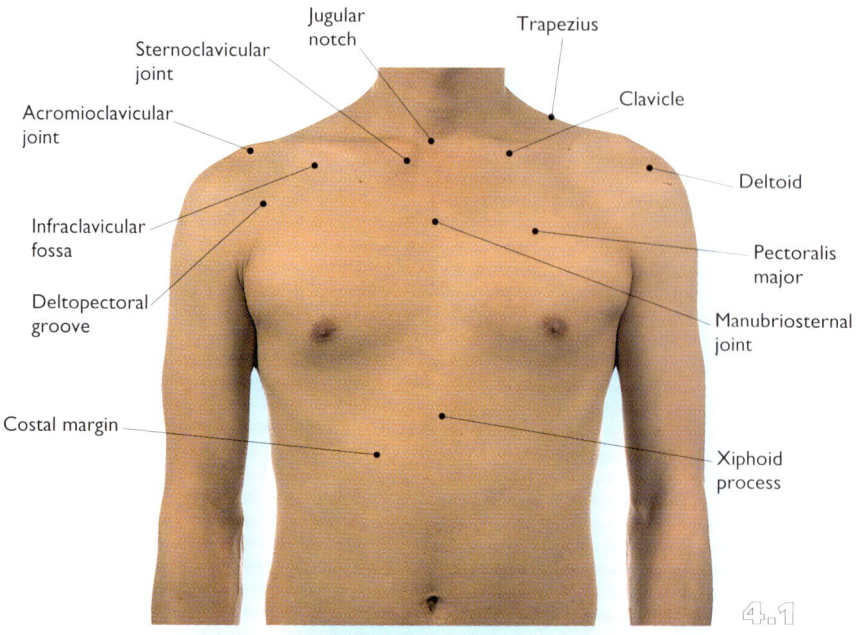

4.1. Surface features of the upper trunk and upper limb, from the front (for the back view see **3.34**)

THE ONLY *bony* connection between the upper limb and the axial skeleton is the small sternoclavicular joint (**4.1, 5.2**). The other connections are *muscular*, mainly pectoralis major at the front, serratus anterior at the side, and trapezius and latissimus dorsi at the back (**4.2, 4.3**). This accounts for the great mobility of the shoulder girdle (clavicle and scapula) compared with the hip girdle (p. 25). Small gliding and rotatory movements take place at the clavicular joints to accompany scapular movements against the chest wall.

Shoulder, axilla and arm

Bony prominences – the clavicle (**4.1, 5.2**) is palpable throughout its length and can be traced from the sternoclavicular joint to its lateral end, where it makes the acromioclavicular joint with the acromion, which is at the lateral end of the spine of the scapula. The acromion lies at a slightly lower level than the clavicle; on palpation there is a small 'step down' from clavicle to acromion. The tip of the coracoid process of the scapula is just under the cover of the anterior border of the deltoid, and can be felt by pressing laterally in the deltopectoral groove (*see below*) about 1 cm below the clavicle.

Sternoclavicular joint – between the bulbous medial end of the clavicle and the manubrium of the sternum, the capsule encloses two joint cavities because a fibrocartilaginous disc separates the two bones. Adjacent to the joint is the costoclavicular ligament, which passes from the first rib and costal cartilage to the under surface of the clavicle, and is important as the fulcrum about which movements of the clavicle take place.

Upper limb

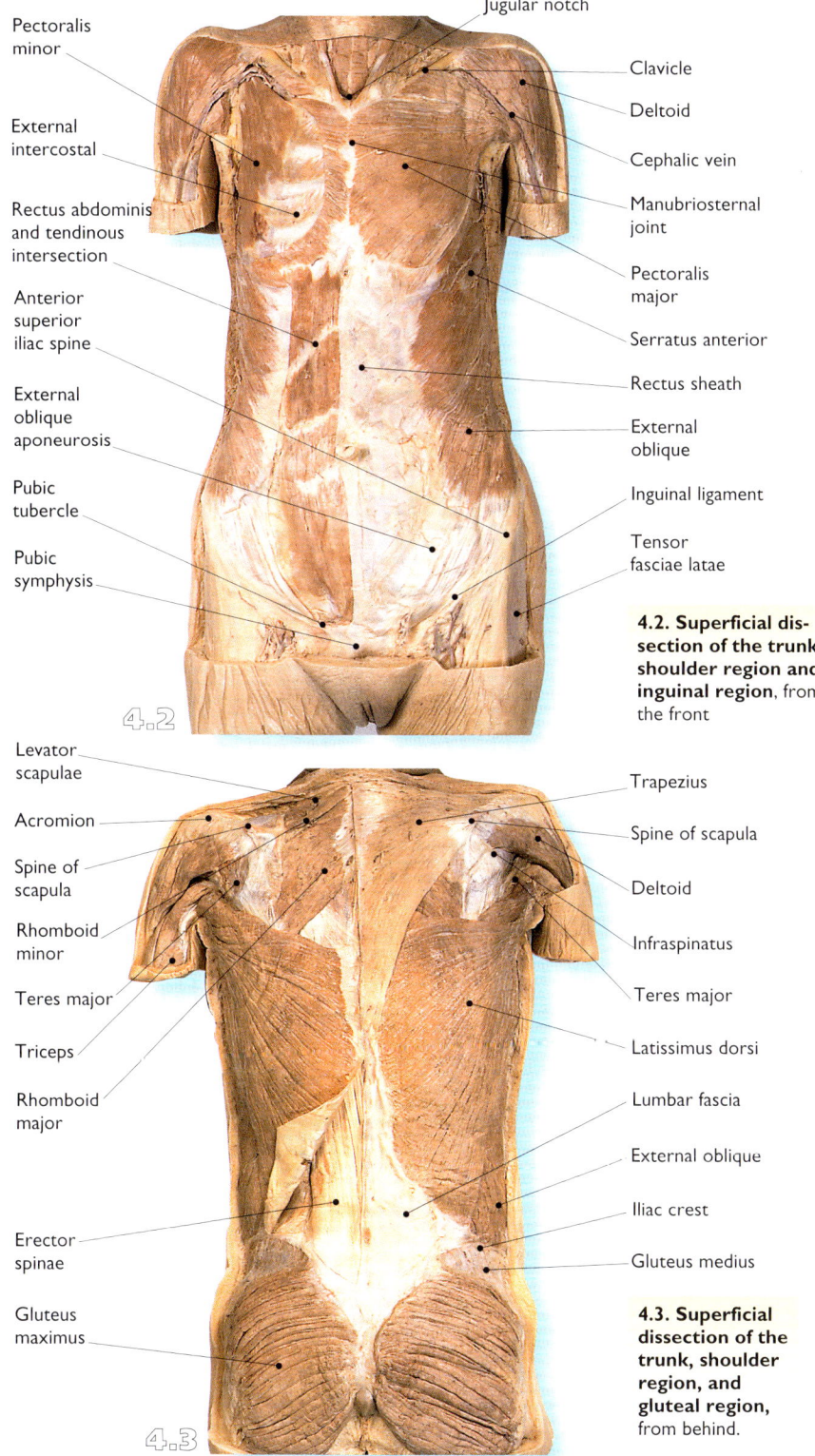

4.2. Superficial dissection of the trunk, shoulder region and inguinal region, from the front

4.3. Superficial dissection of the trunk, shoulder region, and gluteal region, from behind.

Acromioclavicular joint – between the flattened lateral end of the clavicle and the acromion of the spine of the scapula. There is a capsule, but the main factor keeping the bones in place is the coracoclavicular ligament, which runs from the coracoid process of the scapula to the under surface of the clavicle near its lateral end and consists of two parts, the conoid and trapezoid ligaments. These are strong and highly important in maintaining the integrity of the joint; in dislocation, they are torn and the 'step down' from clavicle to acromion is markedly increased.

Pectoralis major – from the medial half of the clavicle and sternum it converges on to the lateral lip of the intertubercular groove of the humerus (**4.2**). It is supplied by medial and lateral pectoral nerves.

Pectoralis minor – small and underlying pectoralis major, it passes from ribs 3, 4, and 5 to the coracoid process of the scapula (**4.2**). Its main importance is that it forms a landmark in the axilla (*see* below).

Serratus anterior – from the upper eight ribs (**4.2**) fibres converge along the length of the medial border of the scapula, but half of them are concentrated on the lower angle to assist in rotation of the scapula (*see* movements of the shoulder, p. 94). It is supplied by the long thoracic nerve.

Trapezius – from a wide origin, from the occipital region of the skull and the spines of all the cervical and thoracic vertebrae, the fibres converge to the lateral third of the clavicle, the inner edge of the acromion, and the spine of the scapula (**4.3**). By its upper fibres it is the main muscle that shrugs the shoulder, and it also helps to rotate the scapula (*see* movements of the shoulder, p. 94). It is supplied by the spinal part of the accessory nerve (p. 82).

Latissimus dorsi – arising from the lower six thoracic vertebrae, lumbar fascia, and the posterior part of the iliac crest (**4.3**), the fibres converge to a narrow tendon which curls around teres major to be inserted into the floor of the intertubercular groove of the humerus. It is a powerful adductor and extensor of the shoulder and is supplied by the thoracodorsal nerve.

Teres major – from the back of the inferior angle of the scapula (**4.3**), it passes *in front of* the long head of triceps to reach the medial lip of the intertubercular groove of the humerus. With the latissimus dorsi tendon curling around in front of it, it forms the lower boundary of the axilla. It is an adductor and medial rotator of the humerus, and is supplied by the lower subscapular nerve.

Rotator cuff muscles – a group of four (subscapularis, supraspinatus, infraspinatus, and teres minor) which fuse with the capsule of the shoulder joint and embrace the head of the humerus, keeping the head in contact with the glenoid cavity of the scapula.

Subscapularis – from the subscapular fossa of the front of the scapula it reaches the lesser tubercle of the humerus. Apart from stabilizing the shoulder joint, it is a medial rotator of the humerus. It is supplied by the upper and lower subscapular nerves.

Supraspinatus – from the supraspinous fossa of the scapula it runs above the shoulder joint to the upper facet of the greater tubercle of the humerus (**4.4A**). Apart from stabilizing the shoulder joint, it acts with the deltoid to abduct the arm. It is supplied by the suprascapular nerve.

Infraspinatus – from the infraspinous fossa (**4.3**) it runs to the middle facet of the greater tubercle of the humerus. Apart from stabilizing the

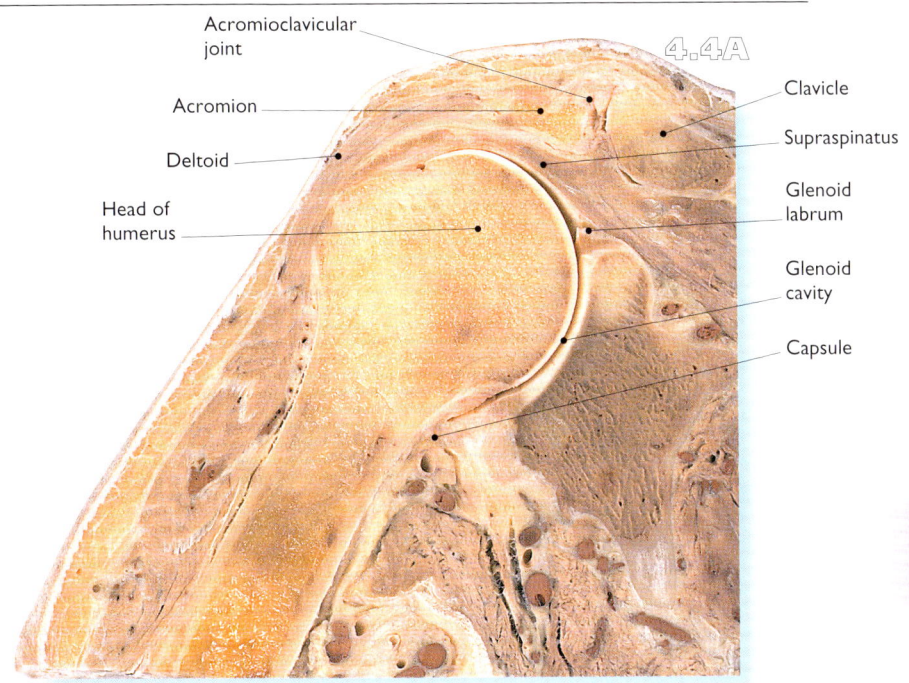

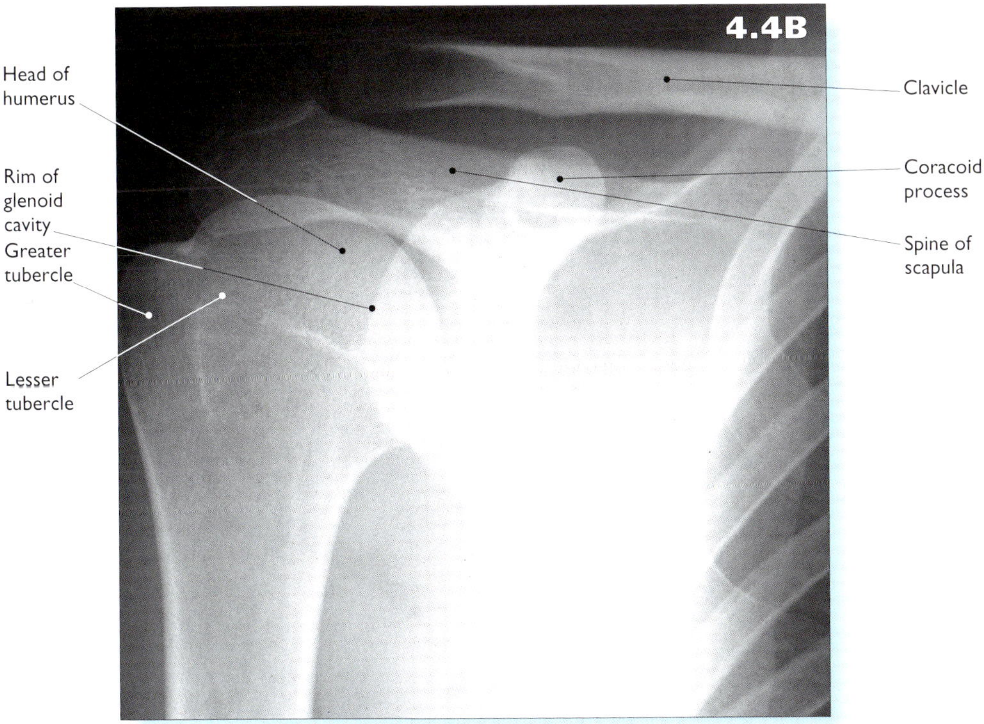

4.4. Right shoulder joint A Coronal section B Radiograph

shoulder joint, it is a powerful lateral rotator of the humerus. It is supplied by the suprascapular nerve.

Teres minor – arising just above teres major, it passes *behind* the long head of triceps to the lower facet of the greater tubercle of the humerus. Apart from stabilizing the shoulder joint, it is a lateral rotator of the humerus. It is supplied by the axillary nerve.

Deltoid – forms the most lateral part of the shoulder, covering the greater tubercle of the humerus (**4.2**, **4.3**). It runs from the lateral third of the clavicle and the acromion and spine of the scapula to halfway down the lateral side of the shaft of the humerus. It is the most important abductor of the shoulder; its anterior fibres also assist in medial rotation of the humerus, and the posterior fibres in lateral rotation. It is supplied by the axillary nerve.

Deltopectoral groove – the gap between the deltoid (attached to the *lateral third* of the clavicle) and pectoralis major (attached to the *medial half* of the clavicle), which allows the cephalic vein to reach the subclavian vein without being compressed by the muscles.

Shoulder joint – between the glenoid cavity of the scapula and the head of the humerus (**4.4**). The glenoid cavity is slightly deepened at the periphery by the fibrocartilaginous glenoid labrum. This is directly continuous with the tendon of origin of the long head of biceps, which runs over the top of the head of the humerus and out of the joint capsule, surrounded by a tubular sleeve of synovial membrane to lie in the intertubercular (bicipital) groove of the humerus.

The capsule is very lax, to allow for the wide range of movement. The lowest part of its attachment to the humerus is to the medial side of the surgical neck; elsewhere, it surrounds the anatomical neck. The rotator cuff muscles compensate for the laxness of the capsule. The coraco-acromial ligament forms a fibrous arch above the joint; between it and the supraspinatus tendon lies the subacromial bursa (sometimes called the subdeltoid, since it projects laterally beyond the acromion). It does not normally communicate with the joint cavity, but if the supraspinatus tendon is torn there will then be a direct communication between the two.

Principal muscles that produce movements at the shoulder joint are:
Abduction – supraspinatus and deltoid.
Adduction – pectoralis major, latissimus dorsi, and teres major.
Flexion – deltoid (anterior part), pectoralis major (sternal part), and biceps.
Extension – deltoid (posterior part), pectoralis major (clavicular part), latissimus dorsi, and teres major.
Lateral rotation – infraspinatus, teres minor, and deltoid (posterior fibres).
Medial rotation – pectoralis major, subscapularis, latissimus dorsi, teres major, and deltoid (anterior fibres).

The amount of abduction possible at the shoulder joint itself (produced by the supraspinatus and deltoid working together) is about 120°. Abduction to 180° (straight up beside the head) requires movement at the joint to be supplemented by rotation of the scapula, tilting the glenoid cavity upwards. This is produced by the upper part of the trapezius (pulling on the acromion and spine of the scapula) and the lower part of serratus anterior (pulling on the inferior angle of the scapula).

Note that the supraspinatus passes right over the centre of the top of the

> The most mobile joint in the body and the most frequently dislocated.

> Cutting the **accessory nerve** in the neck (in operations to remove cervical lymph nodes) paralyses trapezius and limits abduction.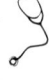

Upper limb

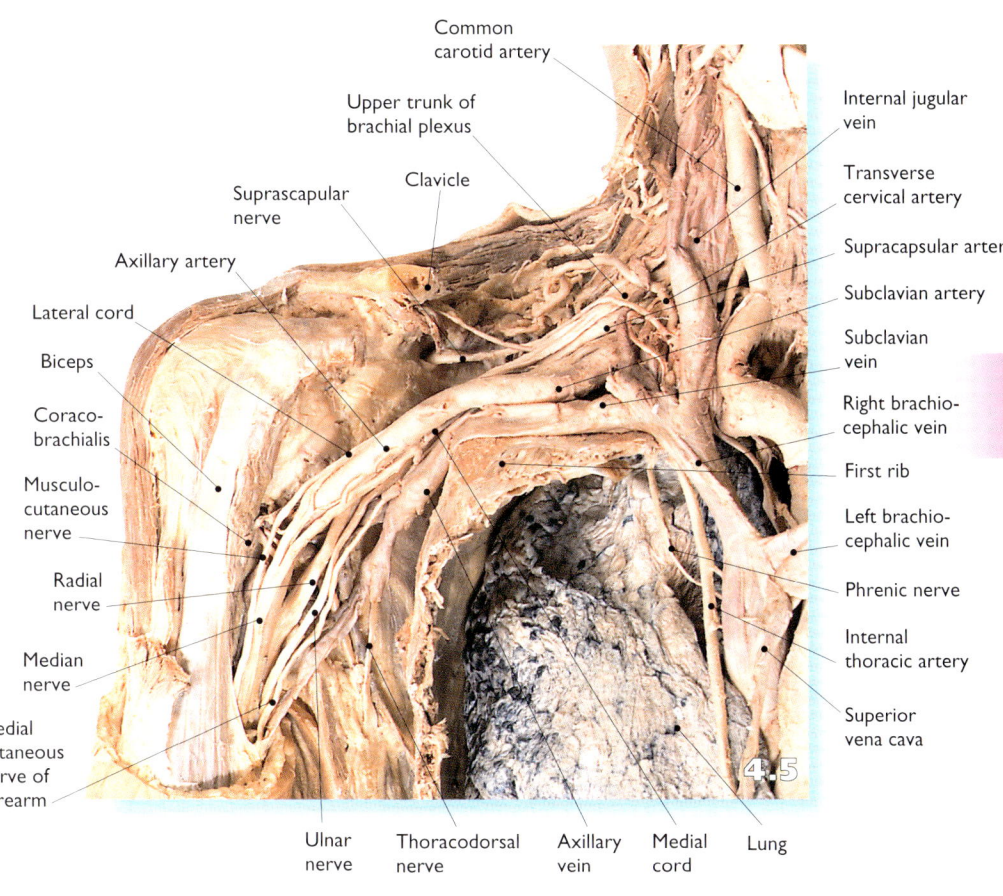

4.5. Right axilla and root of the neck, from the front

joint and is an abductor, not a rotator, despite belonging to the group called 'rotator cuff'.

Axilla – commonly called the armpit, whose anterior wall is formed by pectoralis major and minor, and the posterior wall by subscapularis with latissimus dorsi curling around teres major at the lower border. The main contents are the axillary vessels, cords of the brachial plexus and their branches, lymph nodes, and fat (**4.5**).

Axillary artery – continuation of the subclavian artery, and becoming the brachial artery in the arm. The axillary vein lies medial to the artery. The vessels lie behind pectoralis minor – the guide to the artery and the surrounding cords of the brachial plexus.

Cords of the brachial plexus – arranged around the axillary artery

95

and named according to their positions – lateral, medial, and posterior (**3.18**). To assist in identifying the major branches of the cords, note the capital-M pattern made by the ulnar nerve, the two roots of the median nerve, and the musculocutaneous nerve. (For other parts of the plexus, *see* p. 59 and 80. For the distributions of dermatomes and cutaneous nerves, *see* **3.17, 4.10**.)

Lateral cord – gives rise to the musculocutaneous nerve, lateral root of the median nerve, and lateral pectoral nerve.

Medial cord – gives rise to the ulnar nerve, medial root of the median nerve, medial pectoral nerve, and the medial cutaneous nerves of arm and forearm.

Posterior cord – gives rise to the radial nerve, axillary nerve, subscapular nerves, and thoracodorsal nerve.

Musculocutaneous nerve – most lateral of the large branches, it runs through coracobrachialis, a feature that identifies it from all other branches of the plexus. It supplies biceps, coracobrachialis, and brachialis, and then becomes the lateral cutaneous nerve of the forearm.

Median nerve – formed by its two roots, which unite on the front of the axillary artery, it runs down the arm in front of the brachial artery, overlapped by biceps, and in the cubital fossa lies medial to the artery. There are no muscular branches in the arm.

Ulnar nerve – largest branch of the medial cord, it runs down to the axillary artery and just *behind* the medial cutaneous nerve of the forearm, which is almost as large. Halfway down the arm the ulnar nerve enters the posterior compartment to continue its downwards course in front of the triceps; at the elbow it lies behind the medial epicondyle of the humerus, where it is palpable and most liable to damage. There are no muscular branches in the arm.

Medial cutaneous nerve of the arm – small, lying medial to the axillary vein.

Medial cutaneous nerve of the forearm – almost as large as the ulnar nerve, but lying in front of it (as might be expected since it is heading for skin) and not to be confused with it.

Radial nerve – largest nerve of the whole plexus, from the posterior cord, behind the axillary artery; look for it in front of the white tendon of latissimus dorsi on the lower posterior axillary wall. It is the nerve of the extensor muscles of the arm and forearm. Curling around behind the humerus, between parts of triceps, it enters the forearm on the radial side under cover of brachioradialis, where it divides into an unimportant superficial cutaneous branch and the highly important posterior interosseous nerve, which supplies all the forearm extensor muscles. Remember, therefore, that the radial nerve, which comes from the *posterior* cord of the brachial plexus, is the nerve that supplies the muscles of the *posterior* aspect of the *arm and forearm*.

Radial nerve paralysis, e.g. from fracture of the shaft of the humerus, causes '**wrist drop**' because the extensors are paralysed.

Axillary nerve – large nerve arising high up from the posterior cord, it runs downwards and laterally to disappear backwards below teres major and behind the humerus, to supply the deltoid (and teres minor) and a small overlying patch of skin.

For **ulnar nerve injury** see p. 103.

Axillary lymph nodes – up to about 50 nodes scattered in the axillary fat and mainly located near the axillary vessels and their branches. Apart from receiving lymph from the upper limb, they are of supreme importance because most of the lymphatic drainage from the breast passes to these nodes.

> The nodes are commonly invaded by cancerous spread (**metastases**) from the breast – one of the commonest sites for cancer in females.

Biceps – the prominent muscle of the front of the arm, with a long head continuous with the glenoid labrum within the shoulder joint, and a short head arising from the coracoid process with coracobrachialis. At the elbow its tendon is attached to the *back* of the tuberosity of the radius. It is not only a flexor of the forearm, but also (with the elbow flexed) the most powerful supinator of the forearm (p. 106). It is supplied by the musculocutaneous nerve.

Brachialis – behind the biceps, from the front of the humerus to the front of the coronoid process and tuberosity of the ulna, and a powerful flexor of the forearm. It is supplied by the musculocutaneous nerve.

Coracobrachialis – from the coracoid process of the scapula (with the short head of biceps) to halfway down the medial side of the humerus. Only important because the musculocutaneous nerve, which supplies it, runs through it – a useful identifying feature.

Triceps – extensor of the elbow, the only muscle on the back of the arm, with heads of origin from the scapula below the glenoid cavity (long head), the upper part of the back of the humerus (lateral head), and the rest of the back of the humerus (medial head). All unite in a tendon inserted into the back of the olecranon of the ulna. It is supplied by the radial nerve.

> **Radial nerve injury** from fracture of the humerus (see above) does not usually paralyse triceps because the branches that supply it arise high in the axilla above the level of injury.

Brachial artery – runs down the arm just under cover of the medial border of biceps. In the upper part of the arm the brachial pulse can be felt by pressing *laterally, not backwards,* because at this level the artery lies *medial* to the humerus, not in front of it. This is the artery that is compressed for taking blood pressure; the stethoscope used for listening to the pulsation sounds is placed over the *lower* end of the artery (**4.6**) in the cubital fossa (*see* below), just above where it divides into the radial and ulnar arteries.

Elbow, forearm and hand

Bony prominences – at the elbow the medial and lateral epicondyles of the humerus are easily palpable at the sides, and so at the back is the olecranon of the ulna and the whole length of the posterior border of the ulna (**2.3**). The medial epicondyle gives origin to several flexor muscles and forms the common flexor origin; similarly, the lateral epicondyle forms the common extensor origin. Any of these bony prominences are frequently hit against things. With the elbow straight (extended), the head of the radius can be felt at the back of the elbow (at the bottom of a small depression lateral to the olecranon), where it articulates with the capitulum of the humerus.

At the sides of the wrist, the styloid process of the radius extends 1 cm lower than the styloid process of the ulna. Near the distal skin crease at the wrist on the radial side is the tubercle of the scaphoid,

> In the common fracture of the lower end of the radius (**Colles' fracture**) the two styloid processes come to lie at the same level because the lower broken end is forced upwards.

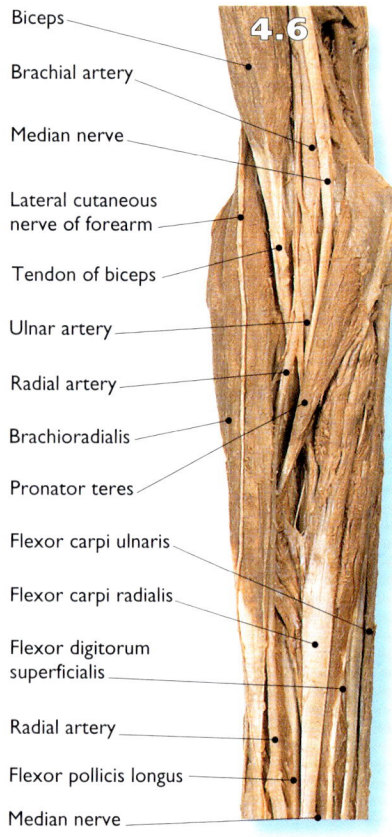

4.6. Superficial dissection of the right cubital fossa and forearm

Labels (top to bottom):
- Biceps
- Brachial artery
- Median nerve
- Lateral cutaneous nerve of forearm
- Tendon of biceps
- Ulnar artery
- Radial artery
- Brachioradialis
- Pronator teres
- Flexor carpi ulnaris
- Flexor carpi radialis
- Flexor digitorum superficialis
- Radial artery
- Flexor pollicis longus
- Median nerve

this bulge is the anterior surface of the head of the ulna (confirm this on an articulated skeleton). Muscles named with the word 'carpi' (meaning 'of the carpus' or wrist), such as flexor carpi radialis and extensor carpi radialis, are usually attached to the bases of metacarpals and can move the wrist, while those with the word 'digitorum' (of the digits) have longer tendons that run beyond the wrist to phalanges of the fingers and so can move the fingers as well as the wrist. The thumb has its own muscles, indicated by 'pollicis', from the Latin for 'thumb'.

Cubital fossa – a descriptive triangular region at the front of the elbow, bounded by pronator teres medially, brachioradialis laterally, and above by a line that joins the humeral epicondyles (4.6). Brachialis and supinator form the floor. Contents from lateral to medial are the tendon of biceps, brachial artery, and median nerve. The radial nerve is under cover of brachioradialis on the lateral side and so is not visible unless the muscle is displaced laterally, when the nerve can be seen dividing into its superficial (cutaneous) and deep (posterior interosseous) branches.

Pronator teres – arising mainly from the common flexor origin, the muscle crosses the forearm obliquely to be attached halfway down the lateral side of the radius. The muscle has a small deep head, and the median nerve, by which it is supplied, passes down between the two heads.

Brachioradialis – from the lateral side of the humerus above the lateral epicondyle, the muscle runs down to the lower end of the radius just above the styloid process. In the commonly used midprone position of the forearm, it helps to maintain the required angle of elbow flexion. It is supplied by the radial nerve.

and on the ulnar side is the pisiform bone with the tendon of flexor carpi ulnaris running into it. On the back (dorsum) of the hand, all the metacarpals are palpable; in a clenched fist, the heads of the metacarpals make the knuckles. In the thumb and fingers, all the phalanges are easily felt.

The hand is essentially attached to the radius, which bears the brunt of upward pressure applied to the hand. When the hand is in the anatomical position with the palm facing forwards, the forearm is in the position of supination (p. 16). When the forearm is pronated, the head of the ulna makes a prominent bulge; note that

Upper limb

Supinator – a deep muscle that arises partly from the supinator crest of the upper ulna, it wraps itself around the upper end of the radius from behind, thus helping to 'unwind' the pronated radius. It is supplied by the posterior interosseous (radial) nerve, which runs through the muscle.

Brachial artery – in the cubital fossa the artery is located with the elbow straight by palpating on the medial side of the biceps tendon (the median nerve lies medial to the artery); the artery is not quite in the centre of the fossa, but a little towards the medial side.

> Used for taking the **blood pressure**, the stethoscope is placed over the artery in the fossa, medial to the biceps tendon.

Superficial veins – commonly make an H or M pattern at the front of the cubital fossa (**4.7**). The cephalic vein on the lateral side and the basilic vein on the medial side both begin from the dorsal venous network on the dorsum of the hand. The cephalic vein runs up into the deltopectoral groove (p. 94), while the basilic vein joins the brachial vein in the middle of the arm.

> Any of these veins are frequently used for **intravenous injections** and to collect blood for tests and transfusions.

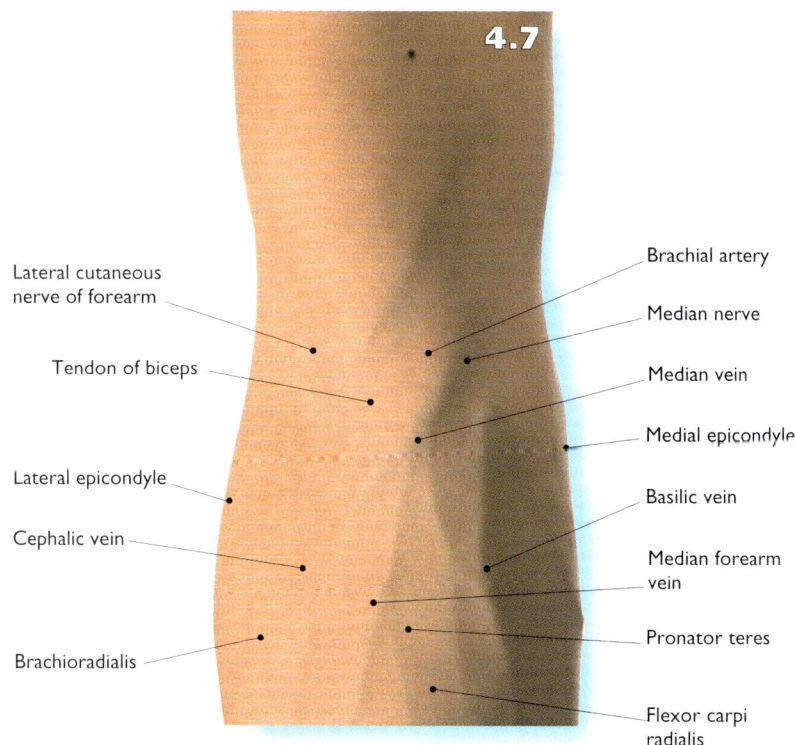

4.7. Surface features of the right elbow region (cubital fossa), from the front

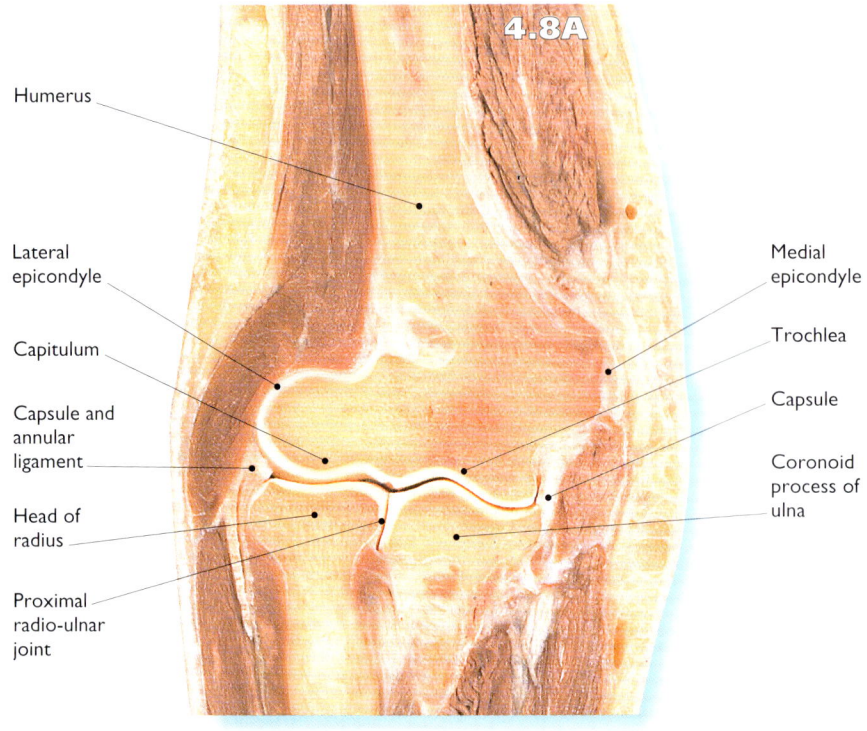

4.8. Right elbow joint A Coronal section B Radiograph

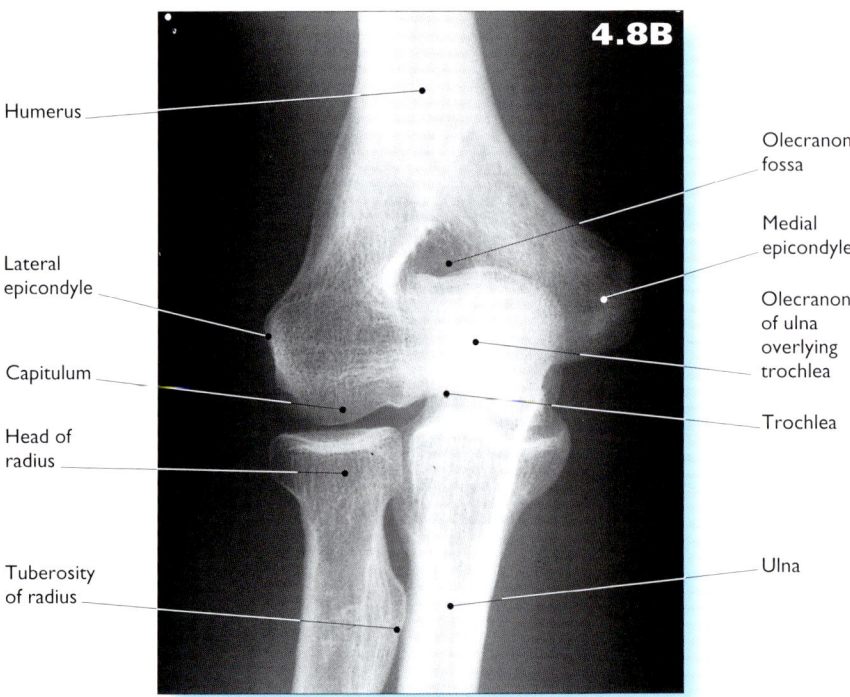

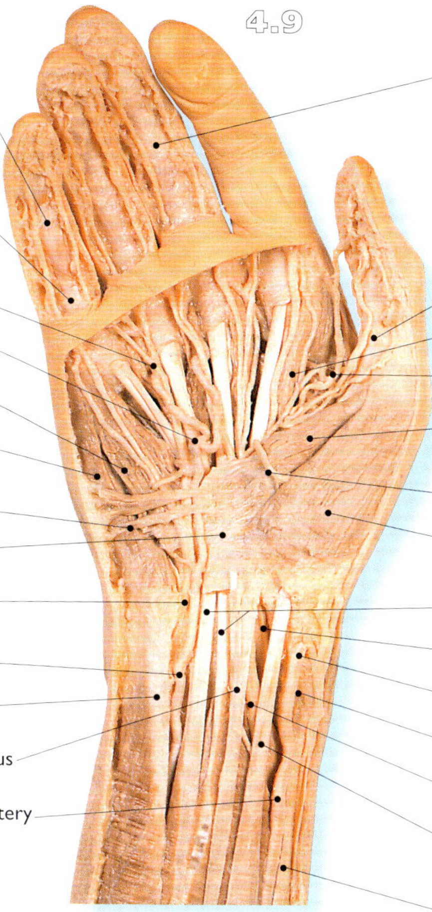

Upper limb

4.9. Superficial dissection of the right lower forearm and palm of the hand

Labels: Flexor digitorum profundus; Flexor digitorum superficialis; Palmar digital artery and nerve; Superficial palmar arch; Flexor digiti minimi brevis; Abductor digiti minimi; Palmaris brevis; Flexor retinaculum; Ulnar nerve; Ulnar artery; Flexor carpi ulnaris; Palmaris longus; Radial artery; Fibrous flexor sheath; Flexor pollicis longus; First lumbrical; Adductor pollicis; Flexor pollicis brevis; Recurrent branch of median nerve; Abductor pollicis brevis; Flexor digitorum superficialis; Flexor pollicis longus; Radial artery; Pronator quadratus; Median nerve; Flexor carpi radialis; Brachioradialis.

Elbow joint – between the trochlea and capitulum of the lower end of the humerus, the trochlear notch of the ulna, and the head of the radius (4.8). The capsule is reinforced by medial and lateral ligaments, with the annular ligament holding the head of the radius in contact with the ulna (*see* Proximal radio-ulnar joint, below).

Principal muscles that produce movements at the elbow joint are:
Flexion – brachialis, biceps, and brachioradialis.
Extension – triceps.

The only movements possible at the elbow joint itself are flexion and extension (pronation and supination occur at the radio-ulnar joints – *see* p. 106).

Radial artery – runs down under cover of brachioradialis and, where subcutaneous at the wrist, is the common site for feeling the pulse (4.9). Lower down, the artery

The **radial pulse** is felt by pressing the artery against the lower end of the radius, on the radial (lateral) side of the tendon of flexor carpi radialis.

101

passes dorsally through the anatomical snuffbox (p.106) and into the palm through the first dorsal interosseus muscle, to become the deep palmar arch, uniting with the deep branch of the ulnar artery. This arch lies at a level 1 cm proximal to the superficial arch (*see* below) and is deep to the long flexor tendons.

Ulnar artery – usually smaller than the radial artery, it enters the hand superficial to the flexor retinaculum. The artery continues into the palm as the superficial palmar arch (**4.9**); it extends no farther into the hand than the level of the web of the outstretched thumb. It is usually J-shaped; only in one-third of hands is the arch completed by union with the superficial palmar branch of the radial artery. The arch lies deep to the palmar aponeurosis, in front of the

> The **ulnar pulse** can usually be felt (though less easily than the radial pulse) on the radial side of the tendon of flexor carpi ulnaris, just before it becomes attached to the pisiform bone.

long flexor tendons, and its branches become those that run up the sides of the fingers, joining with corresponding vessels from the deep arch.

Median nerve – runs down under cover of flexor digitorum superficialis and supplies most of the long flexor muscles of the wrist and fingers. At the wrist it lies on the *ulnar* side of the flexor carpi radialis tendon, partly overlapped by the palmaris longus tendon (if present) (**4.9**). This subcutaneous position is the most common site for median nerve injury, e.g. cuts of the wrist by broken glass. The nerve enters the hand by running *deep* to the flexor retinaculum and then gives off the highly important muscular (recurrent) branch, which supplies the three small muscles of the base of the thumb (p. 106). Other cutaneous branches supply palm and finger skin, including that of

> **Injury** here interferes with gripping (p. 107) and causes loss of sensation at the tips of the thumb and adjacent fingers.

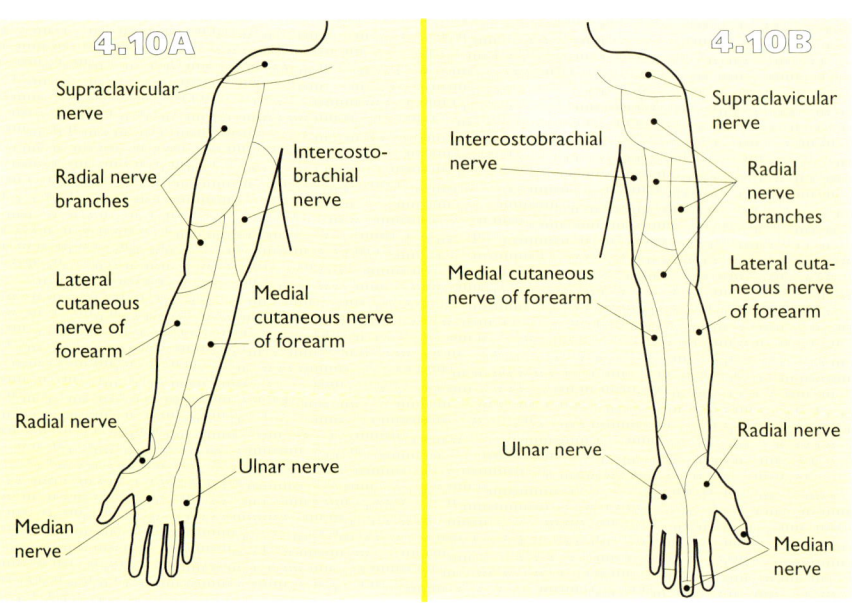

4.10. Cutaneous nerves of the right upper limb A Front **B** Back

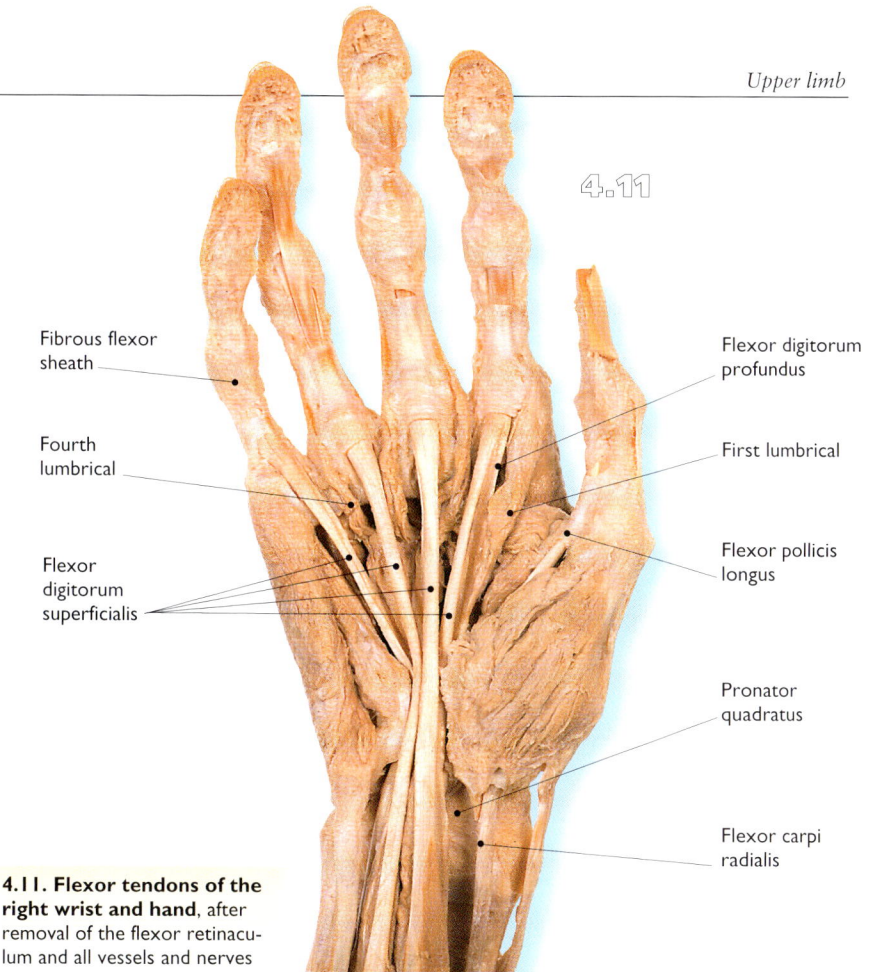

4.11. Flexor tendons of the right wrist and hand, after removal of the flexor retinaculum and all vessels and nerves

the pulps of the thumb, index, and middle fingers – among the most important sensory areas in the body (4.10).

Ulnar nerve – after passing behind the medial epicondyle of the humerus it runs down between the long flexor muscles on the medial side of the forearm to enter the hand *superficial* to the flexor retinaculum (4.9). It supplies flexor carpi ulnaris and half of flexor digitorum profundus, and all the small muscles of the hand [except for the three at the base of the thumb (supplied by the median nerve)], which are so important for intricate movements of the fingers (p. 107). Cutaneous branches supply skin of the ulnar side of the palm and of the little and ring fingers.

Flexor tendons – the prominent superficial tendons at the front of the wrist are those of the flexor carpi radialis (reaching the bases of metacarpals 2 and 3) towards the radial side, palmaris longus (attaching to the flexor retinaculum) almost in the midline (although this muscle is missing in about 13% of limbs), with those of flexor digitorum superficialis behind it, and that of the flexor carpi ulnaris running to the pisiform bone on the ulnar side (4.9, 4.11). At a deeper level (not palpable) are flexor pollicis longus and flexor digitorum profundus, whose lower ends pass in front of the

> Injury to the ulnar nerve at the elbow gives rise to '**claw hand**' due to the inability to extend the fingers, and interferes with sensation on the ulnar side of the hand.

quadrangular-shaped pronator quadratus, which occupies the lower quarter of the front of the ulna and runs straight across to the lower quarter of the radius. The pollicis longus and profundus tendons are attached to the *base* of the *distal* phalanx of the respective digits; the superficialis tendons split into two to become attached to the *sides* of the *middle* phalanx of each finger, thus allowing the profundus tendons to pass through to the distal bone (**4.11**).

Flexor retinaculum – tough fibrous tissue (**4.9**), the size of a small postage stamp, passing from the pisiform and hamate to the scaphoid and trapezium, and forming with them and other carpal bones the carpal tunnel, through which run the tendons to the thumb and fingers, *and the median nerve*. The ulnar nerve and artery lie superficial to the retinaculum.

Fibrous flexor sheaths – form with the phalanges of each digit a sheath that prevents the flexor tendons from bowing forwards when the digits are flexed (**4.11**).

Synovial sheaths – surround the tendons in the carpal tunnel and within the fibrous sheaths of the fingers, to allow tendon movement without friction.

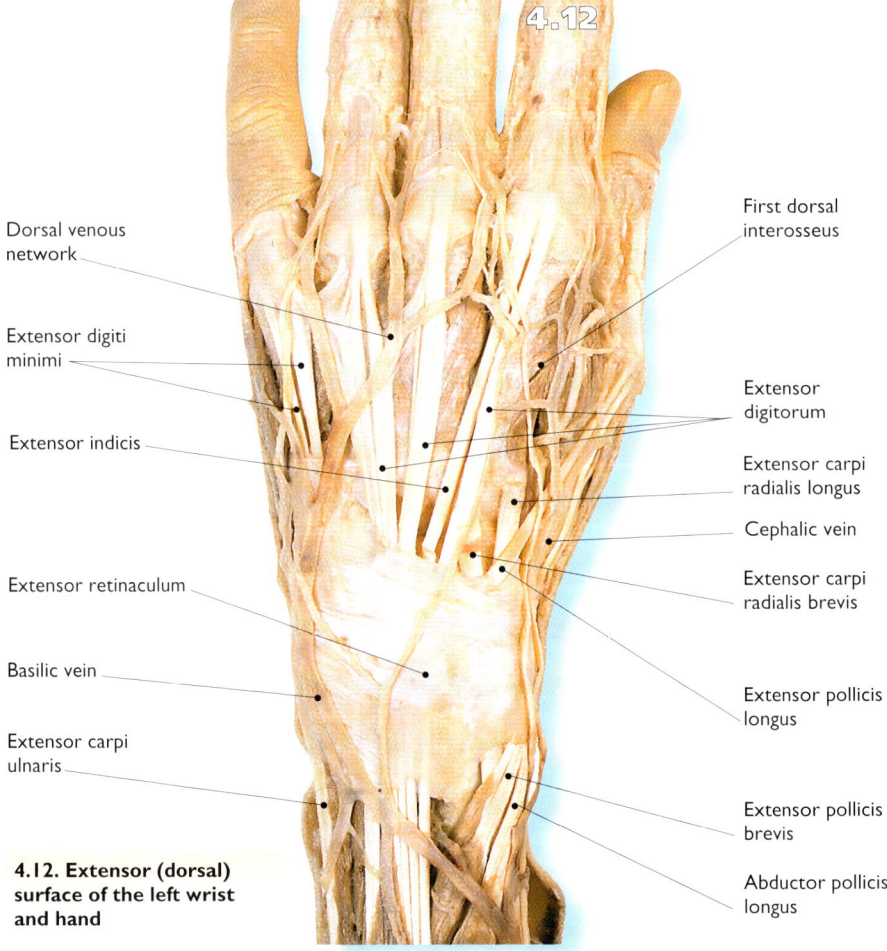

4.12. Extensor (dorsal) surface of the left wrist and hand

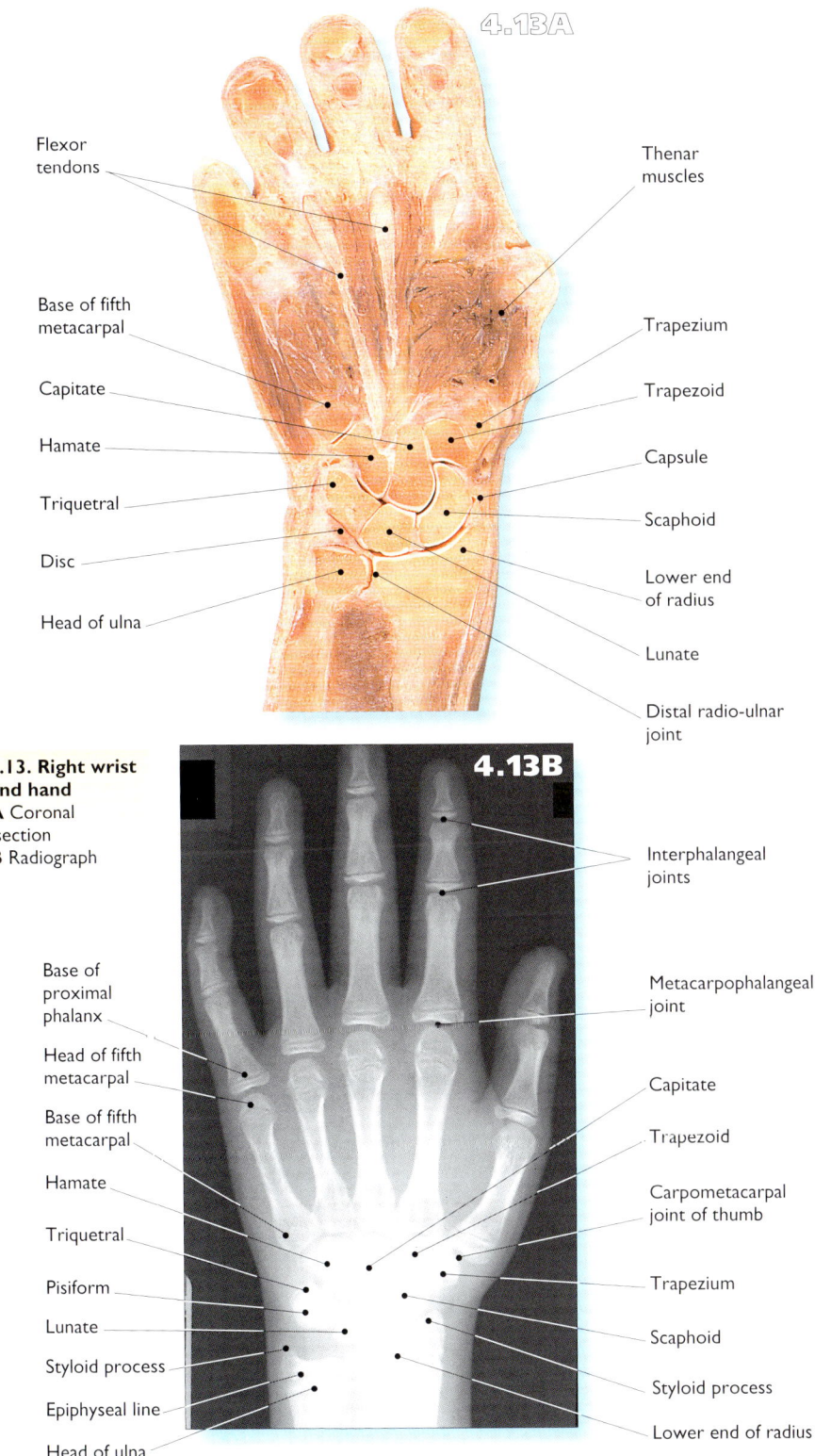

4.13. Right wrist and hand
A Coronal section
B Radiograph

Anatomical snuffbox – the hollow seen distal to the styloid process of the radius on the lateral side of the base of the thumb. Its lateral boundary is formed by two tendons – abductor pollicis longus and extensor pollicis brevis – while the medial boundary is the tendon of extensor pollicis longus. The scaphoid bone and trapezium lie in its floor and the radial artery crosses it to pass into the deep part of the palm.

Extensor muscles and extensor retinaculum – occupy the back of the forearm and hand (**4.12**). The tendons with synovial sheaths are kept in place at the back of the wrist by the extensor retinaculum. Over the metacarpophalangeal joints the extensor digitorum tendons form triangular-shaped dorsal expansions, which wrap around the sides of the joints and receive the attachments of the interosseus and lumbrical muscles. The central parts of the tendons continue on to the bases of the middle and distal phalanges.

Proximal radio-ulnar joint – between the head of the radius and the radial notch of the ulna (**4.8**), held together by the annular ligament (within which the head of the radius can rotate), and sharing the same capsule and joint cavity as the elbow joint.

Distal radio-ulnar joint – between the head of the ulna and the ulnar notch of the radius (**4.13**), the bones are held together by the triangular fibrocartilaginous disc, which normally separates the joint from the wrist joint.

Principal muscles that produce movements at the proximal and distal radio-ulnar joints are:

Pronation – pronator quadratus, pronator teres, and flexor carpi radialis.

Supination – supinator, biceps, and extensor pollicis longus.

Wrist joint – between (proximally) the lower end of the radius and the disc of the distal radio-ulnar joint and (distally) three carpal bones – the scaphoid, lunate, and triquetral (**4.13**). The capsule is reinforced by radial and ulnar ligaments.

Principal muscles that produce movements at the wrist joint are:

Flexion – flexor carpi radialis, flexor carpi ulnaris, and flexor digitorum superficialis and profundus.

Extension – extensor carpi radialis longus and brevis, extensor carpi ulnaris, and extensor digitorum.

Abduction – flexor carpi radialis, extensor carpi radialis longus and brevis, abductor pollicis longus, and extensor pollicis brevis.

Adduction – flexor carpi ulnaris and extensor carpi ulnaris.

The main movements are flexion and extension (which are accompanied by some movement between the two rows of carpal bones – the midcarpal joint), with some degree of adduction and a lesser degree of abduction (because the styloid process of the radius extends lower than the styloid process of the ulna).

Small muscles of the hand – muscles of the thumb and fingers. The bulge on the palmar surface of the base of the thumb, the thenar eminence, is due to flexor pollicis brevis (medially) and abductor pollicis brevis (laterally, **4.9**) overlying opponens pollicis. Arising mainly from the flexor retinaculum and trapezium, they are inserted into the base of the proximal phalanx of the thumb, and are of great importance for opposition of the thumb (see below). They are normally supplied by the median nerve (see above), but flexor pollicis brevis is unique in being the muscle which has the most variable nerve supply of any in the body – median nerve or ulnar nerve, or both.

On the ulnar side of the hand over the fifth metacarpal is the hypothenar eminence, with similar muscles for the little finger (all supplied by the ulnar nerve). There are also interosseus muscles (four dorsal and four palmar) that arise from adjacent metacarpals, and four lumbrical muscles that arise from the tendons of flexor digitorum profundus. All are attached to the dorsal digital expansions (see above), with the interosseus muscles also having attachments to the proximal phalanges; all are supplied by the ulnar nerve, except for the two lateral lumbrical muscles (supplied by the median nerve). For their actions, see below.

First carpometacarpal joint – between the trapezium and the base of the first metacarpal (**4.13B**), it is of great importance. The *saddle-shaped* bone surfaces allow the movement of *opposition* of the thumb – carrying the thumb across the palm towards the bases of the fingers. This is essential for a firm thumb grip, and also allows for more delicate movements, like bringing together the tip of the thumb with the tips of the fingers. Since the first metacarpal lies at right angles to the others, flexion of the thumb means bending it parallel to the rest of the palm and extension implies stretching the 'web' of the thumb, but still in the plane of the palm. Abduction lifts the thumb away from the palm at right angles and adduction restores the normal anatomical position. Opposition involves a mixture of abduction and flexion.

Metacarpophalangeal and interphalangeal joints – all have a similar structure, with a small capsule reinforced on each side by a collateral ligament (**4.13B**).

It is reasonable to guess that the flexor muscles on the front of the forearm and hand will produce flexion of the wrist and/or fingers, and that the extensor muscles on the back will extend them. However, it is unexpected that (as far as finger movements are concerned) extensor digitorum can only produce extension of the metacarpophalangeal joints; it cannot by itself extend the interphalangeal joints. To extend these joints the assistance of the interosseus and lumbrical muscles is required, by pulling on the extensor expansions (although the exact mechanism by which they act is not clear); at the same time, these muscles can help to flex the metacarpophalangeal joints. A less important action of the dorsal interosseus muscles is to fan the fingers out from one another (abduction, with the middle finger as the baseline), and of the palmar interosseus muscles is to bring them together (adduction). These actions are usually remembered by the mnemonics DAB and PAD – Dorsal ABduct and Palmar ADduct. Since all these small muscles are supplied by the ulnar nerve (except for the two lateral lumbrical muscles – median nerve), the ulnar is the all-important nerve for intricate movements of the fingers, such as the upstroke in writing, playing the violin, etc. Contrast this with the median nerve, which supplies the small muscles of the thumb for grosser movements, such as gripping a hammer.

Summary

• The **shoulder joint** is the most mobile in the body and the one most frequently dislocated. Abduction (by supraspinatus and deltoid – suprascapular and axillary nerves respectively) depends not only on movement at the joint itself but is accompanied by rotation of the scapula on the chest wall, tilting the glenoid cavity upwards (by the lower fibres of serratus anterior – own nerve, from roots of the brachial plexus – and the upper fibres of trapezius – accessory nerve).

• At the **elbow joint** only flexion and extension can occur; the forearm movements of pronation (mainly by pronator teres and pronator quadratus – median nerve) and supination (mainly by biceps – musculocutaneous nerve – when the elbow is flexed) take place at the two radio-ulnar joints.

• Fine **finger** movements depend on the interossei and lumbricals, mainly supplied by the ulnar nerve. The small muscles of the thumb, essential for gripping, are supplied by the median nerve.

• The skin of the pulp of the thumb, index and middle fingers, so necessary for the appreciation of touch, is supplied by the **median nerve**. The skin of the ulnar edge of the hand and the little finger is supplied by the **ulnar nerve**.

• The **radial nerve**, from the posterior cord of the brachial plexus, supplies muscles on the posterior surface of the arm and forearm; its skin supply on the hand is negligible.

• The **blood pressure** is taken by occluding the brachial artery by an inflatable cuff placed round the arm above the elbow. The artery is palpated on the front of the elbow (in the cubital fossa) medial to the tendon of biceps.

• The **radial pulse** is felt by pressing the radial artery against the lower end of the radius, lateral to the tendon of flexor carpi radialis.

• Injury to the **radial nerve** is commonest in the upper arm (from fracture of the humerus) and causes 'wrist drop' due to paralysis of the extensors of the wrist and hand.

• Injury to the **ulnar nerve** is commonest at the elbow (where it is subcutaneous behind the medial epicondyle of the humerus), and causes 'claw hand' due to inability to extend the fingers, with anaesthesia on the ulnar side of the hand.

• Injury to the **median nerve** is commonest at the wrist (due to cuts) and interferes with opposition of the thumb, with anaesthesia over the pulps of the thumb and adjacent fingers.

• The segments of the spinal cord mainly concerned in supplying major limb muscles are: C5 – deltoid; C6 – biceps; C7 – triceps; C8 – wrist and finger flexors and extensors; T1 – small muscles of the hand.

Part 5

Thorax

The bony thoracic cage and its associated muscles form an air-tight container which protects the heart and lungs, though the main purpose of the ribs is to assist with respiration. The principal muscle is

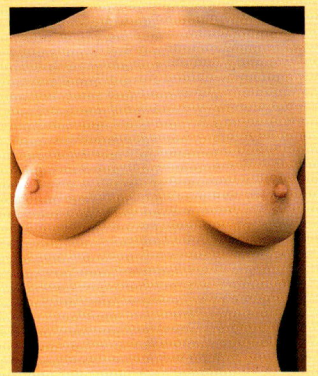 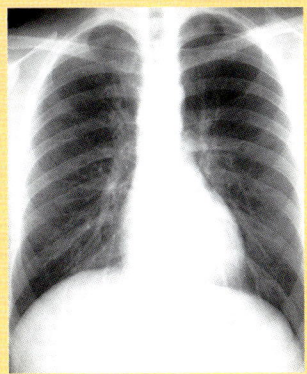

the diaphragm, the muscular and tendinous partition separating the thorax and abdomen.

Perhaps the most unexpected feature of the thorax is the height to which the right and left domes of the diaphragm rise; the capacity of the thorax is much smaller than would be imagined from looking at the outside, and the width of the shoulders obscures the small size of the uppermost part.

THE SKELETON of the thorax (2.2) is covered superficially by the pectoral girdle and its attached muscles (4.2, 4.3), with the overlying breasts at the front. The intercostal spaces (between adjacent ribs and costal cartilages, and numbered from the rib below which they lie) are filled in by three layers of thin intercostal muscles (5.1), with the main intercostal vessels and nerves running between the middle and inner layers along the *lower border* of each rib. The diaphragm, with the liver immediately below it, bulges upwards from the abdomen to a level (viewed from the front) as high as the fifth rib and costal cartilage on the right and the fifth intercostal space on the left (4.1). The gap between the upper border of T1 vertebra, the two first ribs and costal cartilages, and the upper border of the manubrium of the sternum is the thoracic inlet (although sometimes also known as the thoracic outlet); through it pass the trachea and oesophagus, phrenic and vagus nerves, and the sympathetic trunks, great vessels of the neck, and the thoracic duct on the left.

Needles or **drainage tubes** are inserted through the chest wall immediately above a rib, to keep away from the main vessels and nerves.

The central region of the thoracic cavity is the mediastinum, which contains principally the heart and great vessels, while at each side is a lung (5.1). The pleura is a smooth membrane that adheres to the surface of the lung as the visceral pleura; it is continuous at the root of the lung with the parietal pleura, the part that lines the inside of the thoracic wall (costal pleura), the upper surface of the diaphragm (diaphragmatic pleura), and the surface of the mediastinum (mediastinal pleura). The whole pleura thus forms a closed sac, the pleural cavity, though over most of their surfaces the visceral and parietal

If the **negative pressure** in the pleural cavity is destroyed, e.g. by a penetrating wound of the chest wall, the lung collapses (**pneumothorax**).

layers adhere to one another by the surface tension of a thin layer of pleural fluid; the slight negative pressure within the pleural sac keeps the lung expanded.

Manubriosternal joint (angle of Louis) – a most important landmark on the front of the thorax (5.2). It lies about 5 cm below the jugular notch and is always palpable, if not always visible. It indicates the level of the second costal cartilages and ribs on each side. The body of the sternum is opposite the middle four thoracic vertebrae (T5–T8).

From the palpable **second costal cartilages and ribs**, the others can be identified by counting downwards from them. The first rib is too high under the clavicle to be felt.

Breasts

Each breast (mammary gland) lies on the anterior chest wall, largely in front of pectoralis major (5.2). Despite the variations in size of the non-lactating female breast (due to its fat content, not the amount of glandular tissue), the extent of the *base* of the breast is very constant: from near the midline to near the midaxillary line, and from the second to the sixth rib. About 15 lactiferous ducts open on the nipple, which projects from the central pigmented area of skin, the areola. The blood supply is from the internal thoracic and adjacent intercostal arteries. Since the breast is such a common site for cancer in the female, the lymph drainage is of *supreme clinical importance*. Most lymph drains to axillary nodes (which may become palpable and enlarged), but it may also pass through lymph channels that penetrate the chest wall to parasternal nodes within the thorax, beside the internal thoracic vessels (and therefore not palpable). The male breast normally remains very small and rudimentary.

Palpation of axillary lymph nodes is an important part of clinical examination.

Thorax

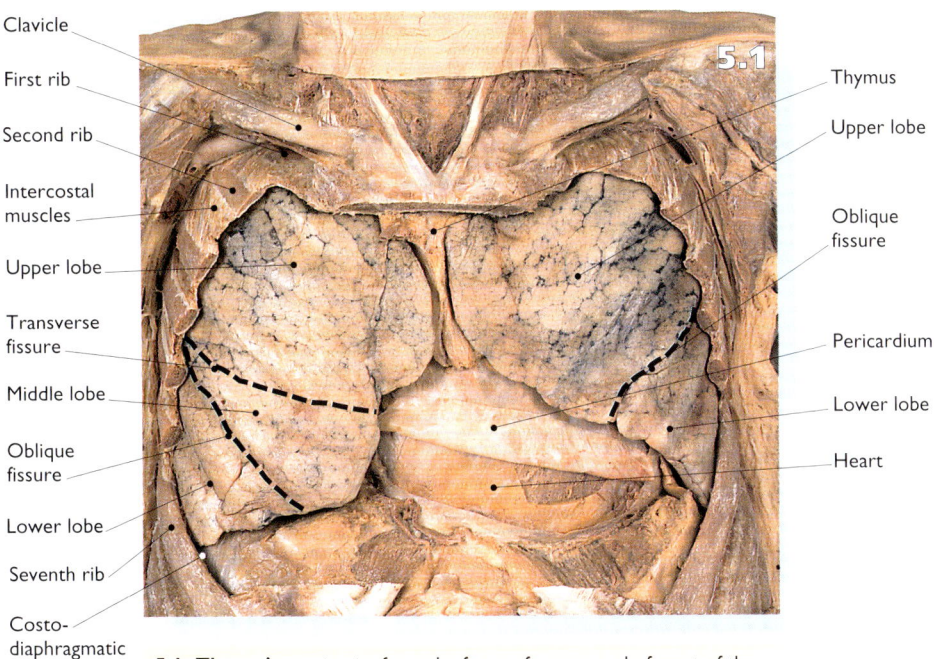

5.1. Thoracic contents, from the front, after removal of most of the sternum and ribs. The pericardium has been incised and turned upwards

5.2. Surface features of the front of the female thorax. The solid line indicates the borders of the heart

111

Diaphragm

The diaphragm is the muscular and tendinous partition between the thorax and abdomen. Muscle fibres arise from the front of the upper two lumbar vertebrae on the left (to form the left crus) and the upper three on the right (right crus, plural crura, **6.13**), from tendinous bands in front of the psoas major and quadratus lumborum muscles (p. 132), and from the inner surfaces of the lower six ribs, with a few fibres from the xiphoid process of the sternum. All these fibres converge on the central tendon, which has the shape of a trefoil leaf, has no bony attachment, and fuses above with the pericardium. Each half of the muscular part receives its motor nerve supply from the phrenic nerve (C3, C4, and C5).

 The phrenic nerves are the only **motor supplies** to diaphragmatic muscle fibres, though they also carry sensory fibres from parts of the diaphragm, pleura, pericardium and peritoneum (p. 116).

The diaphragm contains three large openings and several smaller ones, for the passage of structures between the thorax and abdomen.

Aortic opening – not *in* the diaphragm, but *behind* the union of the two crura, at the level of the T12 vertebra, for the aorta, thoracic duct, and perhaps the azygos vein (which may make its own hole in the right crus).

The **main openings** are at vertebral levels T12 (aortic), T10 (oesophageal) and T8-9 (vena caval).

Oesophageal opening – in the *muscular* part, usually just to the *left* of the midline, but embraced by fibres of the *right* crus, at the level of the T10 vertebra, for the oesophagus, branches of the left gastric vessels and the vagal trunks.

Vena caval foramen – in the *tendon*, at the level of the disc between T8–T9 vertebrae, for the inferior vena cava and the right phrenic nerve.

Smaller openings – in the crura, for thoracic splanchnic (sympathetic) nerves.

The sympathetic trunks pass behind the diaphragm, in front of psoas major, and the subcostal vessels and nerves also run behind it, but more laterally, in front of quadratus lumborum.

Mediastinum

The mediastinum (5.3–5.5) is the central region of the thoracic cavity (between the two pleural sacs). The superior mediastinum is the part above the level of a line drawn from the manubriosternal joint (*see* above) to the lower border of the body of the T4 vertebra. The principal structures in it are the arch of the aorta with its branches (the brachiocephalic, left common carotid, and left subclavian arteries), the right and left brachiocephalic veins uniting to form the superior vena cava, the phrenic and vagus nerves, and the trachea and oesophagus (and thoracic duct on the left) at the back.

The region at the back, behind the heart and below the level of T4 vertebra, is the posterior mediastinum, continuous with the superior mediastinum and containing principally the bifurcation of the trachea into the two main bronchi, the oesophagus with the plexus of vagus nerves around it, and the thoracic duct. The heart and its covering pericardium (see below) lie in the middle mediastinum, although this term is not often used. The narrow gap in front of the heart and behind the sternum is the anterior mediastinum, and may contain the lower part of the thymus.

Any infection of the mediastinum (**mediastinitis**) is highly dangerous because it is deeply seated and can spread widely in the connective tissue between the main structures.

Thorax

5.3

Labels (image):
- Thyroid gland
- [In]ternal jugular vein
- [In]ferior thyroid veins
- Right common carotid artery
- Subclavian vein
- Right subclavian artery
- Brachiocephalic trunk
- Right brachiocephalic vein
- Superior vena cava
- Upper trunk of brachial plexus
- Suprascapular nerve
- Scalenus anterior
- Trachea
- Phrenic nerve
- Left subclavian artery
- Left brachiocephalic vein
- Left common carotid artery
- Arch of aorta
- Upper lobe of lung
- Pulmonary trunk

5.3 Great vessels of the superior mediastinum and root of the neck

Trachea – begins in the neck as the continuation of the larynx at the level of C6 vertebra. It is palpable above the jugular notch of the manubrium of the sternum (3.5, 3.35, 5.3), with the oesophagus behind it (but not palpable). The lumen is kept open as the airway by bands of cartilage in the front and side walls (but not at the back, which contains smooth muscle); although called tracheal rings they are U-shaped and never completely circular. The trachea divides into the two main bronchi just below the level of the manubriosternal joint (5 cm below the jugular notch).

Oesophagus – begins in the neck as the continuation of the pharynx at the level of the C6 vertebra, then continues down in front of the vertebral column through the superior and posterior mediastinum (5.4, 5.5), to pass through the oesophageal opening in the diaphragm, which is usually just to the left of the midline at the level of the T10 vertebra.

> The **trachea** is about 10 centimetres long; the **oesophagus** is about 10 inches (25 centimetres) long.

Aorta – leaves the left ventricle of the heart above the aortic valve as the ascending aorta, which gives off the left and right coronary arteries. Then it curves backwards and slightly left as the arch of the aorta (5.3), giving off the brachiocephalic trunk (which divides into the right common carotid and right subclavian arteries) and the left

> The arch gives the characteristic **'aortic knuckle'** in radiographs of the chest (p. 120).

113

Human Anatomy

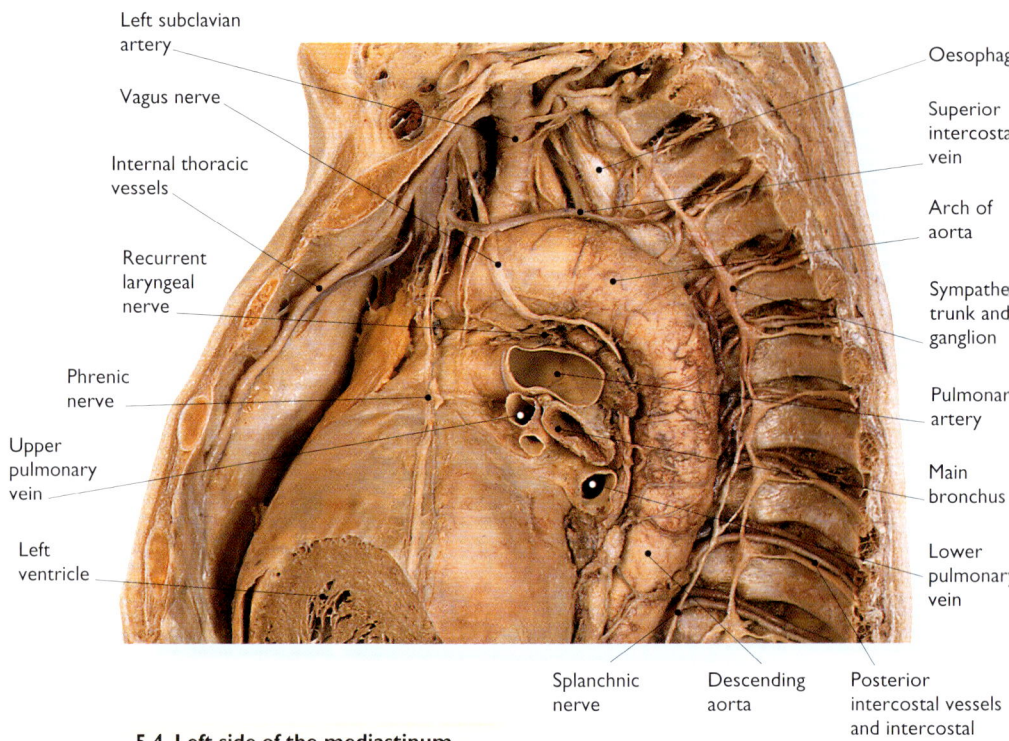

5.4. Left side of the mediastinum

common carotid and left subclavian arteries. The arch rises as high as the midpoint of the manubrium, then continues downwards as the descending (thoracic) aorta, which passes behind the diaphragm at the level of the T12 vertebra to become the abdominal aorta.

Superior vena cava – on the right of the ascending aorta, it is formed by the union of the right and left brachiocephalic veins (**5.3, 5.6**) behind the lower border of the right first costal cartilage, and runs down to enter the right atrium of the heart at the level of the lower border of the right third costal cartilage. At the level of the second costal cartilage it receives the azygos vein which drains intercostal spaces and arches over the right lung root.

Brachiocephalic veins – each is formed by the union of the internal jugular and subclavian veins behind the sternoclavicular joints. The left brachiocephalic vein thus runs from left to right behind the upper half of the manubrium crossing the three large branches from the aortic arch (**5.3**).

Pulmonary trunk – beginning from the right ventricle of the heart to the left and slightly in front of the ascending aorta, it runs upwards and backwards to divide under the aortic arch (**5.3**) into the right and left pulmonary arteries. The left pulmonary artery is joined to the arch by a fibrous cord, the ligamentum arteriosum, the

> A patent ductus arteriosus is the commonest **congenital defect** of the heart and great vessels, and must be closed surgically.

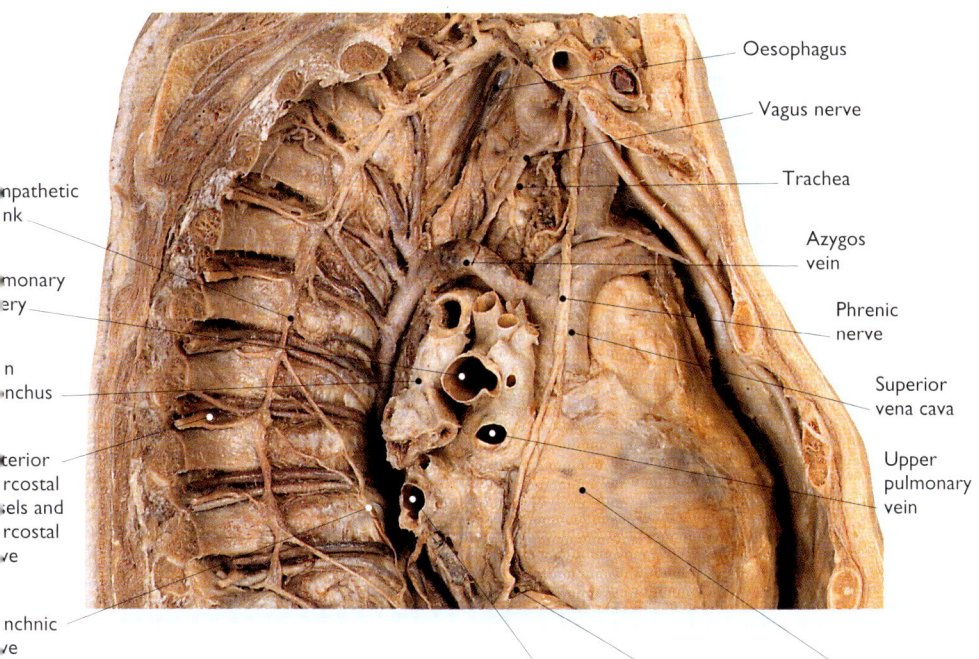

5.5. Right side of the mediastinum

remains of the embryonic ductus arteriosus which short-circuited blood into the aorta to prevent it going through the then non-functioning lungs. The ductus closes within hours of birth.

Thoracic duct – beginning in the abdomen from the cisterna chyli, a sack-like dilatation under the *right* crus of the diaphragm at the level of the L1 vertebra, it passes upwards immediately in front of the vertebral column and reaches the *left* side of the neck to run into the left side of the junction between the subclavian and internal jugular veins (5.6). It drains lymph from the whole body, except for the three right-sided areas that drain to the right lymphatic duct (p. 80).

Thymus – the source of production of T lymphocytes, it lies in front of the great vessels and upper pericardium (5.1), and usually extends into the root of the neck. It may appear to be a single structure, but in fact is two lobes closely applied to one another. It is maximal in size in childhood and thereafter regresses, but remains active throughout life. The function of thymic hormones is still being elucidated.

Sympathetic trunk – each enters the thorax by crossing the neck of the first rib and then runs vertically down through the thorax beside the vertebral column (5.4, 5.5), giving off from its ganglia various branches which join intercostal nerves or provide splanchnic nerves for thoracic and abdominal viscera and blood vessels.

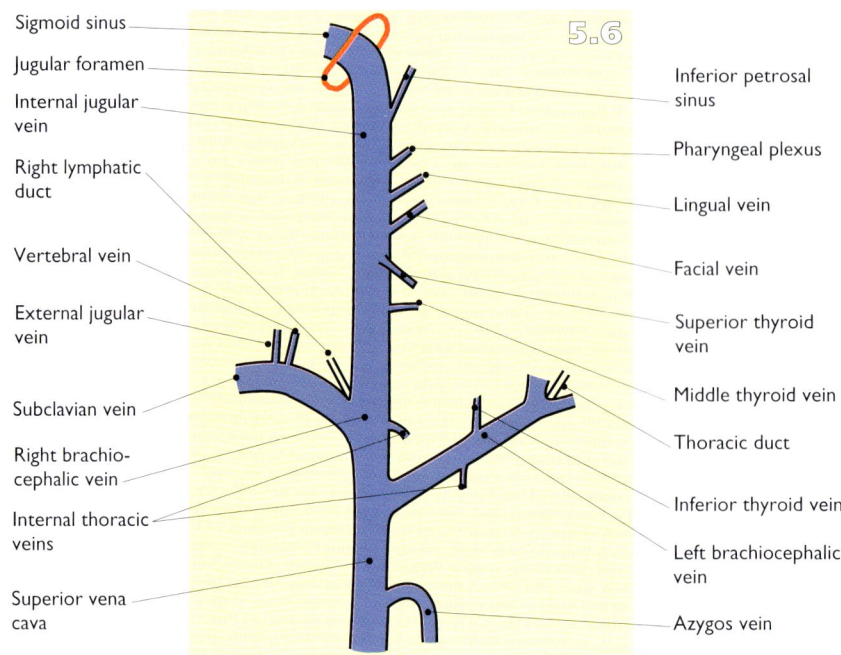

5.6. The superior vena cava and tributaries

Vagus nerves – from the neck (p. 80), the left vagus crosses the aortic arch (**5.4**) and the right runs down the right side of the trachea (**5.5**). Both give branches to the cardiac plexus (the left vagus also gives off the left recurrent laryngeal nerve, p. 82) and pass behind the lung roots to unite and form the oesophageal plexus around the lower oesophagus. From this plexus are formed the left and right vagal trunks which supply the stomach (p. 137).

Phrenic nerves – from the neck (p. 79), the left phrenic nerve (**5.4**) runs down over the arch of the aorta and the pericardium overlying the left ventricle, to pierce the *muscular* part of the diaphragm. The right phrenic nerve (**5.5**) runs down beside the superior vena cava and the pericardium overlying the right atrium to pass through the vena caval foramen in the *tendon* of the diaphragm. Both phrenic nerves spread out on the abdominal surface of the diaphragm as the motor supply to the muscle fibres of their own half. Although the peripheral part of the diaphragm receives fibres from lower intercostal nerves, these are afferent only; *the only motor supply is from the phrenic nerves*. The phrenic nerves also have a large *afferent* area of supply: diaphragm, mediastinal and diaphragmatic pleura, pericardium, and subdiaphragmatic peritoneum (hence referred pain to the C4 dermatome above the shoulder, **3.17**).

Heart

The heart (**1.3, 5.6–5.13**) is the muscular pump of the cardiovascular system, and has four chambers – right and left atria, and right and left ventricles (**5.7, 5.8**). The pulmonary circulation (which involves the right-sided chambers of the heart) is the part of the cardiovascular system that conveys blood to the lungs and brings it back to the

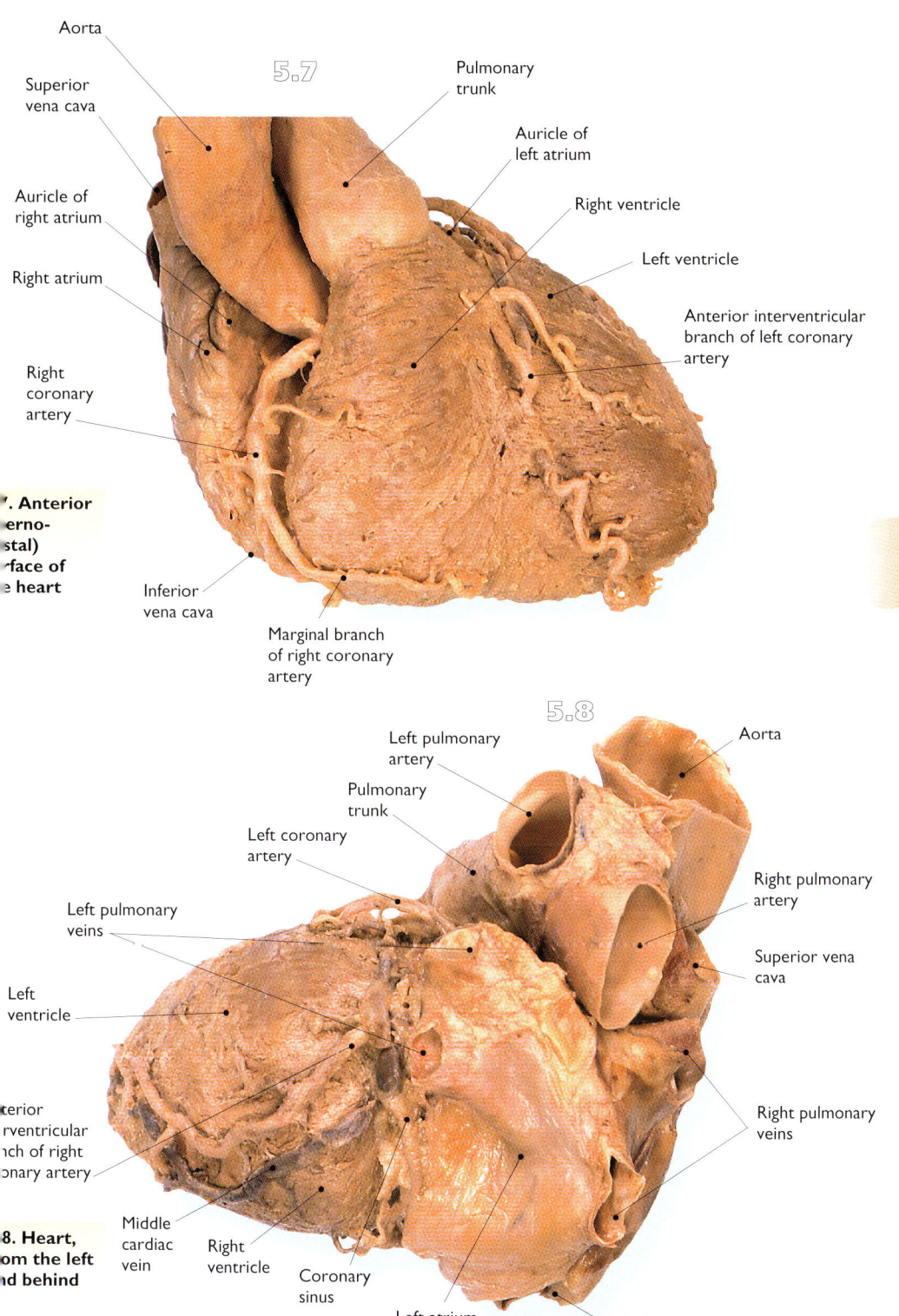

5.7 Anterior (sterno-costal) surface of the heart

5.8 Heart, from the left and behind

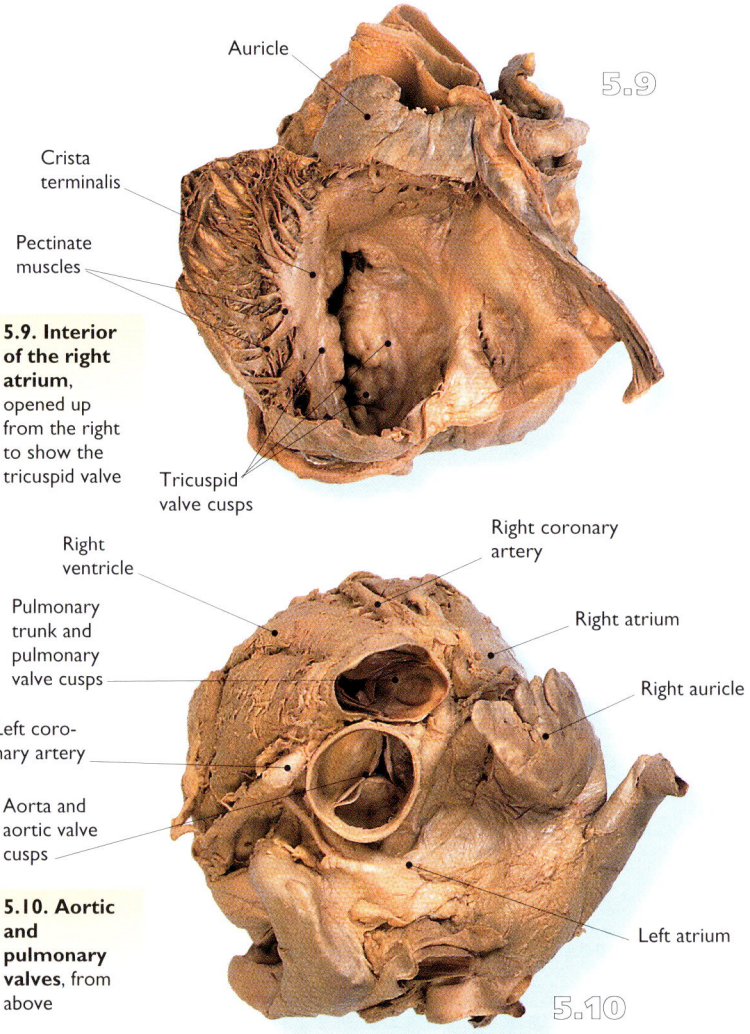

5.9. Interior of the right atrium, opened up from the right to show the tricuspid valve

5.10. Aortic and pulmonary valves, from above

heart, and is distinct from the systemic circulation (which involves the left-sided chambers of the heart) which takes blood to and from the rest of the body. The portal venous system is the part of the systemic circulation concerned with taking blood from the digestive tract (and the spleen) to the liver, so that the absorbed products of digestion can be delivered directly to the liver for chemical processing.

The heart lies within a tough fibrous sac, the fibrous pericardium, lined internally by the serous pericardium, which, like the pleura, has a parietal layer lining it and a visceral layer adhering to the heart and adjacent parts of the great vessels.

Chambers and great vessels – the right atrium (5.7) receives venous blood from the superior vena cava and the inferior vena cava, and also from the coronary sinus (1.3), the main vein of the heart itself. The blood passes through the tricuspid valve (5.9) into the right ventricle, then through the pulmonary valve (5.10) into the pulmonary trunk, and so to the right and left pulmonary arteries, conveying the

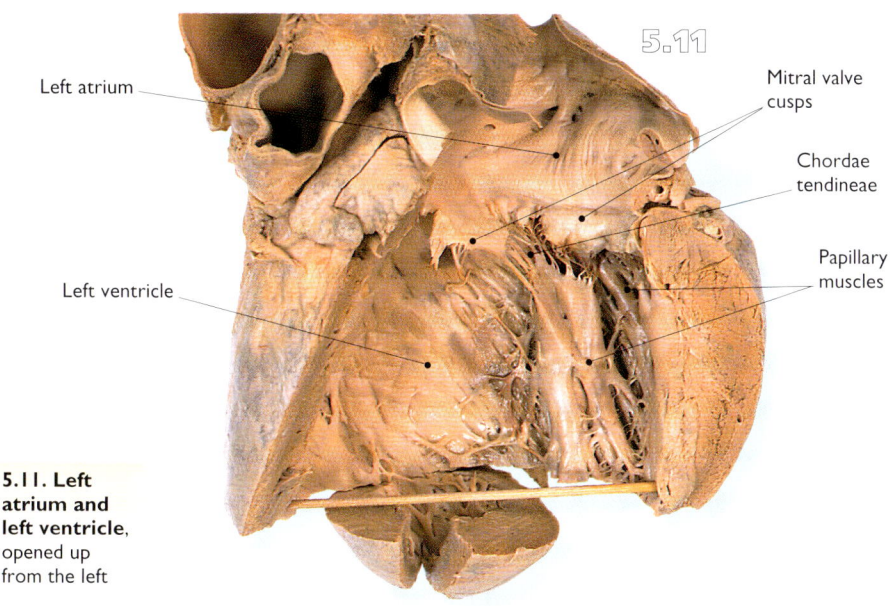

5.11. Left atrium and left ventricle, opened up from the left

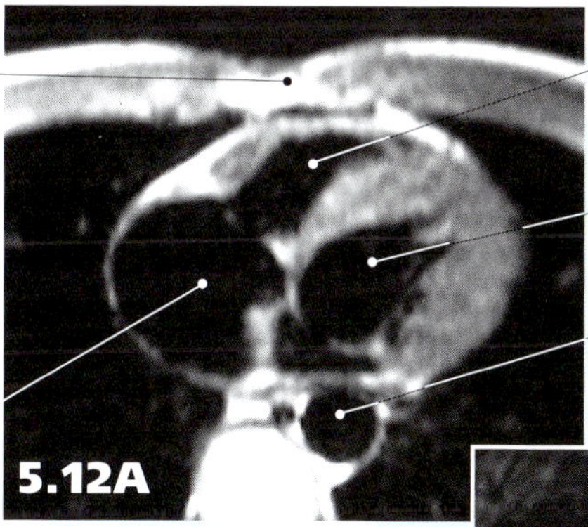

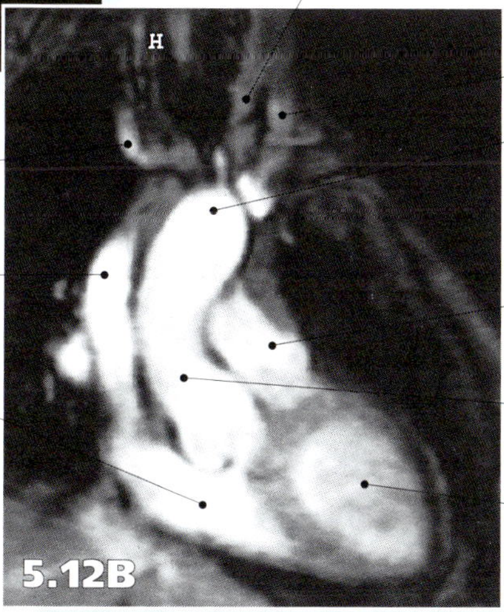

Labels: Left atrium; Mitral valve cusps; Chordae tendineae; Papillary muscles; Left ventricle

5.12. Images of the heart
A Axial magnetic resonance image
B Coronal magnetic resonance image

5.12A labels: Right ventricle; Left ventricle; Descending aorta

5.12B labels: Left common carotid artery; Left subclavian artery; Arch of aorta; Pulmonary trunk; Ascending aorta; Left ventricle; Brachiocephalic artery; Right atrium; Right ventricle

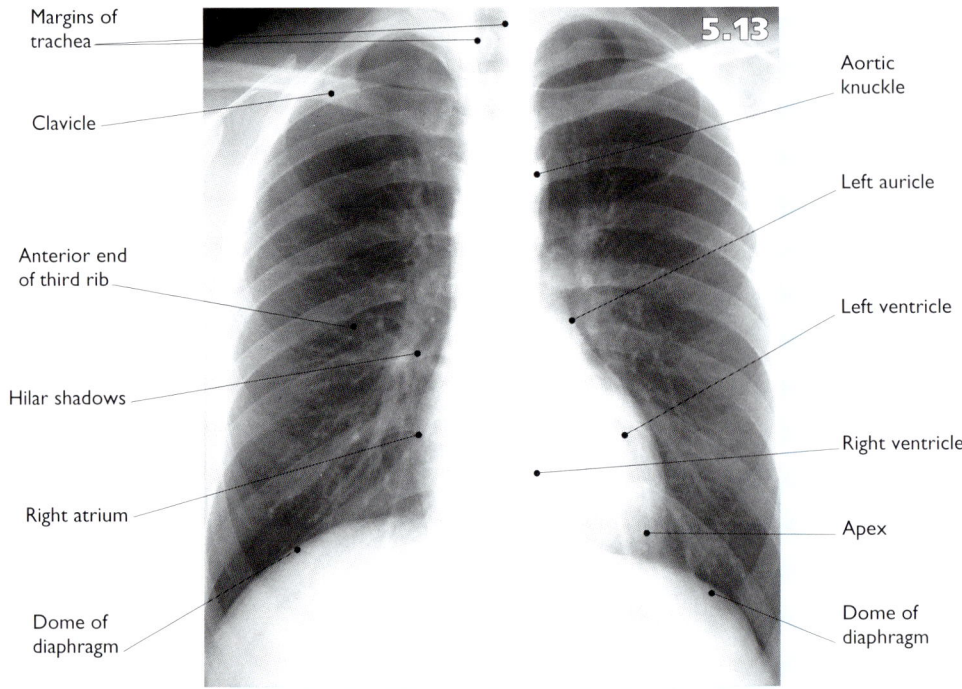

5.13. **Postero-anterior radiograph of the thorax** – the standard 'straight radiograph of the chest'

deoxygenated blood from the right ventricle to the lungs.

From the lungs, oxygenated blood is carried by the pulmonary veins (two on each side) to the left atrium and then passes through the (bicuspid) mitral valve into the left ventricle (**5.11**), from which it leaves through the aortic valve to enter the aorta, the body's largest vessel. The wall of the left ventricle is thicker than that of the right ventricle (**5.12**), because the pressure of blood in the systemic circulation is much greater than that in the pulmonary circulation.

Fibrous chordae tendineae (**5.11**) attach the margins of the cusps of the mitral and tricuspid valves to the papillary muscles that project from the ventricular walls. They prevent the cusps from being 'blown back' into the atria when the ventricles contract, so ensuring that the blood passes out through the aortic and pulmonary valves.

Note that the pulmonary trunk and pulmonary arteries contain venous (deoxygenated) blood, whereas the pulmonary veins contain arterial (oxygenated) blood; the vessels are named, like all other blood vessels, from the direction of blood flow within them, not from the state of oxygenation of their contained blood. Note also that the left and right atria do not normally communicate with one another, being separated by the

The commonest valvular diseases of the heart are **mitral stenosis** (narrowing of the mitral valve) and **aortic incomptetence** (improper closure leading to backflow through the aortic valve).

Blood clots, commonly from deep venous thrombosis in the legs (p. 178), may become impacted in the pulmonary circulation as **pulmonary emboli**; if large they can cause sudden death.

interatrial septum, nor do the left and right ventricles intercommunicate, being separated by the interventricular septum. The systemic and pulmonary circulations thus remain separate.

> In many **congenital heart diseases** the septa are not properly developed, so the circulations become mixed and require surgical correction.

The heart does not 'hang straight down' from the great vessels at the top, with the right chambers on the right and the left chambers on the left, but projects forwards and is rotated to the left. Thus, most of the anterior or sternocostal surface (**5.7**, **5.12**) is formed by the right ventricle, with the pulmonary trunk leaving its upper end; the right atrium is to the right of the right ventricle, and the left ventricle to the left of, but mostly behind, the right ventricle (**5.12**). The lower left extremity of the left ventricle is the apex of the heart. The aorta leaves the upper part of the left ventricle just behind and to the right of the pulmonary trunk (see **5.7**). Thus, the order of the three great vessels at the top of the heart from right to left is: superior vena cava, aorta, pulmonary trunk. The left atrium is at the back and forms the posterior surface or base of the heart; only the auricle of the left atrium is seen when looking at the heart from the front.

> The **base of the heart** is its posterior surface (left atrium), not the top end where large vessels are attached.

Borders – it is important to appreciate the borders of the heart, as seen when looking from the front (as in a standard chest radiograph, **5.13**), and to visualize them in relation to the surface of the thorax (**5.2**). The right border is formed by the right atrium, which runs from the third costal cartilage to the sixth costal cartilage at the right border of the sternum. The inferior border is formed mostly by the right ventricle, with the left ventricle (apex) at the left edge, and

> **Radiography** of the chest to ascertain whether the heart borders and lung fields are normal is one of the most mportant of all clinical procedures.

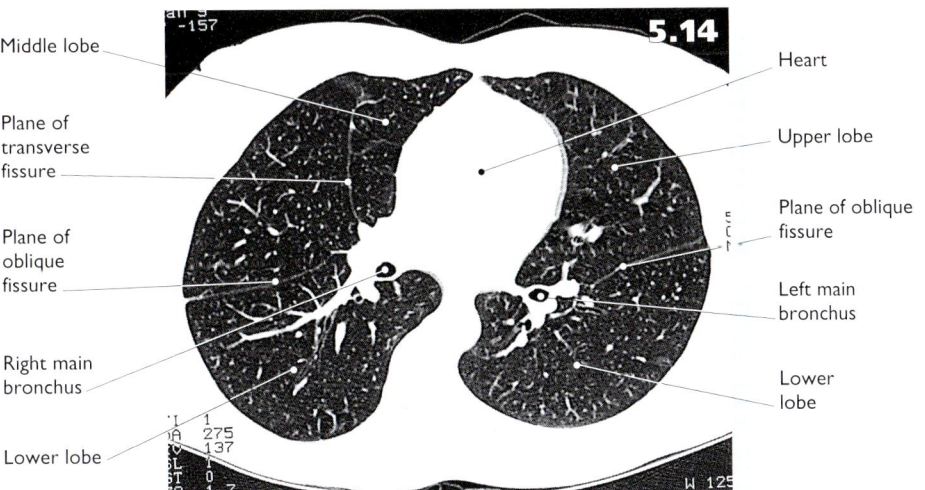

5.14. Computed tomograph of the thorax (lung setting), just below the level of the bifurcation of the trachea into the two main bronchi, viewed from below looking towards the head runs from the right sixth costal cartilage to the left fifth intercostal space, about 9 cm from the midline; this is where the apex beat can be felt on the chest wall. The left border is formed by the left ventricle, with the left auricle at the upper end, and runs from the apex to the left second costal cartilage at the lateral border of the sternum. In a radiograph, above this can be seen the pulmonary trunk and, higher still, the arch of the aorta passes backwards to produce a prominent bulge, the aortic knuckle.

Sound reverberates through the heart and chest wall in such a way that the positions on the chest wall where the sounds of the heart valves are best heard with a stethoscope are not directly over the valves. Generally, the sounds of the pulmonary valve are best heard over the left second intercostal space at the sternal margin, those of the aortic valve over the second right intercostal space at the costal margin, those of the mitral valve at the apex of the heart, and those of the tricuspid valve over the lower right part of the sternum.

Conducting system – the impulse for cardiac contraction begins in a specialized area of heart muscle, the sinuatrial node (SA node), at the top of the right atrium just below the entry of the superior vena cava (5.7). From there the impulse spreads through the ordinary muscle of the atria and reaches another specialized area, the atrioventricular node (AV node), in the lower part of the interatrial septum. The node continues into the interventricular septum as the AV bundle, which sends branches to a network of specialized muscle fibres in each ventricle, thus widely distributing the impulse to the ventricular muscle. These specialized tissues form the conducting or conduction system of the heart.

Blood supply – by two coronary arteries that arise from the ascending aorta just above the aortic valve (5.7). The right coronary artery runs down in the right atrioventricular groove, giving off a large marginal branch, usually near the lower border of the heart, and a posterior interventricular branch on the under surface.

> Disease of the coronary vessels, leading to narrowing and so to reduced blood supply to cardiac muscle (**ischaemic heart disease**) is the commonest cause of death.

The left coronary artery, after a short course *behind* the pulmonary trunk, continues in the left atrioventricular groove as the circumflex branch, after giving off the anterior interventricular branch (sometimes called by clinicians the left anterior descending artery), which runs down in the left interventricular groove.

> This vessel is the one most frequently affected by disease and, being on the front of the heart, is easy to approach surgically for **bypass operations**.

The veins of the heart mostly run with the arteries (although they have different names) and drain into the coronary sinus, in the atrioventricular groove on the back of the heart. The sinus opens into the lower part of the right atrium, near the opening of the inferior vena cava. Unlike the arteries, the veins of the heart are curiously unaffected by disease.

Nerve supply – by numerous sympathetic and parasympathetic (vagal) fibres, which form the cardiac plexus below the arch of the aorta and the bifurcation of the trachea. Increased vagal activity slows the heart rate and sympathetic activity increases it. Pain fibres run with the sympathetic nerves and, because other parts of the same nerves supply other structures, such as blood vessels in the arm and neck, pain due to heart disease may appear to come from elsewhere, especially the left arm and side of the neck (referred pain, p. 59).

> The pain of coronary artery disease is commonly felt behind the sternum, but a patient's complaint of such things as a sore neck, sore arm or indigestion must always alert the medical attendant to the possibility of **referred pain**.

Lungs and pleura

The paired lungs are the principal organs of the respiratory system, where the exchange of gases (oxygen and carbon dioxide) takes place between air and blood. The other parts of the respiratory system (respiratory tract), consisting of the nose and paranasal sinuses, pharynx, larynx, trachea, and main bronchi, are simply conducting pathways with no gaseous exchange. The trachea, bronchi and their branches are often collectively called the 'bronchial tree'.

> Cancer of the lung invariably means cancer of one of the larger bronchi, hence the more correct technical term **bronchial carcinoma**.

By repeated divisions the bronchi become progressively smaller and eventually form the bronchioles, from which the air sacs (alveoli) bud off to form the sponge-like mass of aerated tissue where the exchange of gases (oxygen and carbon dioxide) takes place between the air in the air sacs and the red blood cells in the capillaries of the alveolar walls.

Lobes – the left lung has upper and lower lobes, separated by an oblique fissure, but the right lung has upper, middle, and lower lobes, separated by oblique and transverse fissures (**5.1**, **5.14**). The pleura that covers the outer surface of the lobes dips down into the fissures.

Surface markings – the surface marking of the oblique fissure of both lungs is on a line from the spine of the T3 vertebra round to the sixth costal cartilage, and is approximately level with the medial border of the scapula when the arm is abducted to 180° (**3.34**). The surface marking of the transverse fissure of the right lung is on a line drawn horizontally from the right fourth costal cartilage to where it meets the line of the oblique fissure.

> When listening with the **stethoscope** on the front of the chest, it is mainly breath sounds in the upper lobes (and middle right lobe) that are heard; when listening on the back it is mainly the lower lobe sounds that are heard.

The lower parts of the lower lobes do not completely fill the pleural cavities, even with the deepest respiration. From the sixth costal cartilage level on the front of the chest, the lower level of the pleura extends back to the tenth rib in the midaxillary line and the twelfth rib at the lateral border of the erector spinae (**6.4**), but the lower limit of the lung only extends to the level of the eighth rib in the midaxillary line and the tenth rib at the lateral border of the erector spinae. The part of the pleural cavity without any lung (at the periphery of the diaphragm) is the costodiaphragmatic recess of the pleura (**6.9**).

Hilum – the hilum of each lung (where the great vessels and main bronchus enter or leave it, to form the lung root, **5.4**, **5.5**, **5.14**) lies behind costal cartilages 3 and 4 (level with T5, T6, and T7 vertebrae). Remember the numbers 3, 4, 5, 6, 7 – 3 and 4 for costal cartilages and 5, 6, and 7 for vertebrae. The main bronchus is the most posterior structure in each lung root and the lower pulmonary vein the lowest structure. The upper pulmonary vein lies in front of the pulmonary artery. Remember the sequence vein, artery, bronchus from front to back (compare with vein, artery, ureter in the hilum of the kidney).

> The right main bronchus is more vertical than the left, so **foreign bodies** (such as extracted teeth and peanuts) are more likely to enter the right lung than the left.

Pleura – the two pleurae (pleural sacs) are in contact in the midline of the sternum between the levels of the second to fourth costal cartilages. The pleura and lung on the right side continue down to the level of the sixth costal cartilage, but on the left the presence of the heart causes an indentation (cardiac notch) in the lung and overlying pleura.

On each side, the apex of the pleura (cervical pleura) and lung extends for about 3 cm above the medial third of the clavicle (5.2).

By repeated divisions the bronchi become progressively smaller and eventually form the bronchioles from which the air sacs (alveoli) bud off as the sponge-like mass of aerated tissue where the exchange of gases takes place through the blood capillaries in thin alveolar walls.

Blood supply – although the pulmonary arteries and veins concerned with oxygenation of blood are the largest vessels in the lung, the lung tissue itself is supplied by its own very small vessels (bronchial arteries and veins).

Nerve supply – the smooth muscle of the blood vessels and bronchi of the lungs are supplied by various autonomic nerves, which also provide the important pathways for the cough reflex, enabling the bronchial tree to be cleared of excess mucus and other debris. The visceral pleura is insensitive but the parietal pleura is supplied by spinal nerves such as the intercostals and the phrenics.

Stab wounds of the lower neck may injure the pleura and lung.

Spasm of smooth muscle in the bronchial walls is a feature of **asthma**, with constriction of bronchi and particular difficulty with expiration.

Pleurisy (inflammation of the pleura) may be intensely painful because the normally smooth adjacent surfaces become roughened and rub against one another, irritating the part supplied by spinal nerves.

Summary

- The **bony thorax** consists of the 12 thoracic vertebrae, 12 pairs of ribs and costal cartilages, and the 3 parts of the sternum – manubrium, body and xiphoid process.

- The most important landmark on the surface of the thorax is the **manubriosternal joint**, palpable about 5 cm below the jugular notch at the level of the second costal cartilages and ribs. By counting down from these cartilages and ribs the surface markings of the heart, pleura and lungs can be identified.

- The **manubrium** of the sternum lies opposite the middle 4 thoracic vertebrae (T5-T8).

- The **apex beat** of the heart (left ventricle) is normally in the left fifth intercostal space about 9 cm from the midline; the **left border** of the heart (left ventricle with left atrium at the top) extends from the apex to the left second costal cartilage; **right border** (right atrium) from the right third to sixth costal cartilages; and the **inferior border** (mostly right ventricle) from the right sixth costal cartilage to the apex (left fifth intercostal space).

- The order of the **great vessels** at the top of the heart from right to left is: superior vena cava, aorta, pulmonary trunk.

- The right and left **coronary arteries** arise from the ascending aorta just above the aortic valve.

- The arch of the **aorta** rises as high as the midpoint of the manubrium, and from right to left gives origin to the brachiocephalic, left common carotid and left subclavian arteries.

- The **tricuspid valve** lies between the right atrium and right ventricle, with the **pulmonary valve** between the right ventricle and pulmonary trunk; the **mitral valve** is between the left atrium and left ventricle, with the **aortic valve** between the left ventricle and ascending aorta.

- The **hilum** of the lung is on a level with the third and fourth costal cartilages and the order of the principal structures from front to back in the hilum is: vein, artery, bronchus.

- At the back the **pleura** extends as low as the twelfth rib at the lateral border of erector spinae, but the lung only as low as the tenth rib; the empty part of the pleural cavity is the costodiaphragmatic recess.

- The **trachea** divides into the two main bronchi just below the level of the manubriosternal joint.

- The **oesophagus** runs down through the thorax immediately in front of the vertebral column, with the thoracic duct passing upwards first behind the right margin of the oesophagus and then crossing over to enter the neck behind its left margin.

Part 6

Abdomen

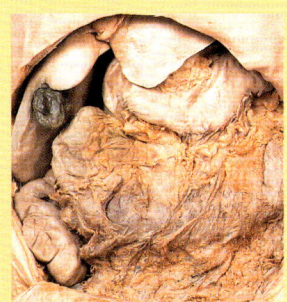

In popular parlance the abdomen or abdominal cavity is the tummy, and abdominal pain is one of the common reasons for seeking medical advice. The anterior abdominal wall is a site where excess fat is deposited, as many discover when trousers or skirt become more difficult to get into!

Most of the digestive system lies within the abdomen, and associated with it is the portal system of veins which conveys to the liver the absorbed products of digestion. The kidneys and adrenal glands 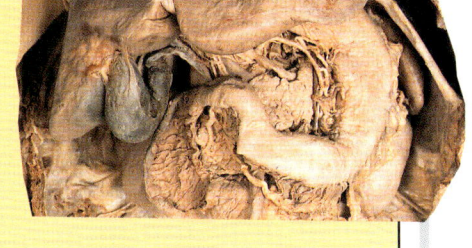 also lie in the upper abdomen, together with the spleen, the largest of the lymphoid organs.

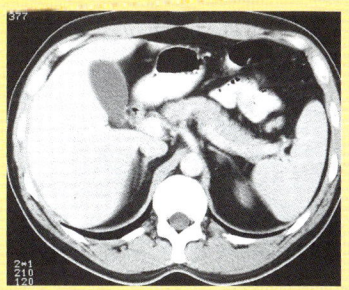

The possibility of disease or injury affecting so many organs makes abdominal surgery one of the commonest reasons for filling hospital beds.

127

THE ABDOMEN, or abdominal cavity, is the part of the trunk below the diaphragm, which separates it from the thoracic cavity. The lowest part of the abdominal cavity, below the pelvic brim (p. 150), is the pelvic cavity or pelvis. Because of the way the diaphragm bulges upwards into the thorax, the abdominal cavity is larger than might be expected when looking at the outside of the trunk, but lower down it is less capacious than might be expected because of the way the lumbar part of the vertebral column projects forwards in the middle of the posterior abdominal wall. Muscles form the rest of the posterior wall, as they do the anterolateral wall.

The peritoneum is a smooth membrane which lines the abdominal and pelvic walls, and forms supporting folds for various abdominal organs. The peritoneum that lines the abdominal and pelvic walls is the parietal peritoneum, while that covering abdominal and pelvic viscera is the visceral peritoneum. Some organs, such as the kidneys, ureters, and pancreas, are plastered onto the posterior abdominal wall by parietal peritoneum (i.e. they are retroperitoneal), while others, such as the stomach and much of the small and large intestines, are suspended by folds of peritoneum. This shiny, lubricated membrane allows free movement between viscera that change size and shape.

Infection of the peritoneum (**peritonitis**) is highly dangerous because of the rapidity with which it can spread over large areas. It gives rise to a characteristic 'board-like rigidity' on palpation of the affected parts of the abdominal wall.

Anterior abdominal wall

The muscles that form the front part of the abdominal wall on each side (**4.2**) are the rectus abdominis, external and internal oblique (abdominis), and transversus abdominis.

Rectus abdominis – runs upwards from the pubic crest (between symphysis and tubercle) to the fifth, sixth, and seventh costal cartilages. It is enclosed by the rectus sheath (*see* below), and usually has three tendinous intersections which adhere to the anterior wall of the sheath. The two sheaths meet in the midline as the linea alba. The muscle is supplied by T7–T12 nerves.

In thin muscular individuals the **intersections** may be seen as transverse depressions on the surface.

External oblique, internal oblique, and transversus abdominis – lie in that order from outside inwards between the iliac crest and lower ribs. The aponeurotic medial part of the internal oblique splits to form the rectus sheath, with the aponeuroses of the external oblique and transversus joining the anterior and posterior layers of the sheath, respectively, except in the lowest part where all three aponeuroses lie in front of the rectus muscle. The lowest part of the external oblique aponeurosis forms the inguinal ligament, stretching between the anterior superior iliac spine and the pubic tubercle. The external oblique is supplied (like rectus abdominis) by T7–T12 nerves, and the others by T7–T12 and L1 (iliohypogastric and ilio-inguinal) nerves.

The **anterior superior iliac spine** is at the anterior end of the iliac crest and easily palpable; the **pubic tubercle** is felt 2.5 cm lateral to the top of the midline pubic symphysis.

Inguinal canal – an oblique gap, about 4 cm long, through the muscle aponeuroses above the medial end of the inguinal ligament (**4.2**), which forms the floor of the canal. The *lowest* muscular fibres of the internal oblique and transversus muscles arch over the canal obliquely and medially from front to back, to form much of

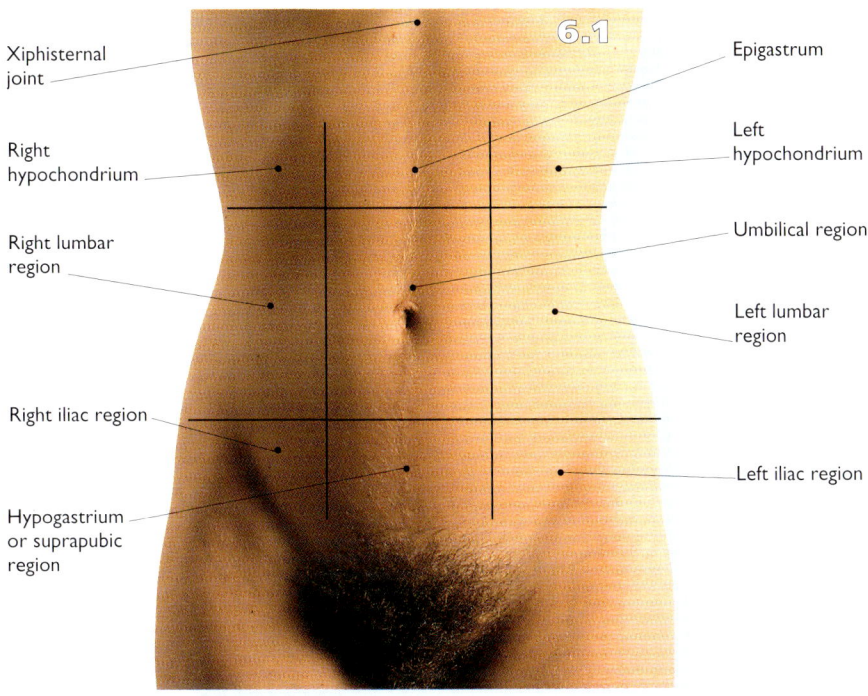

6.1. Regions of the abdomen. The upper transverse line is the transpyloric plane, level with the lower part of L1 vertebra and about a handsbreadth below the xiphisternal joint

its anterior wall and roof; they unite to form the conjoint tendon of the posterior wall. The intactness of the nerve supply of these muscle fibres, from the iliohypogastric and ilio-inguinal nerves (L1), is important to maintain the canal's integrity, which otherwise depends largely on its obliquity. The canal is occupied by the spermatic cord (p. 157) in the male and the round ligament of the uterus in the female, with the ilio-inguinal nerve in both sexes.

The canal is a potentially weak part of the abdominal wall, especially in males (because in fetal life the testis passed through it to reach the scrotum), and may become the site of an inguinal hernia – a protrusion of abdominal contents (usually a loop of small intestine) which may extend into the scrotum. Damage to the ilio-inguinal nerve in the canal (e.g. during the surgical repair of a hernia) does not affect the nerve supply to the muscle fibres guarding the canal, because these motor fibres arise from the nerve well before it reaches the canal; it is incisions in the lateral part of the abdominal wall (e.g. for appendicectomy) that may damage it.

Inguinal hernia is the common hernia in males; **femoral hernia** (p. 167) is the common hernia in females, in whom the inguinal canal is smaller.

Surface features

An imaginary grid of nine squares is used to divide the surface of the abdomen into regions (**6.1**), so that the sites of pain, swellings, palpable

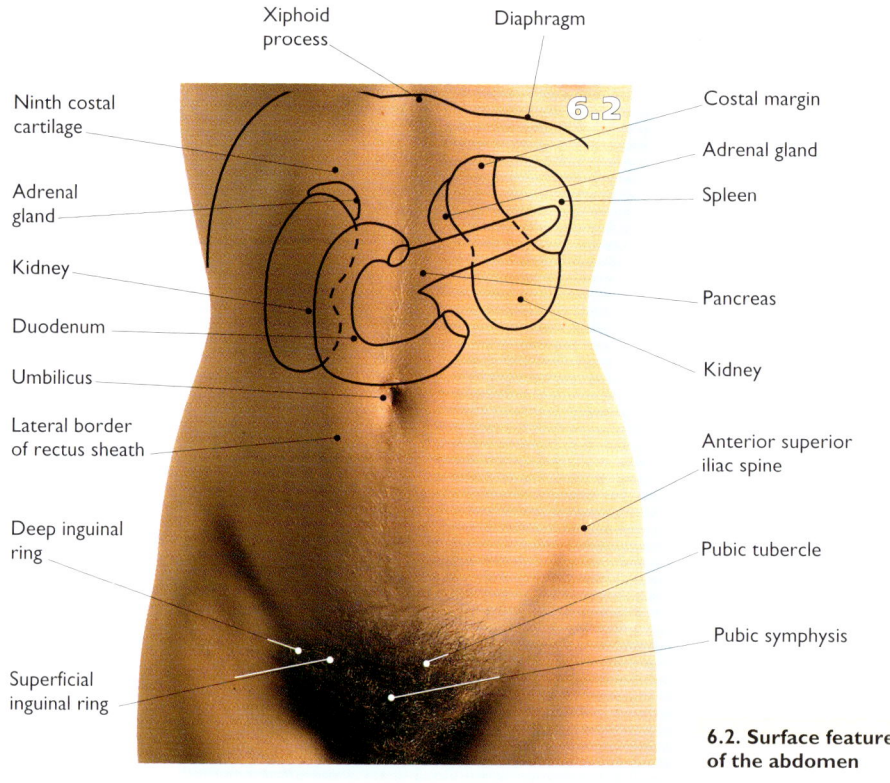

6.2. Surface features of the abdomen

masses, etc., can be described. The central regions are the epigastric, umbilical, and hypogastric (or suprapubic) regions, and at the sides are the right and left hypochondrial, lumbar, and iliac regions. The epigastric and hypogastric regions are sometimes called the epigastrium and hypochondrium, respectively, and the iliac regions the iliac fossae; thus, a gastric ulcer may give rise to pain in the epigastrium and an inflamed appendix to pain and tenderness in the right iliac fossa. A simpler way to divide the abdomen is to draw vertical and horizontal lines through the umbilicus, so dividing it into right and left upper and lower quadrants.

Lateral border of the rectus sheath – meets the costal margin at the ninth costal cartilage (**6.2**). On the right the fundus (lower end) of the gallbladder underlies this point, which is the region of maximal pain and tenderness in gallbladder disease.

Liver – may just be palpable at the right costal margin lateral to the rectus sheath when the patient takes a deep breath, although a liver enlarged and hardened by disease will be much more obvious on palpation.

Umbilicus – the midline puckered scar that indicates the site of attachment of the fetal umbilical cord typically lies at the level of the disc between L3 and L4 vertebrae. The pulsation of the aorta may be felt (and in thin subjects sometimes seen) just above or below the umbilicus by pressure on the overlying coils of the gut.

Duodenum – of the four parts which form the C-shaped curve of the duodenum (**6.2**), which is not normally palpable, the first part lies at the level of the L1 vertebra, the second part at the right edge of the L2 vertebra, the third part crosses the L3 vertebra, and the fourth part lies at the left margin of the L2 vertebra.

Head of the pancreas – lies within the C-shaped curve of the duodenum (often called by radiologists the duodenal loop), and the rest of the pancreas passes slightly upwards and to the right, with its tail reaching the hilum of the spleen. The organ is not normally palpable.

Kidney – the lower pole may be felt in the lumbar region by one hand pressing backwards below the costal margin and the other pressing forwards from behind.

Spleen – not normally palpable, since it is tucked up beneath the left dome of the diaphragm, in the long axis of the tenth rib. It must be 2–3 times its normal size to be palpable at the left costal margin.

An **enlarging kidney** expands downwards towards the iliac crest; an **enlarging spleen** passes more transversely towards the umbilicus.

Urinary bladder – being essentially a pelvic organ it is only palpable, in the suprapubic region, when considerably distended.

A **distended bladder** must not be mistaken for a pregnant uterus (or other pelvic mass such as an ovarian cyst).

Uterus – like the bladder it is a pelvic organ, but enlarges during pregnancy, reaching the top of the pubic symphysis at three months, the umbilicus at the fifth month and appearing to fill the whole abdomen at nine months (full term).

Colon – in the left iliac fossa, faecal material may be palpable in the descending or sigmoid colon ('loaded colon').

Posterior abdominal wall

The lumbar part of the vertebral column, which bulges forwards with the aorta and inferior vena cava in front of it, forms the central part of the posterior abdominal wall (**6.3**), and has the right and left crus of the diaphragm (p. 112) arising from its upper part. At each side is psoas major, with (if

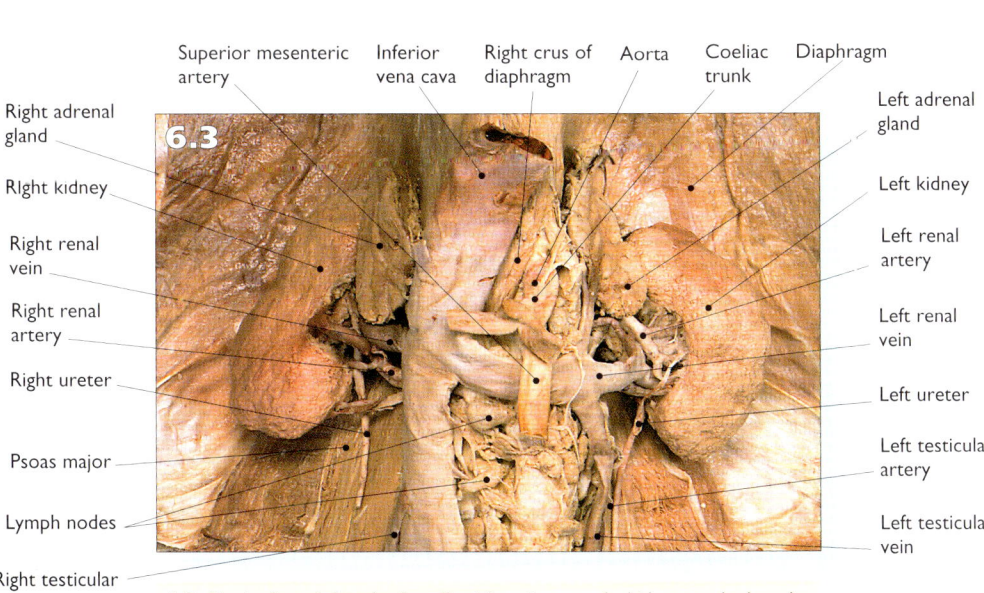

6.3. Posterior abdominal wall, with major vessels, kidneys and adrenal glands left in place

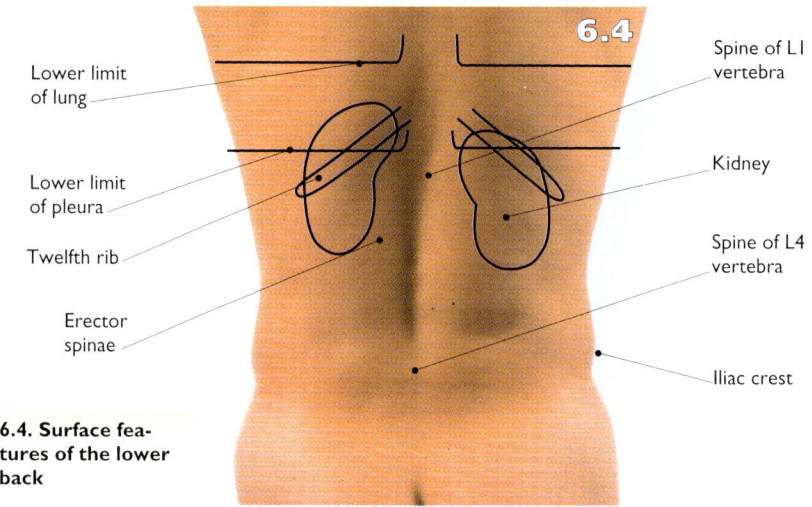

6.4. Surface features of the lower back

present) psoas minor overlying it, and more laterally, filling the gap between the twelfth rib and iliac crest, are quadratus lumborum and transversus abdominis, with the iliacus lower down.

Psoas major – runs down from the sides of the T12–L5 vertebrae and intervening discs to enter the thigh below the inguinal ligament and reach the lesser trochanter of the femur. The lumbar plexus of nerves is embedded within the muscle and the major branches emerge from it (see below), with twigs from L1–L3 nerves supplying the muscle. It is a powerful flexor of the hip (p. 170). The small and unimportant psoas minor (absent in 40% of individuals) arises from the sides of the T12 and L1 vertebrae and the intervening disc and has a long tendon that passes down over psoas major, attaching to the iliopubic eminence of the hip bone.

Quadratus lumborum – lies lateral to psoas major and fills the gap between the medial part of the iliac crest and the medial half of rib 12.

Transversus abdominis – see p. 128.

Iliacus – covers the floor of the iliac fossa and runs down to enter the thigh on the lateral side of psoas major. It is supplied by branches of the femoral nerve.

Surface markings – viewed from behind (6.4), a line drawn between the highest points of the iliac crests passes through the spine of the L4 vertebra; others can be counted upwards from here.

> **Lumbar punctures** (for obtaining specimens of cerebrospinal fluid) and epidural anaesthesia are commonly carried out between the spines of L3 and L4 vertebrae.

The position of each kidney can be visualised as a characteristic kidney shape about 12 cm high and 5 cm broad, with the hilum 5 cm from the midline and centred on the L1 vertebra, the left kidney lying slightly higher than the right. The twelfth ribs are often too short to be palpable through the back muscles; because the costodiaphragmatic recess of the pleura crosses the twelfth rib at the level of the lateral border of erector spinae, it is important not to misidentify the rib.

> The **kidney** is often approached **surgically** from behind, and it is important not to enter the pleural cavity.

Abdominal vessels and nerves

Abdominal aorta – enters the abdomen through the aortic opening at the level of the T12 vertebra (p. 112). It runs down the front of the lumbar vertebrae to end at the level of the L4 vertebra by dividing into the right and left common iliac arteries (**6.5**).

The three large branches that arise from the front of the aorta supply the alimentary tract. Each artery supplies a length of gut that corresponds to three embryonic regions: foregut, from the lower oesophagus to the point where the bile duct enters the duodenum, by the coelic trunk; midgut, from the entry of the bile duct to the transverse colon near the splenic flexure, by the superior mesenteric artery; and hindgut, from near the splenic flexure to the upper part of the anal canal, by the inferior mesenteric artery.

The largest branches from the sides of the aorta are the right and left renal arteries. Smaller paired branches include the gonadal vessels (testicular or ovarian), inferior phrenic and adrenal arteries, and four lumbar arteries.

Coeliac trunk – arises as soon as the aorta enters the abdomen and is usually a very short vessel that divides

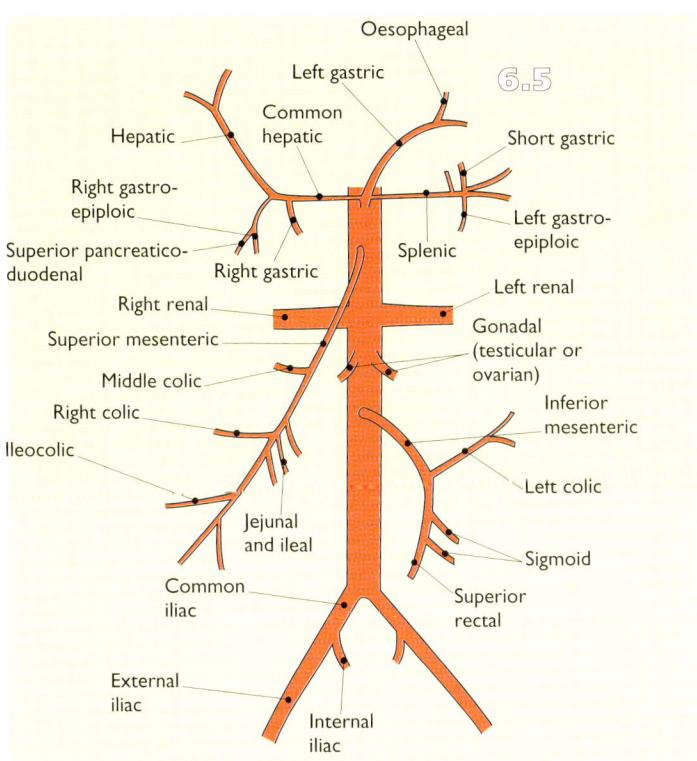

6.5. The principal branches of the abdominal aorta

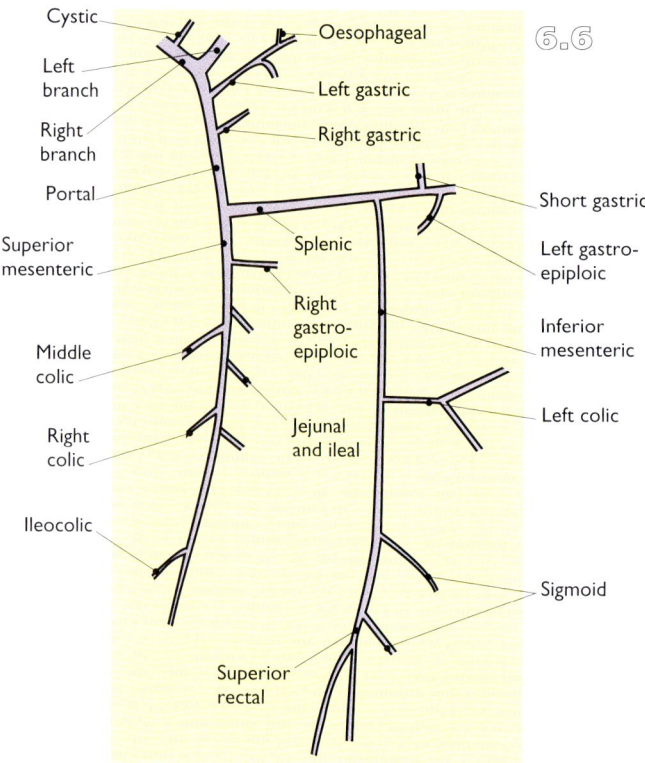

6.6. The principal tributaries of the portal vein.

into three branches: the left gastric, splenic, and common hepatic arteries. The left gastric artery passes upwards and then to the left to reach the lesser curvature of the stomach, and gives off an oesophageal branch. The splenic artery runs to the left along the upper border of the pancreas to the spleen, giving off the left gastro-epiploic and short gastric arteries. The common hepatic artery passes first to the right and gives off the right gastric artery and the gastroduodenal artery (which in turn gives off the right gastro-epiploic and superior pancreaticoduodenal arteries). The common hepatic artery then turns upwards as the hepatic artery in the right free margin of the lesser omentum (p. 142) to reach the liver; note the change of name from common hepatic to hepatic.

Superior mesenteric artery – arises from the aorta behind the pancreas. The principal branches are the numerous jejunal and ileal arteries (from its left side) and the inferior pancreaticoduodenal, ileocolic, right colic, and middle colic arteries (from its right side).

Inferior mesenteric artery – arises from the aorta behind the third part of the duodenum. The principal branches are the left colic and sigmoid arteries; it ends by changing its name to the superior rectal artery, which passes down into the pelvis to reach the rectum and anal canal.

Portal vein – receives the blood from all the structures supplied by the three large aortic branches just described. It is formed behind the pancreas by the union of the superior mesenteric vein with the splenic vein (**6.6**); the inferior mesenteric vein runs into the splenic vein. By the various tributaries of these vessels the portal vein drains the gut from the lower end of the oesophagus to the upper part of the anal canal, thus conveying to the liver substances absorbed from the alimentary tract. The lower end of the oesophagus is the most important site of portal–systemic anastomosis, between veins of the portal system and systemic veins.

> Enlarged veins at this site (**oesophageal varices**) may burst and give rise to dangerous haemorrhage.

Inferior vena cava – the principal vein of the body below the diaphragm, it lies on the right side of the aorta. It begins at the level of the L5 vertebra by the union of the right and left common iliac veins (**6.7**) and runs up to pierce the tendon of the diaphragm behind the liver at the level of the T8–T9 vertebrae. The largest tributaries are the right and left renal veins. The gonadal vein (testicular or ovarian) drains directly into the vena cava on the right, but on the left it enters the left renal vein. The highest tributaries of the vena cava are the hepatic veins, which enter the vena cava as that vessel lies in the deep groove on the back of the liver (the hepatic veins therefore have no extrahepatic course). A number of small lumbar veins also enter the vena cava at various levels.

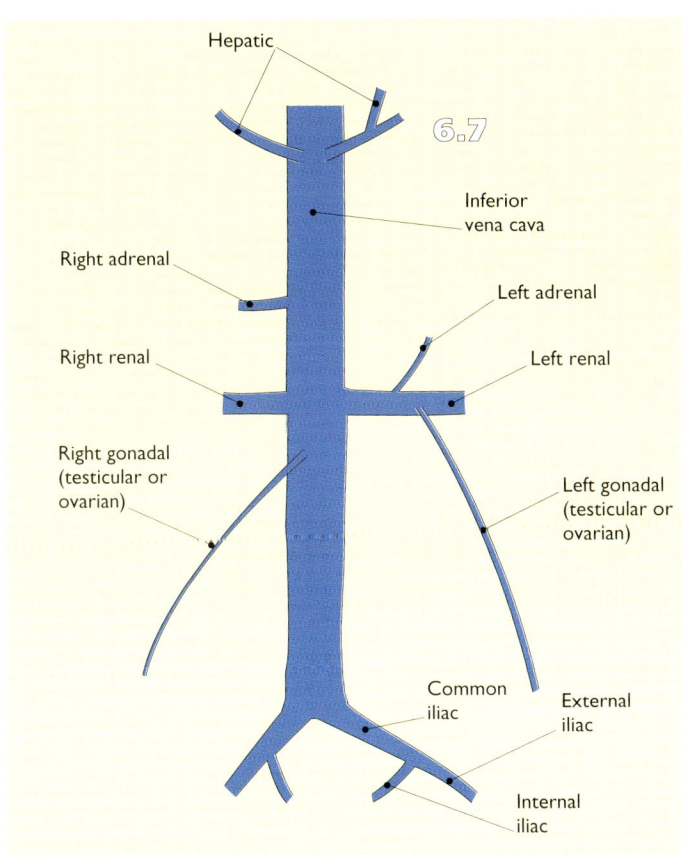

6.7. The principal tributaries of the inferior vena cava

They connect with pelvic veins and with venous plexuses around the vertebral column.

Femoral nerve (L2, L3, L4) – the largest nerve on the posterior abdominal wall and the largest branch of the lumbar plexus (**3.19**), which is within psoas major, it emerges from the *lateral* side of psoas low down and runs down to enter the front of the thigh beneath the inguinal ligament on the lateral side of the external iliac artery (which becomes the femoral artery in the thigh).

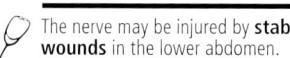
The nerve may be injured by **stab wounds** in the lower abdomen.

Lateral femoral cutaneous nerve (L2, L3) – smaller than the femoral nerve and emerging from psoas higher up, it curls down over iliacus to enter the thigh beneath the lateral part of the inguinal ligament.

Iliohypogastric and ilio-inguinal nerves (L1) – smaller than the last named and emerging from psoas above it, they run laterally to enter the lower anterior abdominal wall. They are important because these first lumbar nerve fibres are the ones that supply the parts of the anterior abdominal wall muscles that guard the inguinal canal.

Lumbosacral trunk – emerges from the deep *medial* border of psoas to join the anterior ramus of the S1 nerve in front of piriformis on the posterior pelvic wall.

Obturator nerve – also emerges from the deep medial border of psoas to tun along the side wall of the pelvis (p. 151) to enter the medial part of the thigh.

Sympathetic trunks – continuing down from the thorax behind the diaphragm, these run on the lumbar vertebral column, the left trunk *at* the left margin of the aorta, and the right trunk *under cover of* the right margin of the inferior vena cava. Branches from the ganglia join lumbar nerves and supply adjacent viscera and blood vessels.

Abdominal viscera

Most of the abdomen is occupied by viscera that belong to the digestive system (digestive tract, alimentary tract). The whole system comprises the mouth and pharynx (in the head and neck), oesophagus (mainly in the thorax), and the stomach, small intestine, and large intestine, which occupy the abdomen, and its lower part, the pelvis. In the upper abdomen are the liver and pancreas, which are the largest of the digestive glands, and also the kidneys, which are the principal organs of the urinary system, the adrenal glands (belonging to the endocrine system), and the spleen (part of the lymphatic system).

The viscera and their blood supplies are considered individually. Although all receive autonomic nerve supplies, only a few details are important:

Sympathetic nerves (vasoconstrictor) carry pain fibres.

Parasympathetic (vagal) fibres to the stomach stimulate motility and secretion (also controlled by the hormone gastrin).

Movement of the rest of the gut (peristalsis) depends on its own intrinsic nerve networks and not on the external supply.

Lymph drainage is to adjacent nodes, which eventually reach para-aortic nodes, which in turn drain to the cisterna chyli (p. 115). Lymph drainage is most important for the stomach and colon (the common sites for cancer) and, as far as the small intestine is concerned, for the transport of fat molecules, which are absorbed by the lacteals (lymphatic capillaries) of the gut mucosa and not into the blood capillaries.

Stomach

The stomach, stimulated by the vagus nerves (p. 116), is where protein digestion begins. It is the most dilated part of the alimentary tract, situated between the oesophagus and duodenum and lying in the epigastrium and left hypochondrium (6.8, 6.9). It is roughly J-shaped, with the upper opening at the cardia or gastro-oesophageal junction to the left of the midline at the level of the T9 vertebra, and the lower opening at the pylorus or gastroduodenal junction to the right of the midline at the level of the L1 vertebra (transpyloric plane). The upper border is the lesser curvature, suspended from the liver by a fold of peritoneum, the lesser omentum (see below). The lower border is the greater curvature, with the greater omentum of peritoneum hanging down from it like an apron in front of coils of intestine. The transverse mesocolon (the peritoneal support for the transverse colon – see below) and the transverse colon adhere to the back of the greater omentum. Behind the stomach (and in front of the pancreas and upper part of the left kidney) there is a recess of peritoneum, the lesser sac (properly called the omental bursa); the opening into it (like the vertical slot in a coin machine) is the epiploic foramen and lies behind the right free margin of the lesser omentum, immediately in front of the inferior vena cava. The recess ensures free movement of the stomach against the structures behind it.

The stomach has three parts: the fundus (the part above the level of entry of the oesophagus), the body (main part), and the pyloric part (pyloric antrum, with the pyloric sphincter at the junction with the duodenum).

> The word **stomach** (as in 'stomachache') is often used by lay people to mean the **abdomen** rather than the specific organ.

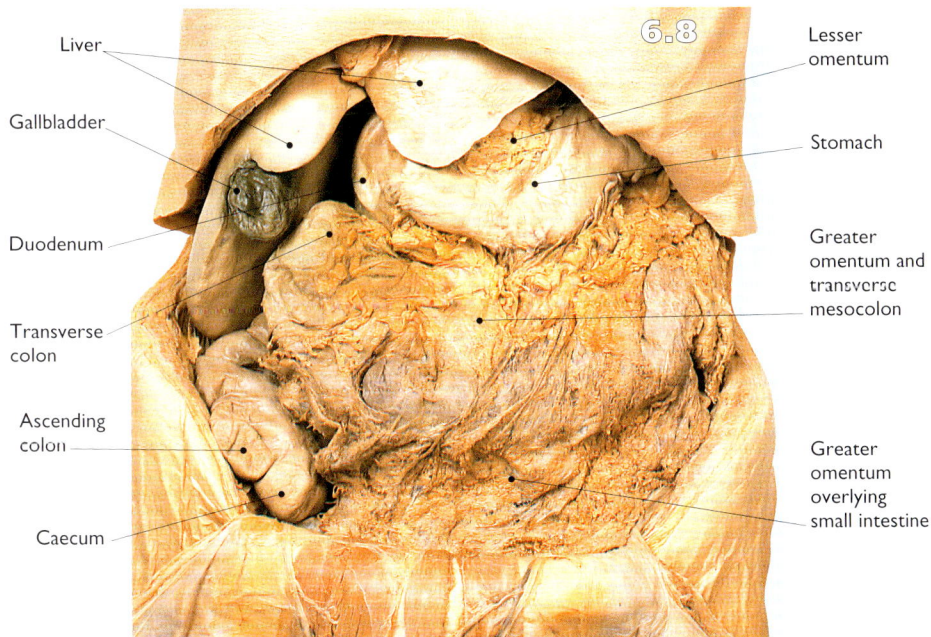

6.8. Upper abdominal viscera, with the anterior abdominal wall turned downwards

Blood supply – from the left and right gastric arteries along the lesser curvature, and from the short gastric and left and right gastro-epiploic arteries along the greater curvature. Accompanying veins drain to the portal system (**6.6**).

Small intestine

The small intestine consists of the duodenum, jejunum, and ileum. It extends from the pylorus to the ileocaecal junction and is a hose-like tube about 4 m long (although longer after death due to relaxation of the muscular wall) concerned with the digestion and absorption of foodstuffs.

Duodenum – 25 cm long, it is plastered onto the posterior abdominal wall by peritoneum (i.e. it is retroperitoneal) and is C-shaped, with four parts (usually called first to fourth) which run respectively up to the right, down, across to the left, and up, embracing the head of the pancreas and lying at the levels of L1–L3 vertebrae (**6.2, 6.9**). It receives the bile and pancreatic ducts, which join at the hepatopancreatic ampulla embedded in the posteromedial wall of the second part and opening at the major duodenal papilla (**6.12**). The adjacent minor duodenal papilla receives the opening of the accessory pancreatic duct.

> Clinically the term **small intestine** usually excludes the duodenum.

> **Duodenal ulcers** occur in the first part, where acid gastric contents first impinge after passing through the pylorus.

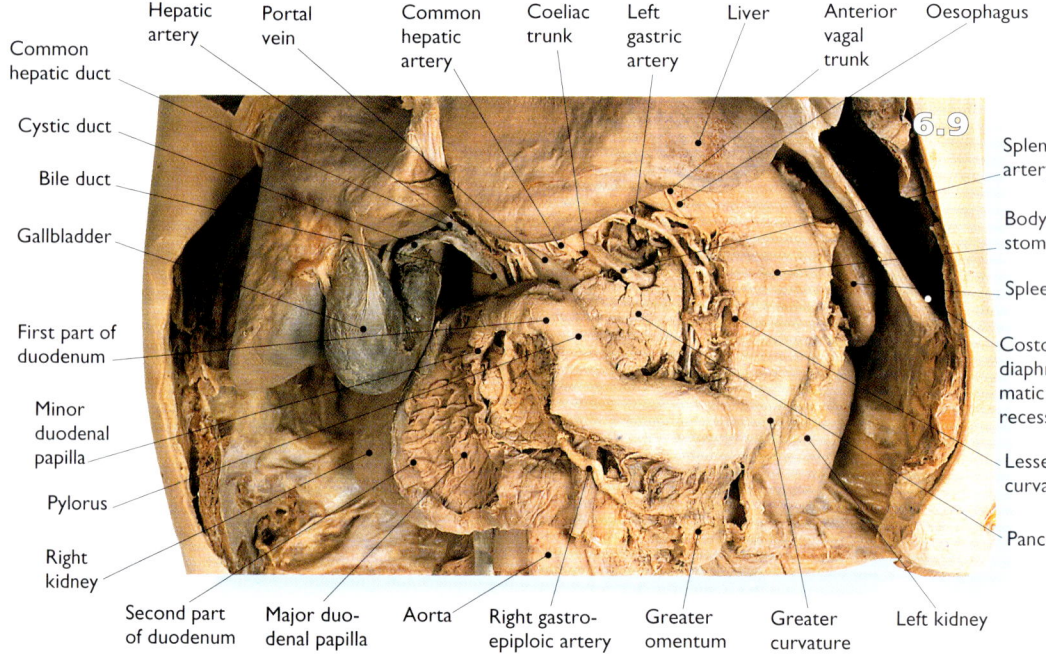

6.9. Upper abdominal viscera. The lesser omentum (between the liver and stomach) and most of the greater omentum have been removed, together with part of the anterior wall of the duodenum

Abdomen

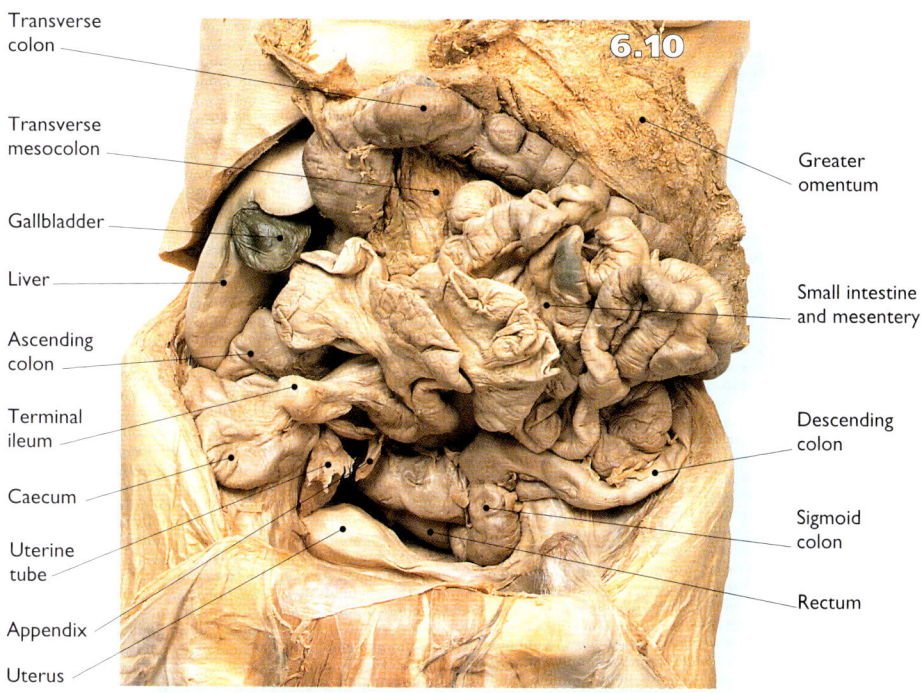

6.10. Small and large intestines. The greater omentum, transverse colon, and transverse mesocolon have been lifted upwards (over the stomach), so the posterior surfaces of these structures are seen here. Some coils of small intestine have also been displaced upwards to show female pelvic structures

Jejunum and ileum – suspended from the posterior abdominal wall by a fold of peritoneum, the mesentery (**6.10**) is only about 15 cm long at its attachment to the posterior abdominal wall, but becomes immensely frilled at the intestinal attachment. There is no clear junction between jejunum and ileum; the slightly thicker jejunum, the proximal two-fifths of the whole tube, is continuous with the fourth part of the duodenum at the duodenojejunal flexure, and the rest is the ileum, which joins the large intestine at the ileocaecal junction. The mesentery contains blood vessels, lymphatics and lymph nodes, nerves, and fat.

Blood supply – of the duodenum down to the opening of the bile and pancreatic ducts by branches of the common hepatic artery (**6.5**), the rest of the duodenum and the jejunum and ileum by the superior mesenteric artery (**6.11**). Veins drain to the portal system (**6.6**).

Large intestine

The large intestine is concerned with water absorption and the storage and evacuation of the waste products of digestion. It consists of the caecum (with the appendix), colon, rectum, and anal canal, and is about 1.5 m

> **Cancer** of the small intestine is rare; cancer of the stomach, colon and rectum is common. The reason for the difference is not known.

Human Anatomy

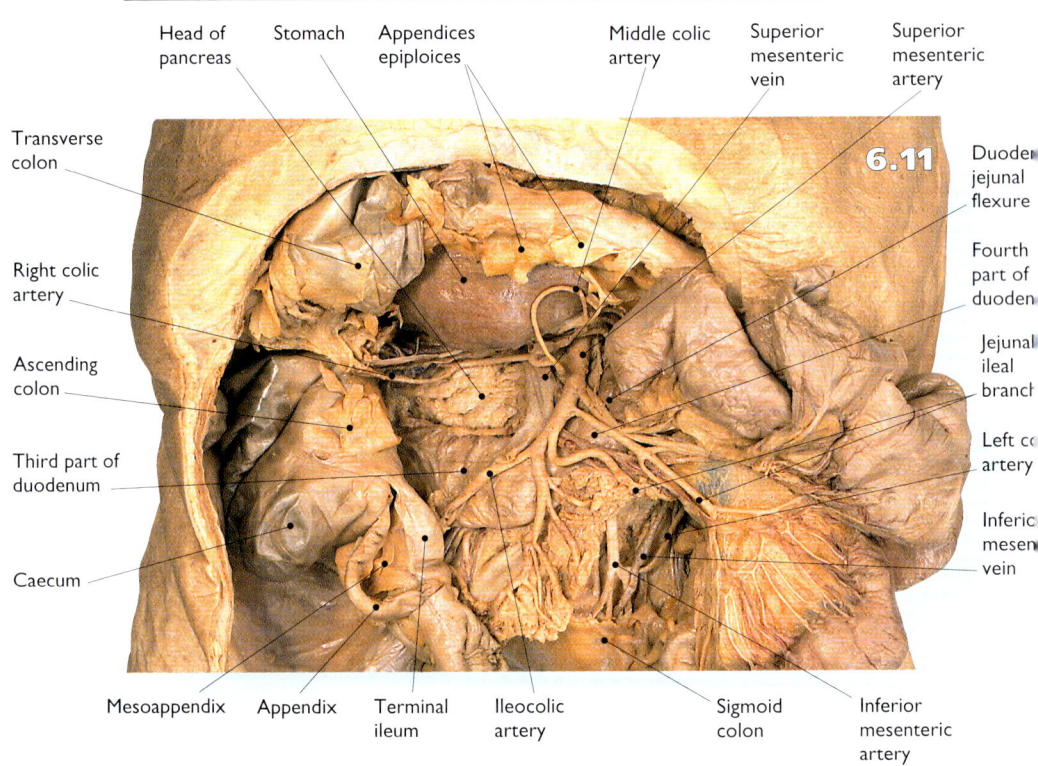

6.11. Mesenteric vessels and adjacent viscera. The transverse colon has been lifted upwards and coils of small intestine have been displaced to the left, with the mesentery of the small intestine dissected away

long from the end of the ileum to the lower opening of the anal canal (anus). Of larger diameter than the small intestine, most of it (caecum and colon) has three longitudinal bands of muscle on the outer surface (taeniae coli) and small fatty tags (appendices epiploices), both of which features instantly distinguish it from the small intestine (**6.10, 6.11**).

Caecum – the blind rounded start of the large intestine (**6.10, 6.11**), it continues upwards as the colon and is joined at the left side by the ileum at the ileocaecal junction. It lies in the right iliac fossa.

Appendix – (properly called vermiform appendix – worm-like) a narrow blind-ended tube (the narrowest part of the whole alimentary tract), with its base opening into the caecum 2 cm below the ileocaecal junction (**6.10, 6.11**). Its length varies, but is often about 8 cm, with the tip in any position from behind the caecum to hanging over into the pelvis. It has its own small mesentery, the mesoappendix, containing the appendicular artery (**6.12**). The three taeniae coli (longitudinal muscle) of the caecum all converge onto the base of the appendix – a useful

> **McBurney's point**, a third of the way along a line from the anterior superior iliac spine to the umbilicus, is a landmark for the opening of the appendix into the caecum.

> **Appendicitis** (of unknown cause) is the most common reason for emergency abdominal surgery.

guide to finding it if hidden behind coils of gut.

Colon – consists of ascending, transverse, descending, and sigmoid parts (**6.8–6.10**). The ascending colon, which is retroperitoneal, continues upwards from the caecum to the liver, where it turns medially at the right colic flexure (hepatic flexure) to become the transverse colon. This is suspended by peritoneum (transverse mesocolon) from the lower border of the pancreas. At the spleen it turns down at the left colic flexure (splenic flexure) as the descending colon (retroperitoneal) to the left iliac fossa, where it regains a mesentery (sigmoid mesocolon) to become the sigmoid colon.

• The sigmoid part is the commonest site for **colonic cancer**.

Rectum and anal canal – see p. 155 and 158.

Blood supply – from caecum to near the splenic flexure by branches of the superior mesenteric artery, then by the inferior mesenteric artery (**6.5**). One of the caecal branches of the superior mesenteric gives off the appendicular artery. Veins drain to the portal system (**6.6**).

Liver

The liver is the largest gland in the body, with many metabolic and storage functions, including the secretion of bile which assists in fat digestion. It is wedge-shaped, tapering and extending to the left, largely under the right dome of the diaphragm (**6.13**); it thus lies mostly in the right hypochondrial and epigastric regions. It has peritoneal attachments to the diaphragm and

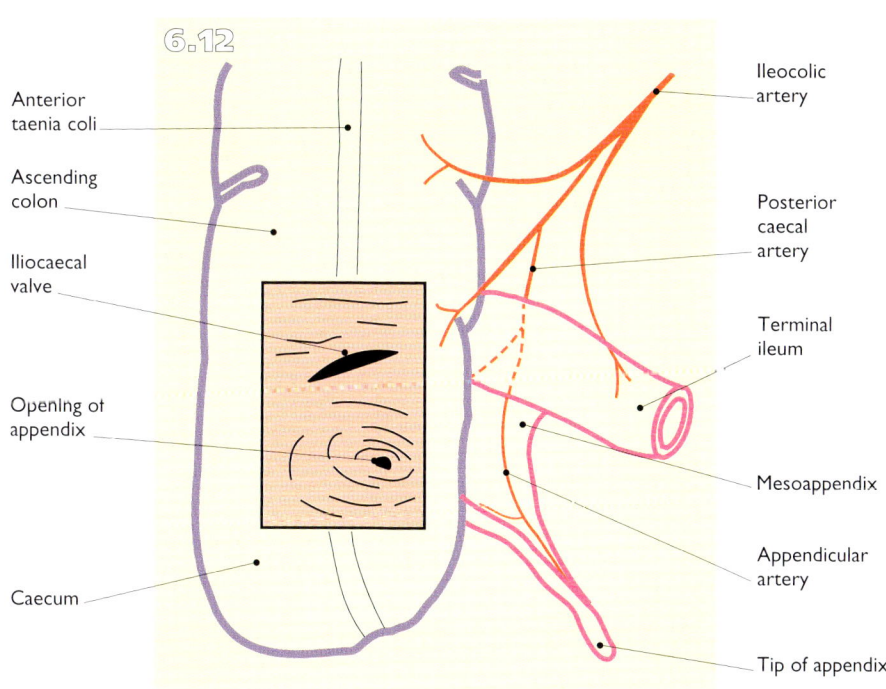

6.12. **The caecum and appendix**, with a window cut in the anterior wall of the caecum

141

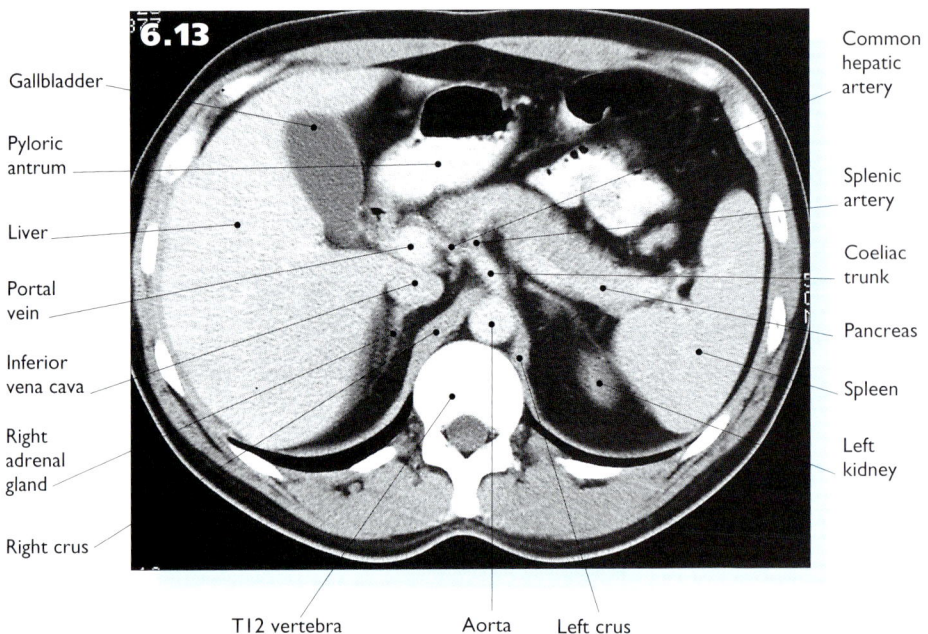

6.13. Axial computed tomograph of the upper abdomen at the level of the T12 vertebra, from below

anterior abdominal wall, but is kept in place mainly by the hepatic veins which run into the inferior vena cava, lying in a deep groove at the back of the liver. It has a large right and a small left lobe, but the caudate and quadrate lobes, which are part of right lobe, are *functionally* part of left lobe because, like the left lobe, they receive blood from *left* branches of the hepatic artery and portal vein; the main part of the right lobe receives blood from the right branches of these vessels. Near the centre of the liver at the back is the porta hepatis, where vessels and ducts enter and leave. The lesser omentum, the peritoneal fold that runs between the stomach and liver, is attached to the margins of the porta hepatis, and running in the right margin of the lesser omentum are the portal vein, hepatic artery, and bile duct (below and **6.9**).

Blood supply – by the hepatic artery for arterial blood (20%) and by the portal vein for portal blood (80%) from the alimentary tract and spleen (**6.5, 6.6**). The right and left branches of these vessels enter at the porta hepatis. Three or more hepatic veins drain to the inferior vena cava (not via the porta hepatis) and are hidden from sight unless the liver is removed.

Gallbladder and biliary tract

Bile from liver cells reaches the right and left hepatic ducts, which leave the liver at the porta hepatis and unite to form the common hepatic duct, which is joined by the cystic duct from the gallbladder to form the bile duct (**6.9, 6.14**).

Gallbladder – where bile is concentrated, stored, and released under the influence of an intestinal hormone. The gallbladder is pear-shaped and about 10 cm long, attached to the under surface of the right lobe of the liver, with the lowest part, the fundus, lying against the anterior abdominal wall, where the right margin of the rectus sheath meets the costal margin (ninth costal cartilage).

Behind, the fundus overlaps the junction of the first and second parts of the duodenum (hence the green post-mortem staining of this part of the gut by bile that seeps through the gallbladder wall), while a high transverse colon may lie just below the fundus.

Bile duct – about 8 cm long and 8 mm diameter, it lies in the right margin of the lesser omentum, where it is in front of the portal vein, with the hepatic artery on the duct's left side. Correct identification of the bile duct and adjacent structures is vital to the understanding of diseases of, and operations on, the stomach, duodenum, pancreas, liver, and biliary tract. The bile duct then passes behind the

> Stones (calculi) in the gall bladder (**gallstones**) may escape into the cystic and bile ducts and cause spasms of pain (**biliary colic**).

> This is the region of abdominal pain and tenderness in **gallbladder disease** (p. 130).

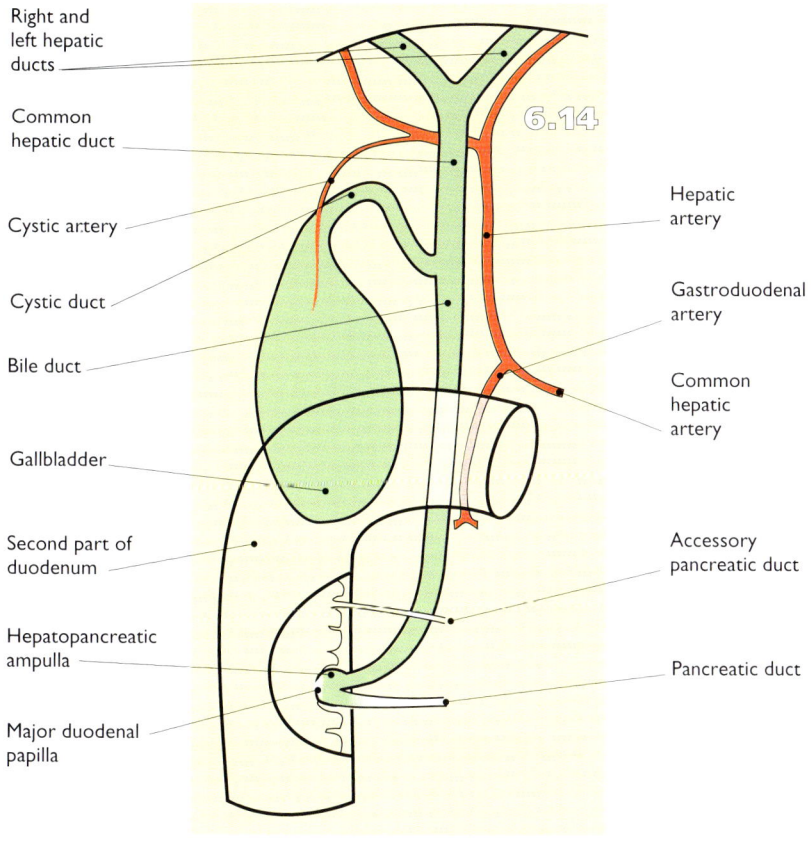

6.14. **The biliary tract**, with a window cut in the second part of the duodenum

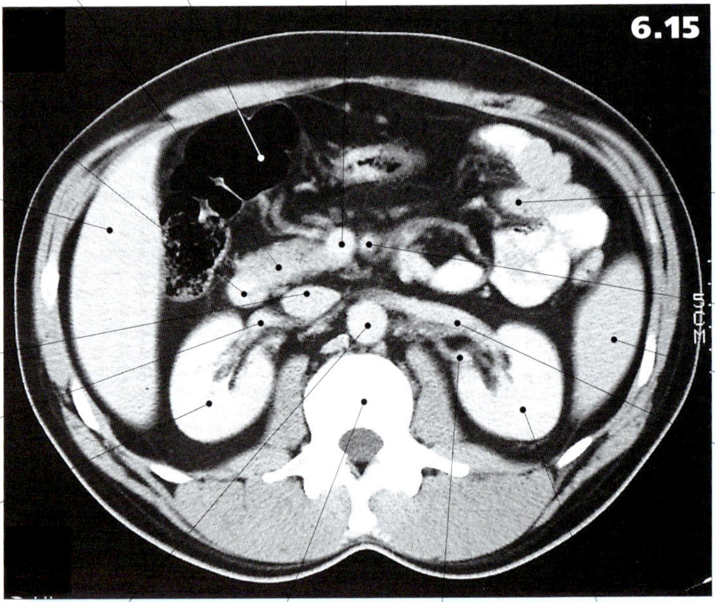

6.15. Axial computed tomograph of the upper abdomen at the level of the LI vertebra, from below

first part of the duodenum to reach the second part, where it enters the posteromedial part of the wall to join the pancreatic duct at the hepatopancreatic ampulla, which opens at the major duodenal papilla (about 10 cm beyond the pylorus).

Blood supply – the gallbladder receives the cystic artery (from the hepatic), which supplements small vessels from the gallbladder bed of the liver, into which most of the venous blood drains (a cystic vein draining to the right branch of the portal vein is uncommon) (6.5, 6.6). The bile duct is supplied by branches from the gastroduodenal and hepatic vessels.

This is one of the most important areas in the whole abdomen. Obstruction of the bile duct (e.g. by a gallstone or cancer of the head of the pancreas) is one cause of **jaundice** (yellow pigmentation of the skin and cornea).

Pancreas

The pancreas secretes (under the control of intestinal hormones) digestive enzymes and also has endocrine cells (in the islets of Langerhans) whose products, mainly insulin and glucagon, are essential for carbohydrate metabolism. It is a hook-shaped gland, about 15 cm long, that lies transversely across the upper abdomen, with the head in the C-shaped curve of the duodenum (**6.9, 6.13**), extending to the left as the body behind the stomach and ending as the tail lying against the hilum of the spleen. It is retroperitoneal, with the transverse mesocolon hanging down from the lower border.

Pancreatic duct – runs from the tail to the lower part of the head and joins the bile duct at the hepatopancreatic ampulla. A small accessory pancreatic duct runs from the upper part of the head into the duodenum, about 2 cm proximal to the main duct (**6.14**). The ducts convey the pancreatic enzymes concerned with digestion; the endocrine secretions from the islets leave in the venous blood.

Blood supply – mainly from the splenic artery, which runs just behind the upper border of the pancreas, with some superior mesenteric branches to its head (**6.5**). Veins drain to the portal system (**6.6**).

Kidneys and ureters

The urinary system in both sexes consists of the kidneys, ureters, urinary bladder, and urethra, all concerned with the production, storage, and elimination of urine in order to maintain the body's proper content of water and dissolved substances.

The main function of the kidneys is to produce urine, so maintaining the body's fluids and electrolytes in their proper concentrations and helping to keep blood pressure within normal limits. Each kidney is about 12 cm long, 6 cm wide, and 4 cm thick, and lies behind the peritoneum in the 'gutter' at the side of the vertebral column (**6.3, 6.15**), the top (upper pole) of the left kidney rising as high as the eleventh rib, with the diaphragm and the lowest part of the pleura intervening; the right kidney only rises as high as the twelfth rib (due to the bulk of the liver on the right). The hilum of the kidney (the groove on the medial aspect, where vessels and ureter enter or leave) is on a level just above the transpyloric plane (p. 137) on the left and just below it on the right; on each side it lies 5 cm from the midline. The second part of the duodenum overlies the hilum on the right side; the body of the pancreas crosses the left hilum. The ureter, which conducts urine from the kidney to the bladder, runs down behind the peritoneum (but adhering to it) on psoas major to enter the pelvis by crossing the external iliac vessels. The expanded upper end of the ureter (the part that leaves the hilum of the kidney) is the renal pelvis.

> The order of structures in the **hilum** is vein, artery, ureter from front to back; compare with the hilum of the lung – vein, artery, bronchus.

Blood supply – from the single large renal artery which leaves the aorta at a right angle and runs into the hilum, dividing into several branches (**6.5**). Occasionally, an accessory renal artery may leave the aorta to run to the lower pole. Veins unite in the hilum to form the single renal vein that drains to the inferior vena cava (**6.7**); the left renal vein crosses in front of the aorta. Branches from the renal, gonadal, iliac, and vesical vessels supply the ureter, depending on the level.

Adrenal glands

The adrenal (suprarenal) glands (**6.3**) are endocrine organs with two distinct parts: an outer cortex that produces hormones, such as cortisol, concerned with blood and fluid volumes and their electrolyte contents, and an inner medulla that secretes the hormones noradrenaline and adrenaline (catecholamines), which supplement the activity of the sympathetic nervous system. The right suprarenal gland is rather like a three-sided pyramid, about 3 cm high and thick, which lies partly behind the peritoneum against the top of the right kidney, but with its uppermost part in contact with the liver. The left gland, often more crescentic in shape, is behind the peritoneum of the lesser sac (behind the stomach), on the medial side of the left kidney above the hilum. The glands are unique in that their medullary cells receive preganglionic sympathetic fibres directly from lateral horn cells (p. 15).

Blood supply – several small arteries from the aorta, renal, and inferior phrenic arteries. There is usually only one vein on each side; on the right it is very short and runs into the inferior vena cava, which is just beside the gland, but on the left it is longer and drains into the left renal vein (**6.7**).

Spleen

The spleen, the largest of the lymphoid organs, lies tucked up against the left half of the diaphragm (which separates it from the pleura and ribs 9–11), along the outer border of the upper part of the left kidney and behind the stomach (**6.13, 6.15**). It is surrounded by peritoneum whose folds (lienorenal ligament and gastrosplenic ligament) anchor it to the kidney and stomach, respectively.

Blood supply – by the splenic artery, often a tortuous vessel that runs behind the upper border of the pancreas (**6.9**). The splenic vein runs behind the pancreas to join the superior mesenteric vein and form the portal vein (**6.6**). Thus, although the spleen is not part of the alimentary tract, its blood unexpectedly drains to the portal system.

Summary

- The **umbilicus** normally lies at the level of the disc between L3 and L4 vertebrae, and most of the important abdominal structures lies above this level. The other important area is the **right iliac fossa**, where the pain of appendicitis becomes localised.

- The **hilum of each kidney** is about 5 cm from the midline, just above and just below the transpyloric plane on the left and right respectively. The usual order of structures in the hilum is vein, artery, ureter from front to back. The **adrenal glands** are found against the upper and medial part of each kidney.

- The C-shaped curve of the **duodenum** lies between the levels of L1 and L3 vertebrae, and embraces the head of the pancreas whose body passes to the left across the left kidney to the hilum of the spleen.

- The **lesser omentum** of peritoneum runs from the liver to the lesser curvature of the stomach, and contains in its right free margin the portal vein with the bile duct in front of the right edge of the vein and the hepatic artery on the left of the duct.

- The **bile duct** is formed above the first part of the duodenum by the union of the cystic duct from the gall bladder with the common hepatic duct, which results from the union of the right and left hepatic ducts that emerge from the liver.

- The **caudate** and **quadrate lobes of the liver** belong functionally to the left lobe; they receive blood from the left branches of the hepatic artery and portal vein, and drain bile to the left hepatic duct. The right branches supply the right lobe, and bile drains to the right hepatic duct.

- The three large branches from the front of the abdominal aorta are those that supply gut: **coeliac trunk** (from lower oesophagus to where the bile duct enters the duodenum), **superior mesenteric artery** (from duodenum to near the splenic flexure of the colon) and **inferior mesenteric artery** (from splenic flexure to the upper part of the anal canal). The above areas of supply, supplemented by the splenic vein, comprise the drainage area of the portal vein.

- Of the main tributaries of the inferior vena cava, those most frequently forgotten are the **hepatic veins**; they have no extrahepatic course and cannot be seen unless the liver is removed.

- The most important site of **portal-systemic anastomosis** is the lower end of the oesophagus, where enlarged veins may burst.

Continued overleaf ...

> ... *Continued from previous page*
>
> - The left and right **gastric arteries** anastomose along the lesser curvature of the stomach, and the left and right **gastro-epiploics** along the greater curvature; the short **gastric arteries** supply the fundus.
>
> - The main blood supply of the pancreas is the **splenic artery**, with the smaller pancreaticoduodenal vessels passing to the head of the pancreas.
>
> - The root of the **mesentery of the small intestine** runs from the duodenojejunal flexure downwards and to the right towards the right iliac fossa, and is only 15 cm long.
>
> - The transverse colon and sigmoid colon have their own mesenteries (**transverse mesocolon** and **sigmoid mesocolon**), but the ascending and descending colon are retroperitoneal.
>
> - **McBurney's point**, a third of the way along a line from the anterior superior iliac spine to the umbilicus, indicates the position of the base of the appendix, where it opens into the caecum; the tip of the appendix is very variable in position.

Part 7
Pelvis and perineum

The word pelvis, as in bony pelvis, means a basin, but it can also be used as a term to mean the lower part of the abdominal cavity and can be called the pelvic cavity.

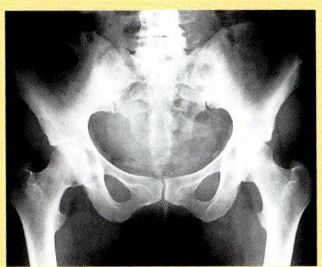

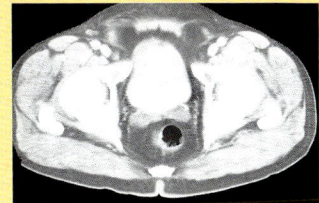

The bony pelvis is so structured that in the anatomical position the body weight is transmitted from the vertebral column to the lower limbs.

In the female the lower part must provide sufficient accommodation for the passage of a fetus on its birth-journey to become a newborn child. The very lowest part in both sexes is the perineum containing the external genital organs and some small perineal muscles, the most important of which are the external anal and urethral sphincters.

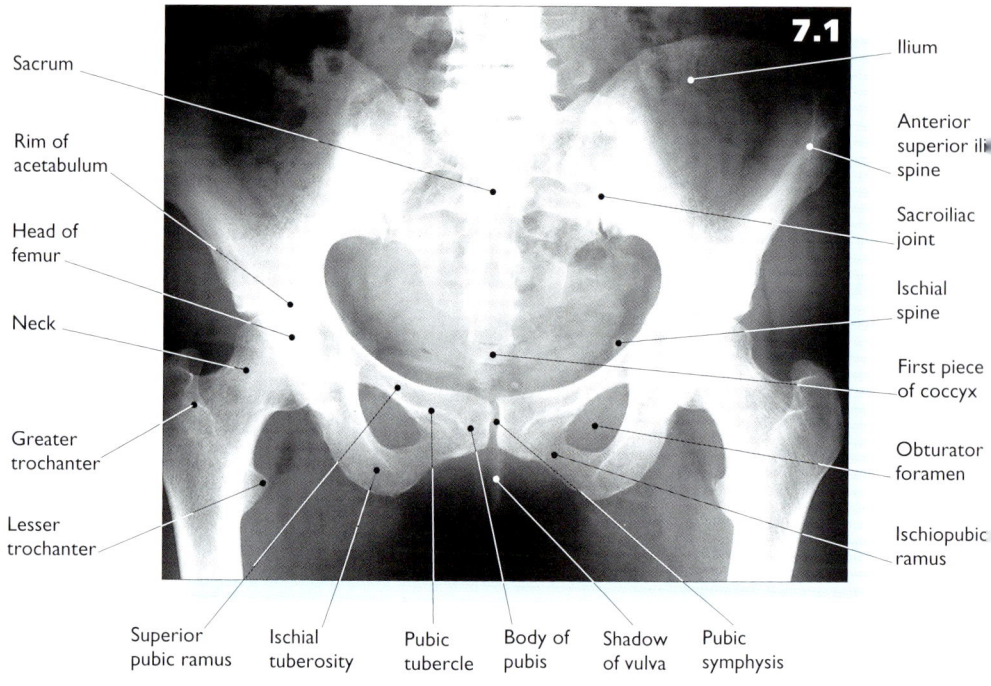

7.1. Radiograph of the female pelvis

THE BONY PELVIS consists of the sacrum and coccyx at the back, which unite at each side with the hip bone at the sacroiliac joint (7.1); at the front the two hip bones are joined at the pubic symphysis. The pelvic brim is formed by the top edge of the sacrum (with the sacral promontory in the midline), the arcuate line of the ilium and the top of the pubic bone and pubic symphysis; it is the boundary between the true pelvis or pelvic cavity, below the brim, and the false pelvis which is the part above the brim and really belongs to the abdominal cavity. It is important to note that when the bony pelvis is correctly orientated, i.e. tilted forwards so that the anterior superior iliac spines and the top of the pubic symphysis are in the same vertical plane (as when holding the pelvis against a wall with these bony points touching the wall), the pelvic cavity runs backwards almost at a right angle to the abdominal cavity. The pelvic muscles of each side are piriformis at the back and obturator internus at the side (these muscles also belong to the gluteal region of the lower limb), while coccygeus and levator ani form the highly important pelvic floor or pelvic diaphragm. The sacral plexus lies in front of the piriformis; most of its branches are examined in dissections of the gluteal region (8.5). The sacral parts of the sympathetic trunks lie medial to the anterior sacral foramina and S2–S4 nerves give off parasympathetic branches. The inter-

> The **pelvic diaphragm** must not be confused with the urogenital diaphragm (p. 155) whose main muscle is the external urethral sphincter.

nal iliac vessels and their branches lie in front of the nerves and supply the pelvic viscera (7.2, 7.3), although the ovarian artery arises high up from the abdominal aorta and reaches the ovary through its own fold of peritoneum, the suspensory ligament of the ovary. The corresponding testicular artery runs through the spermatic cord in the inguinal canal.

The perineum is the lowest part of the trunk of the body, roughly 'the bit between the legs', and is below the pelvic floor. Viewed from below it is diamond-shaped, bounded by the pubic symphysis at the front, the ischial tuberosities at the sides, and the coccyx at the back (7.4, 7.5). The back part, containing the opening of the anal canal (anus), is the anal region and the front part, containing the external genital organs, is the genital region. The male external genital organs are the scrotum (containing the testis, epididymis, and start of the ductus deferens) and penis.

The female external genital organs consist of the mons pubis, the paired labia majora and labia minora, the bulb of the vestibule, the vestibule of the vagina, and the clitoris. Collectively, they form the vulva.

Piriformis – arises from the middle three pieces of the front of the sacrum and runs laterally to leave the pelvis through the greater sciatic foramen and become attached to the greater trochanter of the femur. For its importance as a landmark in the gluteal region (p. 168).

Obturator internus – arises from the lateral wall of the inside of the pelvis and the obturator membrane (7.6), and turns at 90° through the lesser sciatic notch to reach the greater trochanter of the femur. The obturator nerve runs below the pelvic brim to pass into the thigh through the obturator foramen.

Coccygeus – is really the muscular part of the sacrospinous ligament, and forms the posterior part of its own half of the pelvic floor.

Levator ani – the pair form most of the pelvic floor (7.3–7.5). The levator ani has two bony attachments: at the front to the body of the pubis, and at the back to the ischial spine. In between, it arises from the fascia that overlies the obturator internus muscle. The front half of the levator ani is often called the pubococcygeus and the rest of it the iliococcygeus. The muscle fibres run downwards and inwards to form a gutter, which converges on the perineal body (see below), the anococcygeal ligament, and the coccyx, but there is a gap between the medial borders of each muscle through which pass the urethra and anal canal in both sexes and also the vagina in the female.

Stretching of the pelvic floor during childbirth (**parturition**) may lead to urinary incontinence (e.g. when coughing, which suddenly increases abdominal pressure).

Some of these medial fibres unite with their fellows of the opposite side, as does the puborectalis muscle, to form a sling at the anorectal junction that maintains an angle of 120° between the rectum and anal canal (*see* below). Other medial fibres form the levator prostatae muscle, below the male prostate; similar fibres in the female constitute the pubovaginalis muscle, which acts as a vaginal sphincter and assists in maintaining urinary continence. The nerve supply of the levator ani is by S3 and S4 nerves.

Pelvic splanchnic nerves – parasympathetic branches from S2-S4 nerves which supply pelvic viscera. In particular they are the motor nerves to the smooth muscle of the bladder, and are also responsible for the vasodilatation that causes erection of the penis (hence their old Latin name, nervi erigentes).

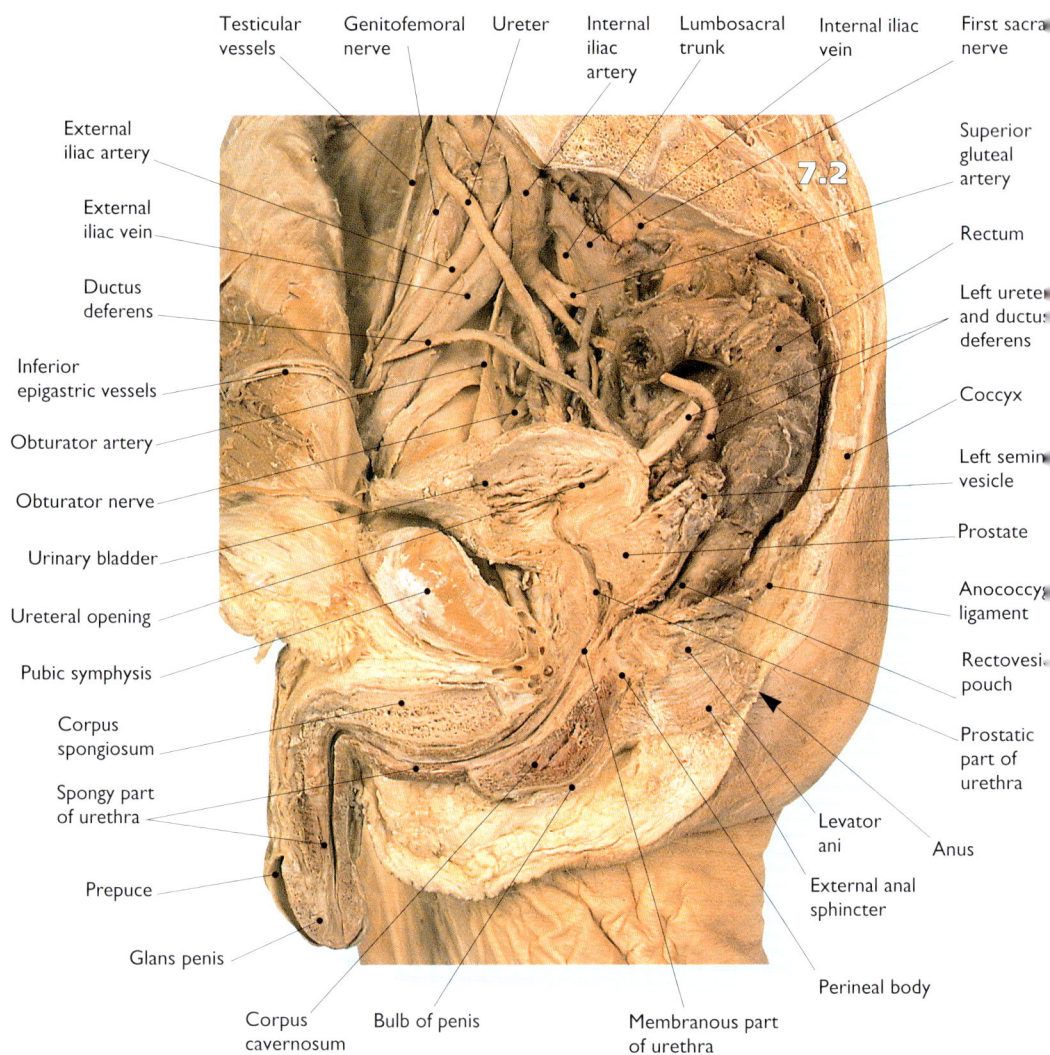

7.2 Right half of a sagittal section of the male pelvis. The cut has passed through the whole length of the urethra, but the rectum and anal canal have not been sectioned and the external anal sphincter covers the left side of the anal canal. The lower ends of the left ureter and ductus deferens are seen, together with part of the left seminal vesicle

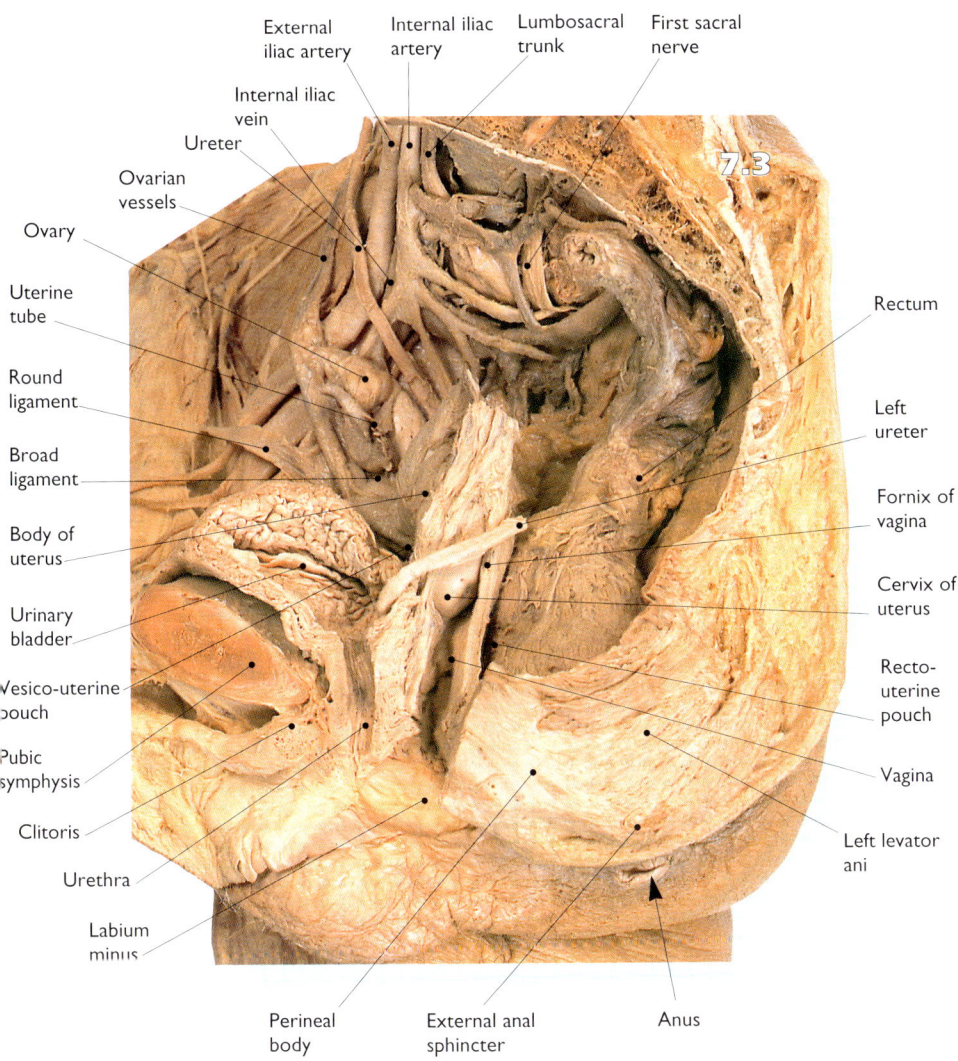

7.3 Right half of a sagittal section of the female pelvis. Part of the left levator ani muscle overlies the lower end of the rectum and blends with the left side of the external anal sphincter. The vagina has been opened to show the cervix of the uterus, and the lower part of the left ureter has been dissected out as it passes through the bladder wall

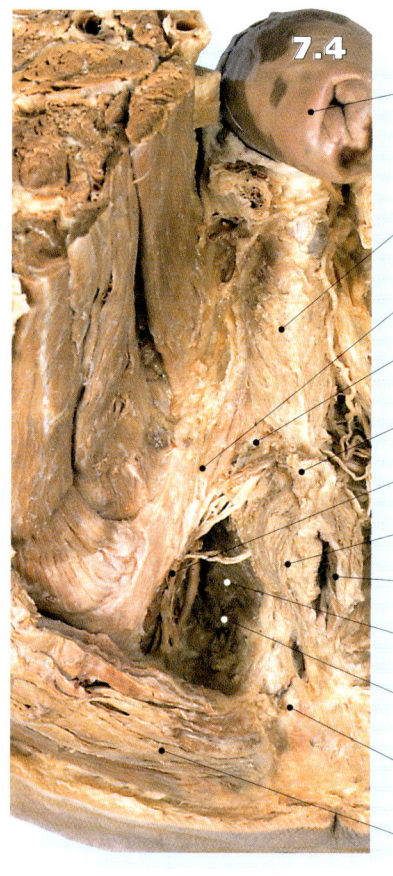

7.4. Dissection of the central and right parts of the male perineum

Labels: Prepuce of penis; Bulbospongiosus muscle overlying corpus spongiosum; Ischiocavernosus muscle overlying corpus cavernosum; Perineal membrane; Perineal body; Pudendal canal with vessels and nerves; External anal sphincter; Anal canal and anus; Levator ani; Ischio-anal fossa; Anococcygeal body; Gluteus maximus

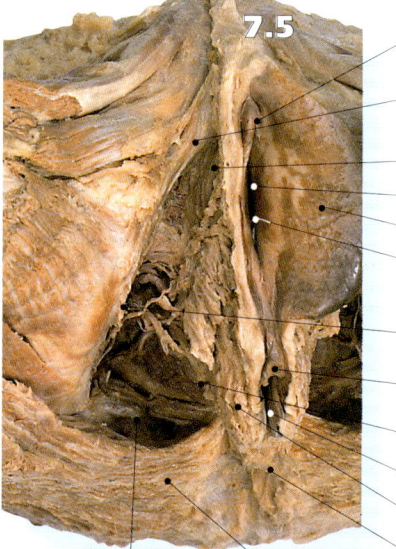

7.5. Dissection of the central and right parts of the female perineum

Labels: Clitoris; Ischiocavernous muscle overlying crus of clitoris; Bulbospongiosus muscle overlying bulb of vestibule; Opening of urethra; Labium minus; Vagina; Pudendal canal with vessels and nerves; Perineal body; Levator ani; Anal canal and anus; External anal sphincter; Ischio-anal fossa; Gluteus maximus; Anococcygeal body

Pelvis and perineum

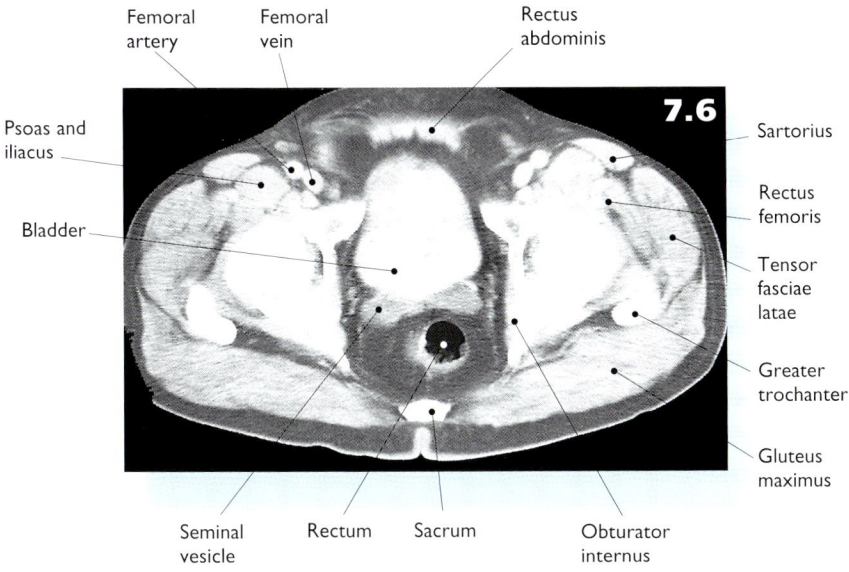

7.6. Axial computed tomograph of the male pelvis at the level of the greater trochanters of the femurs, from below

Perineal body – a mass of midline tissue (properly called the central perineal tendon) at the front of the anus (7.2) and so in the female between the anus and vagina (7.3).

> Obstetricians and gynaecologists use the term '**perineum**' in a restricted sense to mean the perineal body and not the whole of the genital and anal regions, as defined anatomically.

Anococcygeal ligament – similar midline tissue between the anus and coccyx.

Ischio-anal fossa – the fat-filled space (formerly called the ischiorectal fossa) below the pelvic diaphragm on either side of the anal canal (7.4, 7.5). In the lateral wall of the fossa, against the ischial tuberosity, is the pudendal canal, a fascial channel through which run vessels and nerves that supply the perineum. In the female the fossa allows for the great expansion of the vagina during childbirth.

Forming a floor for the anterior part of the fossa is a small muscle mass, the urogenital diaphragm, whose most important part is the sphincter urethrae (external urethral sphincter), with the urethra passing through it.

Male pelvic and genital organs

Rectum and anal canal – the rectum is the continuation of the sigmoid colon, beginning at the third piece of the sacrum and lying in the concavity of the lower sacrum and coccyx (7.2, 7.6). It is about 12 cm long and is retroperitoneal.

The anal canal continues from the lower end of the rectum as the last 4 cm of the alimentary tract, ending at the anus in front of the perineal body. The canal has an internal sphincter of smooth muscle and is surrounded by an external sphincter of skeletal muscle (7.4) (supplied by branches of the pudendal nerve). The junction between rectum and anal canal is marked by the anorectal ring, a palpable landmark on rectal examination (U-shaped rather than a complete ring), due to the sling of the puborectalis muscle (p. 151) which maintains an angle of 120°, important for rectal continence; during defaecation the muscle relaxes and the angle becomes less acute.

Blood supply - branches of the inferior mesenteric artery (superior rectal) supply the rectum and upper part of the anal canal, but the lower part is supplied by branches of the pudendal artery (inferior rectal). There are corresponding veins, so that the upper part of the canal drains to the portal system and the lower part to systemic veins. The anal canal is thus a site for portal-systemic anastomosis (p. 135), and is also an important watershed for lymph drainage - the upper part to pelvic nodes, but the lower to (palpable) inguinal nodes.

Rectal examination - means digital examination by a (gloved and lubricated) index finger inserted through the anus and upwards as far as possible. The anorectal ring, prostate and cancerous growths in the lower rectum or cancerous deposits in the rectovesical pouch of peritoneum (recto-uterine pouch in the female, p. 159) may be detected.

Piles (**haemorrhoids**) are enlarged veins of the lower part of the anal canal.

Ureter – enters the pelvis by *crossing* the external iliac vessels and then running down the back part of the lateral wall *in front of* the internal iliac vessels (7.2) before turning *forwards* to be crossed by the ductus deferens

The pain of renal colic is usually due to a small stone (**calculus**) getting stuck in the ureter on its way between kidney and bladder.

before reaching the upper posterior corner of the bladder.

Urinary bladder – when empty it lies behind the pubic symphysis and in front of the lower part of the rectum (7.2, 7.6). The lowest part of the peritoneal cavity is formed by a fold of peritoneum from the front of the rectum to the upper part of the back of the bladder, the rectovesical pouch. It is highly important since it falls within reach of the examining finger in rectal examination (*see* above). As the bladder fills with urine, it rises above the level of the pubic symphysis behind the lower part of the anterior abdominal wall, pushing the peritoneum off the wall as it rises. It then becomes possible to insert a needle or drainage tube into the bladder just above the pubic symphysis without opening into the peritoneal cavity. The lower posterior part of the bladder is the trigone, the most fixed part and shaped like an inverted triangle with the ureters entering at each upper angle and the urethra leaving at the lower angle (internal urethral meatus). The nerve supply is parasympathetic, from the pelvic splanchnic nerves.

Prostate – consists of glands embedded in a mass of connective tissue and smooth muscle. It secretes about 30% of the seminal fluid (p. 157), is about the size and shape of a chestnut, lies below the bladder (7.2), and is supported by the urogenital diaphragm. The urethra runs through the gland (*see* below) and about 12 minute ducts discharge the secretion into it.

Enlargement of the prostate (**prostatic hypertrophy**) is common after the age of about 50 and may lead to obstruction of urinary outflow and distension of the bladder.

Urethra – the common channel for urine and seminal fluid (semen), it leaves the lowest part of the bladder

(7.2) and runs through the prostate (prostatic urethra) and then through the urogenital diaphragm (membranous urethra, where it is surrounded by skeletal muscle that forms the external urethral sphincter, responsible for urinary continence), and finally enters the root of the penis to become the penile urethra (a total length of about 18 cm). There is a 90° change of direction between the proximal end of the penile part of the urethra and the membranous part. Some smooth muscle at the junction of the bladder and prostatic urethra forms the internal urethral sphincter; it is not concerned with urinary continence, but probably prevents regurgitation of seminal fluid into the bladder during ejaculation.

> This must be remembered when **passing a catheter** through the penis into the bladder.

Testis and epididymis - the testis, roughly egg-shaped and about 3 cm long, contains a mass of seminiferous tubules that manufacture the male germ cells, spermatozoa, which pass into the epididymis, a coiled tubular structures that adheres to the *posterolateral side* of the testis and where spermatozoa are stored and mature. The front and sides of the testis are covered by a closed membranous sac derived from peritoneum, the tunica vaginalis. The testes also contain groups of endocrine cells that produce the male sex hormone, testosterone. The testis and epididymis of both sides are contained within the scrotum. The testicular arteries arise from the abdominal aorta; the corresponding veins drain on the right to the inferior vena cava and on the left usually to the left renal vein. Lymphatic channels accompany the testicular vessels, so that lymph drains to para-aortic nodes and not to the overlying scrotal skin or inguinal nodes.

> The combined testis and epididymis are sometimes called the testicle.

> An accumulation of fluid in the tunica vaginalis (**hydrocele**) produces a swelling surrounding the front and sides of the testis; an enlarged epididymis lies towards the top and back of the testis – an important distinction.

Ductus (vas) deferens – the direct continuation of the epididymis, it leaves the *lower* end of the epididymis to run up in the spermatic cord and through the inguinal canal. Emerging from the lateral end of the inguinal canal (p. 128), it runs down the *front* part of the lateral wall of the pelvis and crosses *superficial to the ureter* to reach the back of the prostate (7.2). Here it joins the duct of the seminal vesicle to form the ejaculatory duct, which enters the prostatic part of the urethra.

> **Vasectomy** (removing a short length of ductus, whose old name was vas deferens, to produce male sterilization) is carried out at the top of the scrotum on each side by dissecting out the ductus from the rest of the spermatic cord structures.

Seminal vesicle – produces much of the seminal fluid and lies lateral to the ductus on the posterior wall of the bladder (7.2), with its upper end just below the point of entrance of the ureter into the bladder. The very short duct leaves the lower end to join the ductus deferens at the edge of prostate and form the ejaculatory duct.

> Normal seminal vesicles are not usually palpable on rectal examination.

Seminal fluid – the fluid vehicle for transport of spermatozoa. It is produced by the seminal vesicles (60%) and prostate (30%), with only a small amount coming from the testes.

Spermatic cord – the collective name for the ductus deferens, the testicular and other vessels and nerves, and various connective tissue coverings derived from the abdominal musculature that form the inguinal canal.

Scrotum – the wrinkled sac of skin and some smooth muscle that enclose the testis, epididymis, and start of the ductus deferens of both sides.

Penis – the male organ of micturition (urination) and copulation (sexual intercourse), whose root lies in front of the anus (7.4). It consists of three columnar masses of vascular tissue: a single corpus spongiosum with an expanded part at the end (glans penis) and a corpus cavernosum on each side, all bound together in a tubular sheath of skin and connective tissue. The fold of skin covering the glans is the prepuce (foreskin, 7.2). The urethra (p. 156) runs through the corpus spongiosum and glans to open at the tip of the glans; it serves at different times for the passage of urine or seminal fluid. Erection is due to (parasympathetic) vasodilatation of the arteries of the corpora and is a necessary prelude to ejaculation, the discharge of seminal fluid (semen) containing sperm (spermatozoa). Ejaculation depends on the (sympathetic) contraction of the smooth muscle of the prostate and each seminal vesical and ductus deferens, supplemented by contraction of the bulbospongiosus (skeletal) muscles that overlie the bulb of the penis.

> **Circumcision** is the operation to remove the foreskin.

Female pelvic and genital organs

Rectum and anal canal – already described (p. 155), but see also Vagina (below).

Ureter – after running down the lateral pelvic wall in front of the internal iliac vessels, it turns forwards, under the broad ligament of the uterus and crossed by the uterine artery, to enter the bladder, crossing the vaginal fornix as it does so (7.3).

Urinary bladder – lies behind the pubic symphysis (7.3), as in the male, and in front of the upper part of the vagina, with the body of the uterus usually lying on its upper surface.

Urethra – is straight, only 4 cm long, and is surrounded by the external urethral sphincter. Most of the urethra is embedded within the anterior wall of the vagina and it opens into the vaginal (7.3) vestibule (*see* below), 2.5 cm behind the clitoris.

> The shortness of the female urethra predisposes to ascending infection into the bladder, leading to **cystitis**.

Ovary – produces the female germ cells, ova, and also the hormones oestrogen and progesterone, which control the female reproductive system. An almond-shaped structure (7.3), it is suspended by a fold of peritoneum, the mesovarium, from the back of the broad ligament. The open end of the uterine tube lies nearby, so that discharged ova may enter it. The ovarian artery arises (like the testicular artery) from the abdominal aorta and reaches the ovary by passing over the pelvic brim in its own fold of peritoneum, accompanied by the ovarian vein which (like the testicular vein) drains on the right into the inferior vena cava and on the left into the left renal vein.

> Cancer of the **ovary** and **uterus** are among the commonest female cancers.

Uterus – the womb, whose lining during reproductive life undergoes the monthly changes of the menstrual cycle, and where the fertil-

> **Bimanual examination of the uterus** involves placing the flat of one hand above the pubic symphysis and pressing downwards while the index and middle fingers of the other hand (as in vaginal examination, below) press the cervix upwards.

ized ovum becomes implanted and develops into a new individual. The uterus (6.10, 7.3) is a pear-shaped, thick-walled organ of smooth muscle, about 8 cm long, usually tilted forwards (anteverted) to overlie the bladder. The main part is the body, whose upper end is the fundus; the lower end is the cervix (about 3 cm long), which projects into the vagina and opens into it through the external os at the lower end of the cervical canal. From the junction of the body and fundus a uterine tube projects at each side towards the lateral pelvic wall. The cavity of the uterus is lined by specialized mucous membrane, the endometrium, which responds to cyclical hormonal changes (although the lining of the cervix does not take part in these changes). Below the tube, the round ligament runs laterally to enter the inguinal canal.

Cancer of the **uterine cervix** has the highest successful treatment rate of any cancer.

The uterine artery runs forwards from the internal iliac, and crosses the ureter superficially; there are corresponding veins. Lymph from the cervix and body of the uterus drains to pelvic nodes, but some from the fundus may travel via lymphatics that accompany the round ligament and so reach inguinal nodes.

Although a loose fold of peritoneum, the broad ligament, attaches the uterus to the side wall of the pelvis, the main factors that hold the uterus in its normal position are condensations of connective tissue under the peritoneum in the region of the cervix and upper vagina, which pass

The **uterosacral ligaments** may be detected on rectal (not vaginal) examination, since they pass backwards on either side of the rectum.

laterally to the lateral pelvic wall, as the lateral or cervical ligaments, and backwards on either side of the rectum to the sacrum, as uterosacral ligaments. These are difficult to appreciate in dissections, but are highly important in the living body.

The hymen is a mucosal fold at the vaginal margin that is usually ruptured at the first sexual intercourse.

If particularly dense or interfering with the discharge of menstrual products, the **hymen** may have to be surgically incised.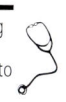

Vagina – the female copulatory organ, and also the birth canal and passage for the discharge of menstrual products (7.3). About 12 cm long when undistended, it lies behind the bladder and urethra, although the urethra is more accurately described as being embedded within the connective tissue of the front wall of the vagina. The cervix of the uterus projects into the upper end of the vagina; the furrow surrounding the cervix here is the vaginal fornix, named anterior, lateral, or posterior. Behind the vagina is the lower part of the rectum, and stretching between the posterior vaginal fornix and rectum is the recto-uterine pouch of peritoneum (pouch of Douglas; despite the name recto-uterine, it passes between the rectum and vagina). This corresponds to the rectovesical pouch in the male and is, likewise, the lowest part of the peritoneal cavity in the female. The lower end of the vagina is the introitus or vestibule, and has the urethra opening into it at the front, 2.5 cm behind the clitoris. There are no glands in the vagina; the moisture that occurs during sexual excitement is largely due to a transudation of fluid through the vaginal walls.

On vaginal examination, using the index and middle fingers, the uterine cervix can be palpated at the top, with the recto-uterine pouch of peritoneum as a possible site for cancerous deposits behind it. At the side the ovary and part of the uterine tube may be palpated.

Mons pubis – the fatty tissue in front of the pubic symphysis, covered by hairy skin, continues backwards on each side of the vaginal opening as the labia majora (singular, labium majus).

Labia minora – smaller, fat-free skin folds (singular, labium minus) internal to the labia majora (7.5), which form the immediate boundaries of the vaginal opening. On either side of the opening is the bulb of the vestibule, an elongated mass of erectile tissue.

Clitoris – the corresponding structure to the penis of the male, but although the male urethra runs through the penis the female urethra does not run through the very much smaller clitoris (7.5), which is an organ concerned only with sexual arousal. The urethra opens into the vestibule of the vagina 2.5 cm behind the clitoris.

Greater vestibular (Bartholin's) glands – small mucous glands under cover of the back part of the bulb of the vestibule. They open on the inside of the labia minora by a single duct on each side, in the 4- and 8- o'clock positions when looking from below with the patient lying on her back.

> Infection of the glands may lead to painful **abscesses** in these positions.

Summary

- The cavity of the **true pelvis**, below the pelvic brim, runs backwards at almost 90° from the abdominal cavity.

- The two levator ani and the two coccygeus muscles form the **pelvic diaphragm** or **pelvic floor** (skeletal muscle, supplied by S3 and S4 nerves), separating the pelvic cavity from the perineum, and must not be confused with the **urogenital diaphragm** which is a much smaller muscle mass (below and separate from the pelvic diaphragm) whose principal component is the **sphincter urethrae** (external urethral sphincter, skeletal muscle, supplied by the pudendal nerve).

- The **ureter** enters the pelvis by crossing the external iliac vessels at the pelvic brim and then runs down the lateral pelvic wall in front of the internal iliac artery before turning forwards (crossed superficially by the ductus deferens or uterine artery) to enter the bladder and open at the upper angle of the trigone. The **ductus deferens** runs down the lateral pelvic wall well in front of the ureter.

- The empty **bladder** is a pelvic organ, lying behind the pubic symphysis, but when distended it may rise above the level of the symphysis. The smooth muscle of the bladder is supplied by the pelvic splanchnic (parasympathetic) nerves.

- The **male urethra** is about 18 cm long and has prostatic, membranous and spongy (penile) parts; the external urethral sphincter surrounds the membranous part. The **female urethra** is straight and only 4 cm long, surrounded by the sphincter.

- Each **seminal vesicle** lies behind the bladder and its duct joins the ductus deferens to form the ejaculatory duct which runs through the prostate to open into the prostatic urethra.

- The junction of the rectum and anal canal is marked by the **palpable anorectal ring** produced by the sling of the puborectalis muscle. The lowest part of the peritoneal cavity (rectovesical or recto-uterine pouch) is in reach of the fingertip during rectal examination.

- The upper part of the **anal canal** is a site of portal-systemic anastomosis and a watershed for the drainage of lymph; from the lower part it drains to inguinal nodes, like other parts of the perineum, including the lower vagina and vulva and the scrotum (but not the testis, whose lymphatics accompany its blood vessels and therefore drain to aortic nodes within the abdomen).

- The **body of the uterus** usually overlies the bladder and the **cervix** projects into the upper end of the vagina. The **ovary** is suspended from the back of the broad ligament of the uterus, and the **round ligament** of the uterus enters the inguinal canal. The main uterine supports are the lateral cervical and uterosacral ligaments. Most uterine lymph drains to pelvic nodes, but some from the fundus may reach inguinal nodes via the round ligament.

Part 8

Lower limb

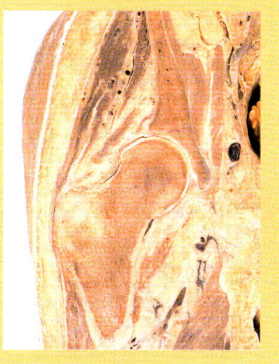

The lower limb accounts for 10% of the body weight. The delicate pirouette of the ballet dancer and the relentless plod of the marathon runner are different examples of lower limb movement and control. When standing upright the centre of gravity of the body passes just behind the axis of movement of the hip joint but in front of the knee and ankle, and various trunk and limb muscles make unconscious adjustments to maintain the upright position.

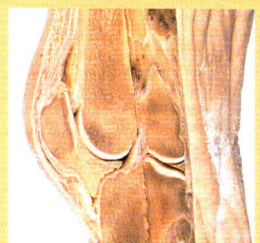

Like so much of normal health, locomotion is taken for granted and only fully appreciated when injury or disease impose a limit on accustomed movement.

The perfect ball-and-socket of the hip joint give it a stability not enjoyed by the shoulder, and the firm union between the tibia and fibula in the lower leg provides a suitable anchor for keeping the weight-bearing foot in place.

THE TWO HIP BONES are firmly united at the front, in the midline pubic symphysis, and at the back each makes a sacroiliac joint with the sacrum (2.4), so forming the bony pelvis (7.1). Although synovial, the sacroiliac joints are atypical in that they allow negligible movement between the bones (although there is a slight increase in the later stages of pregnancy to assist in childbirth). Compared with the shoulder, the hip joint is very stable, since the bones of the hip girdle are firmly united and the head of the femur is lodged deeply in the cup-shaped acetabulum of the hip bone.

Hip and thigh

The front of the thigh is the flexor compartment that contains the femoral vessels and nerve. The main muscle mass is quadriceps femoris, made up of rectus femoris and the three vastus muscles – medialis, lateralis, and intermedius. The medial part of the thigh is the adductor compartment, whose nerve is the obturator nerve. At the back, behind the hip, is the gluteal region, and the back of thigh is the extensor compartment that contains the muscles commonly called the hamstrings and the largest nerve in the body, the sciatic nerve.

Bony prominences – at the junction between the thigh and abdomen (8.1, 2.4A), the two important landmarks are the anterior superior iliac spine, at the front end of the iliac crest, and the pubic tubercle, which is 2.5 cm

> The **anterior superior iliac spine** can be seen and felt easily; the **pubic tubercle** cannot be seen but can be felt.

(1 inch) lateral to the top of the pubic symphysis. The inguinal ligament stretches between them. At the side of the upper thigh, well below the iliac crest, the greater trochanter of the femur can be felt; this forms the most lateral part of the hip. At the back, the ischial tuberosity is under cover of gluteus maximus (8.2); it can be felt when sitting by leaning to one side and slipping a hand under the raised side.

Femoral triangle – a descriptive region (8.3) bounded by the inguinal ligament, medial border of sartorius, and medial border of adductor longus. It contains the femoral nerve, artery, vein, and canal, in that order from

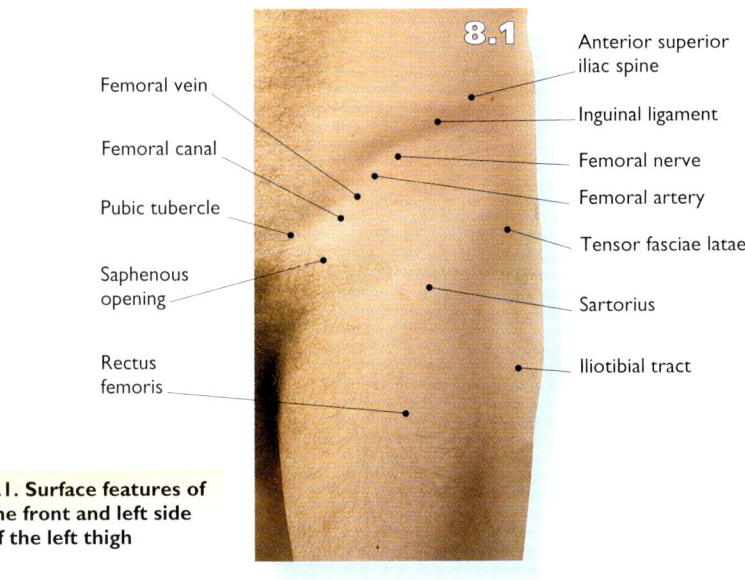

8.1. Surface features of the front and left side of the left thigh

Lower limb

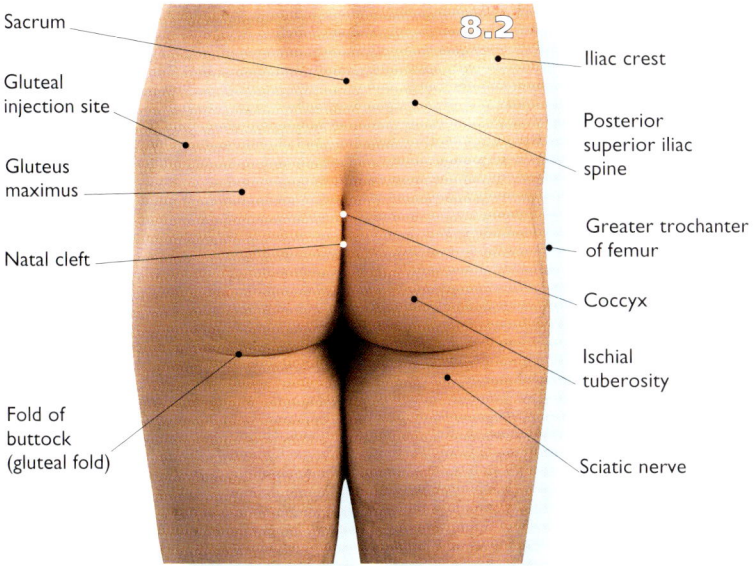

8.2. **Surface features of the lower back and gluteal region**

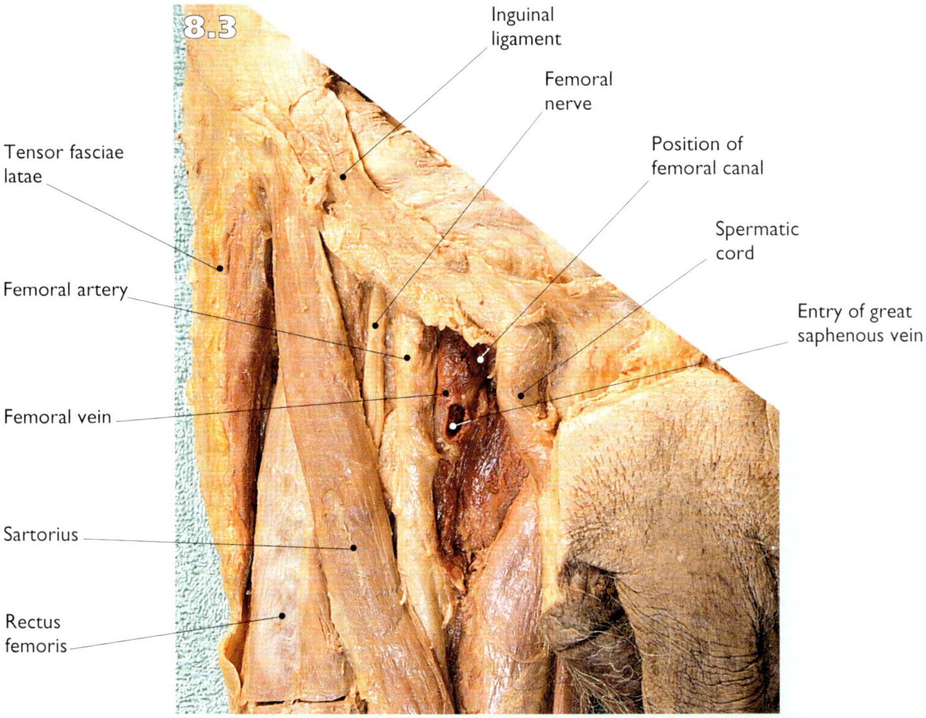

8.3. **Femoral region of the right thigh in the male**

Human Anatomy

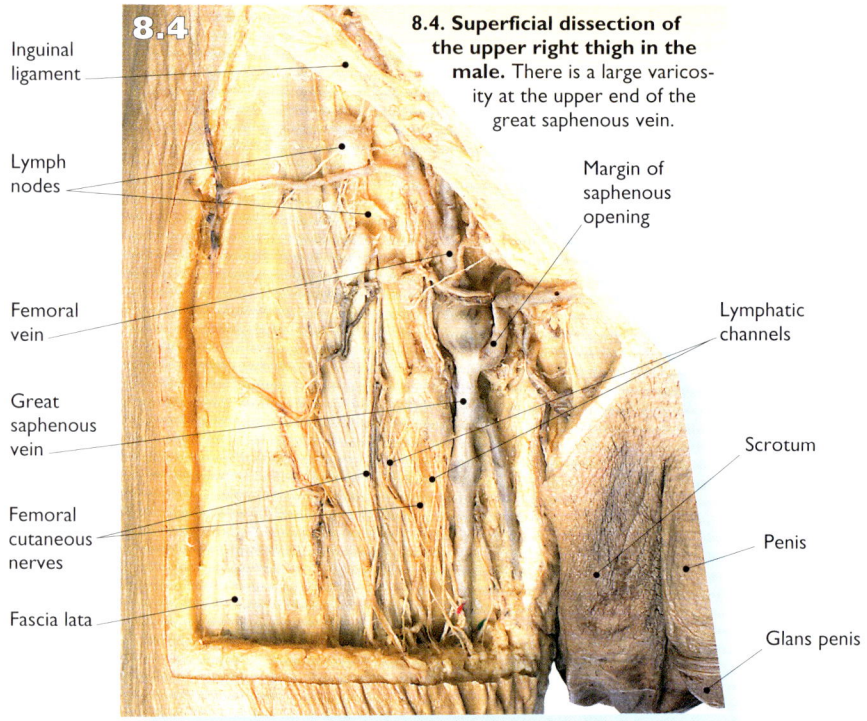

8.4. Superficial dissection of the upper right thigh in the male. There is a large varicosity at the upper end of the great saphenous vein.

Labels: Inguinal ligament; Lymph nodes; Femoral vein; Great saphenous vein; Femoral cutaneous nerves; Fascia lata; Margin of saphenous opening; Lymphatic channels; Scrotum; Penis; Glans penis.

medial to lateral below the inguinal ligament. The upper parts of the artery and vein and the canal are surrounded by the connective tissue femoral sheath, but the nerve is outside the sheath. All are deep to the deep fascia of the thigh, the fascia lata, whose most lateral part forms a particularly thick and strong band, the iliotibial tract (p. 168).

> The **femoral nerve** lies lateral to the palpable artery; the femoral vein lies medial to the artery.

Femoral nerve – lies *lateral* to the artery (8.3) and breaks up into a sheaf of muscular and cutaneous branches, which supply the muscles and skin of the front of the thigh. The saphenous nerve is a large cutaneous branch which runs as far as the base of the great toe – the only femoral nerve branch to reach as far as the foot.

Femoral artery and vein – continuous, under the inguinal ligament, with the corresponding external iliac vessels, the vein lies medial to the artery (8.3). The largest branch of the artery is the profunda femoris artery, whose branches supply muscles on the *front and back* of the thigh. In the lower thigh, the femoral artery pierces adductor magnus to become the popliteal artery.

> The **femoral pulse** can be felt at a point midway between the anterior superior iliac spine and the pubic tubercle.

Great saphenous vein – the largest tributary of the femoral vein, which it enters by passing through the saphenous opening (8.4), a gap in the fascia lata 4 cm below and lateral to the (palpable) pubic tubercle. It receives several tributaries before passing through the opening (see also p. 177).

Lower limb

Femoral canal – the most medial compartment of the femoral sheath (8.3), about 4 cm long, with an opening (femoral ring) into the peritoneal cavity behind the inguinal ligament. The canal exists to allow lymphatics to pass from the lower limb into the pelvis, and also to allow the femoral vein to expand for increased venous return from the lower limb.

A loop of intestine may protrude through the ring into the canal, so forming a **femoral hernia**.

Inguinal lymph nodes – about 15 or so, lying superficially along the great saphenous vein and below the nearby part of the inguinal ligament (8.4), with two or three deep to the deep fascia beside the femoral vein. Efferent channels pass from these deep glands through the femoral canal to external iliac nodes. Apart from draining the whole of the lower limb (including the gluteal region), the nodes receive lymph from the trunk (front and back) below the umbilical level and from the perineum, thus including the lower vagina and anal canal.

Inguinal nodes may become involved from disease in the perineum and gluteal region as well as from the lower limb and lower abdominal wall.

Quadriceps femoris – collective name for rectus femoris and the three vastus muscles. Rectus femoris (8.3) arises from the hip bone above the acetabulum and the anterior inferior iliac spine, and is the most anterior muscle. Vastus medialis, lateralis, and intermedius (the deepest muscle) arise from the front and sides of the femur. All converge onto the quadriceps tendon, attached to the top of the patella, which in turn is anchored to the tuberosity of the tibia by the patellar ligament (8.7, 8.8). Only the rectus can flex the hip, but both it and the vasti extend

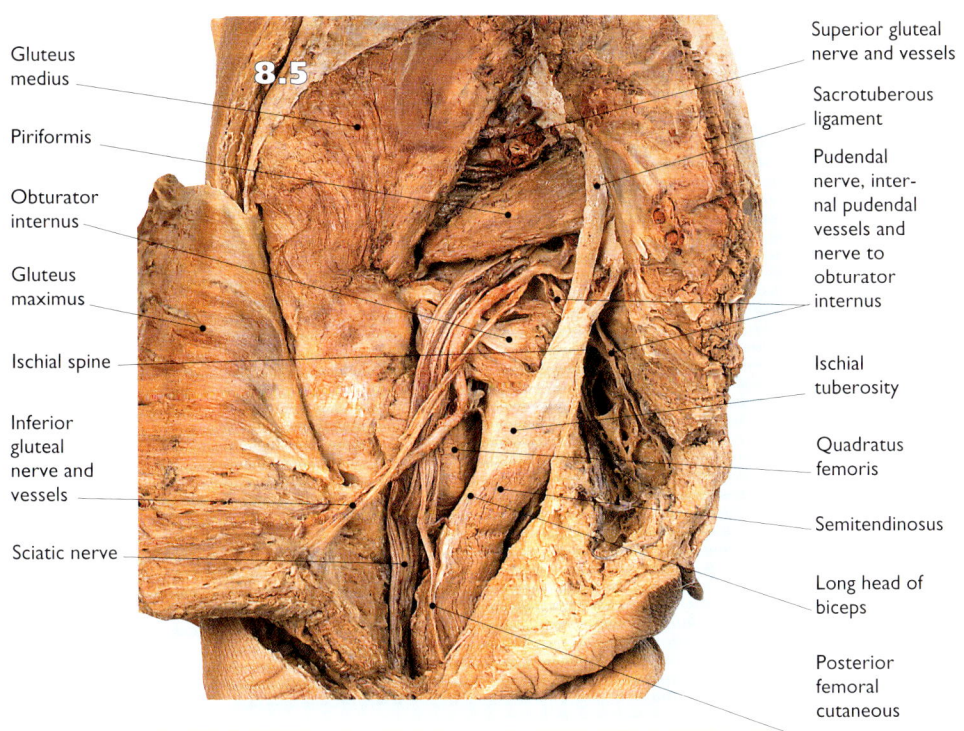

8.5. Dissection of the left gluteal region, with gluteus maximus turned laterally

167

the knee (p. 172). All four muscles are supplied by the femoral nerve.

Tensor fasciae latae – short muscle at the lateral side of the front of the thigh (**8.3**), which arises from the front 5 cm of the outer edge of the iliac crest and runs down to insert into the iliotibial tract. It helps to brace the iliotibial tract and keep the knee extended, and assists in medial rotation of the hip (p. 170). It is supplied by the superior gluteal nerve.

Sartorius – the muscle with the longest parallel fibres in the body, it passes obliquely across the thigh (**8.3**) from the anterior superior iliac spine to the medial surface of the tibia (in front of the gracilis and semitendinosus). It assists in flexion of the thigh and knee and is supplied by the femoral nerve.

Pectineus – in the medial part of the floor of the femoral triangle, it runs from the pectineal line of the pubis to the femur along a line between the lesser trochanter and the linea aspera. It separates the femoral vein and canal from the hip joint, and is usually supplied by the femoral nerve (sometimes by the obturator nerve).

Adductor muscles – the most superficial of the group is gracilis, the most medial muscle of the thigh, with adductor longus adjacent and adductor brevis more deeply placed. All arise from the pubis and its rami; gracilis reaches the medial surface of the tibia (between sartorius and semitendinosus), while the other two are inserted into the linea aspera of the femur. Adductor magnus is the largest and deepest of the group, running from the ischial tuberosity to the whole length of the linea aspera, and to the medial supracondylar line and the adductor tubercle of the femur. The lower part contains the opening through which the femoral artery passes backwards to enter the popliteal fossa. The group is supplied by the obturator nerve, with part of adductor magnus receiving supply from the sciatic nerve.

Gluteal fold – fold of the buttock (**8.2**), a transverse, but downwardly curved, skin crease due to hip joint movement; it does *not* correspond to the lower border of gluteus maximus.

Gluteus maximus – the muscle which forms the bulge of the buttock (**8.2, 8.5**) and whose fibres run down at 45° from part of the ilium, sacrum, coccyx, and sacrotuberous ligament to cross the gluteal fold obliquely. The fibres are mostly inserted into the iliotibial tract of the fascia lata; only one-quarter of them reach the gluteal tuberosity on the back of the femur. The muscle is a powerful extensor of the hip, as in climbing stairs and running, and is supplied by the inferior gluteal nerve.

Gluteus medius and gluteus minimus – arising from the outer side of the ilium, these converge on to the greater trochanter of the femur (**8.6**). They are described as abductors of the hip, but are much more important as preventers of adduction (*see* Hip joint, below). They are supplied by the superior gluteal nerve.

Piriformis – functionally unimportant (p. 151), but the guide to the gluteal region: nerves and vessels coming in from the pelvis do so either above or below this muscle (**8.5**). The only ones above it are the superior gluteal nerve and vessels; all the rest are below it. The muscle arises from the middle pieces of the sacrum and passes laterally through the greater sciatic foramen (p. 33) to the tip of the greater trochanter of the femur. The surface marking of the lower border is along a line from midway between the posterior superior iliac spine and the coccyx to the tip of the trochanter.

Sciatic nerve – the most important structure in the gluteal region, it emerges

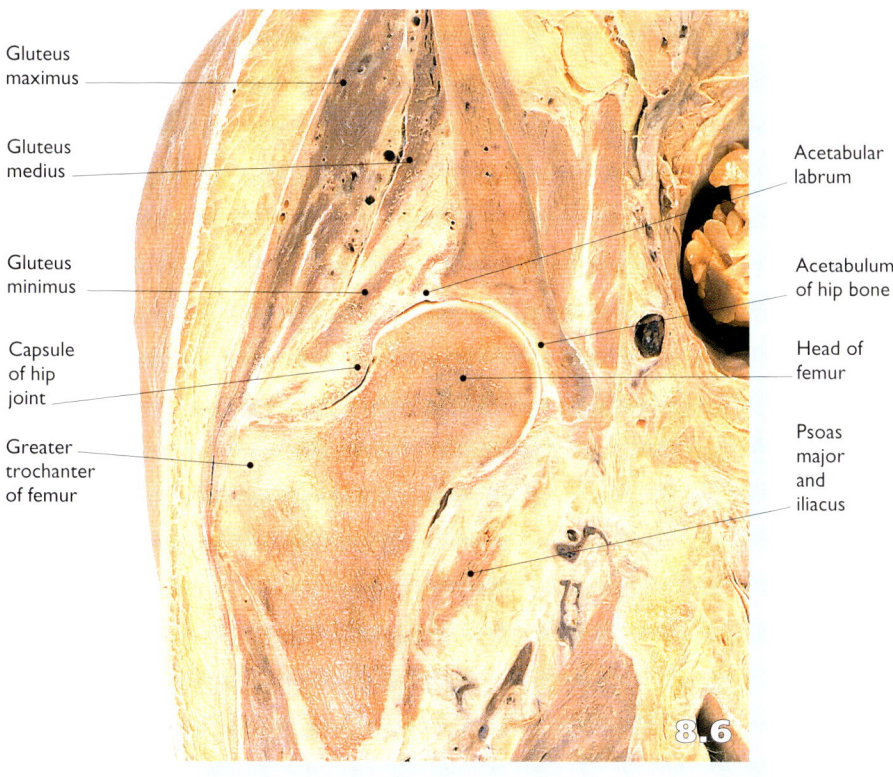

8.6. Coronal section of the right hip joint

from the pelvis below piriformis (8.5) and runs down the back of the thigh deep to the hamstring muscles (biceps laterally and semitendinosus and semimembranosus medially), supplying them and part of adductor magnus. At the upper angle of the popliteal fossa it divides into the tibial and common peroneal nerves (p. 174 and 176).

> The **surface marking** of the nerve at the top of the thigh is midway between the ischial tuberosity and the tip of the greater trochanter of the femur.

Posterior femoral cutaneous nerve – runs down superficial to the hamstrings (8.5) to supply a strip of skin down the middle of the back of the thigh and calf – a long narrow area of supply.

Superior gluteal nerve – supplies gluteus medius and minimus and tensor fasciae latae (8.5).

Inferior gluteal nerve – supplies only gluteus maximus (8.5).

Pudendal nerve, internal pudendal vessels, and nerve to obturator internus – these structures (8.5) have a very short course in the gluteal region, leaving the pelvis through the greater sciatic foramen below the piriformis, then crossing the ischial spine and sacrospinous ligament to enter the perineum through the lesser sciatic foramen.

Gluteal intramuscular injection – the correct site is the *upper outer* *quadrant* of the gluteal region (**8.2**). The quadrants are defined by measuring from the highest point of the iliac crest to the gluteal fold, and from the midline to the outer edge of the greater trochanter. Correctly defined, the upper outer quadrant is well away from the sciatic nerve.

The most common cause of **sciatic nerve injury** is misplaced gluteal injections.

Hamstrings – muscles that span both the hip joint and knee joint, the semitendinosus, semimembranosus, and long head of biceps (**8.9**). All arise from the ischial tuberosity (the *short* head of biceps arises from the back of the femur and hence is not a true hamstring, since it does not span the hip joint). Biceps runs down the lateral side to the head of the fibula, with the common peroneal nerve behind its lower part. The 'semi' muscles run down the medial side, semimembranosus attaching to the medial condyle of the tibia and semitendinosus to the medial surface below the condyle, deep to the gracilis attachment. The hamstrings act as extensors of the hip and flexors of the knee and are supplied by the sciatic nerve.

With the knee flexed to a right angle, the biceps tendon is easily felt on the lateral side behind the knee, with the tendon of semitendinosus overlying the broader semimembranosus on the medial side.

Hip joint – the best example of a ball-and-socket joint: the head of the femur fits snugly into the hip bone's acetabulum (**7.1, 8.6**), which is deepened around the periphery by the cartilaginous acetabular labrum and across the acetabular notch by the fibrous transverse ligament. The ligament of the head of the femur runs from the transverse ligament to the fovea of the head, supplying blood vessels to the head in the young child, but these usually degenerate before adult life. The capsule is attached to the hip bone around the margins of the acetabulum; on the femur, it attaches *at the front* to the intertrochanteric line, but *at the back* it attaches halfway along the neck. Thus, much of the neck is intracapsular and covered by synovial membrane, beneath which blood vessels run to supply the head of the femur.

Fractures of this part of the neck may tear these vessels, causing **avascular necrosis** of the head and delayed healing.

Iliofemoral ligament – most important of the ligaments that reinforce the capsule and one of the strongest in the body (because the body's centre of gravity passes behind the joint, so the ligament resists the tendency to tilt backwards), it is shaped like an inverted V and runs from the anterior inferior iliac spine to the lateral and medial ends of the intertrochanteric line.

Pubofemoral and ischiofemoral ligaments – reinforce the capsule at the front and back, respectively.

Principal muscles that produce movements at the hip joint are:
- **Flexion** – psoas major, iliacus, rectus femoris, sartorius, and tensor fasciae latae.
- **Extension** – hamstrings, gluteus maximus, and ischial part of adductor magnus.
- **Abduction** – gluteus medius and minimus.
- **Adduction** – adductor longus, brevis, and magnus, and gracilis.
- **Lateral rotation** – gluteus maximus, piriformis, obturator externus, obturator internus and gemelli, and quadratus femoris.
- **Medial rotation** – gluteus medius and minimus, and tensor fasciae latae.

The types of movement possible at the hip joint are similar to those at the shoulder, but are more limited because of the shapes of the bones. Note that, in walking, the rather small amount of hip extension is produced by the hamstrings; only with greater ranges of movement, as when climbing stairs or running, does gluteus maximus play an important part. The abducting action of gluteus medius and minimus is less important than the way these muscles *prevent adduction*: during walking those on the side of the leg that is on the ground prevent the pelvis from tilting to the opposite side. They also produce medial rotation of the femur; the long-standing belief that psoas major is a medial rotator is not supported by electromyographic studies.

Knee, leg and foot

Bony prominences – the patella is the obvious feature at the front of the knee, with the tuberosity of the tibia below it (**2.4A, 8.7**). With the knee flexed to a right angle, it is easy to feel at the front the medial and lateral condyles of the femur and tibia and the joint gap in between. On the lateral side, the head of the fibula has the tendon of biceps inserted into it. In the leg the medial surface of the tibia, commonly called the shin, is subcutaneous and can be traced down to the medial malleolus at the ankle (**8.12**). On the lateral side, most of the fibula is covered by muscles, but becomes subcutaneous at the lower end and ends in the lateral malleolus.

Knee joint – the joint between the condyles of the femur and tibia, with the patella also taking part at the front by articulating with the condyles of the femur (but not with the tibia) (**8.8**). The femur and tibia are held together mainly by the lateral, medial, and cruciate ligaments.

The joint capsule is replaced at the front by the patella and patellar ligament; the ligament keeps the patella at a constant distance from the upper end of the tibia, although the position of the patella in relation to the femur changes as the knee joint flexes and extends. The popliteus tendon penetrates the back of the lateral side of the capsule to reach its attachment to the side of the lateral epicondyle. Although intracapsular, it remains

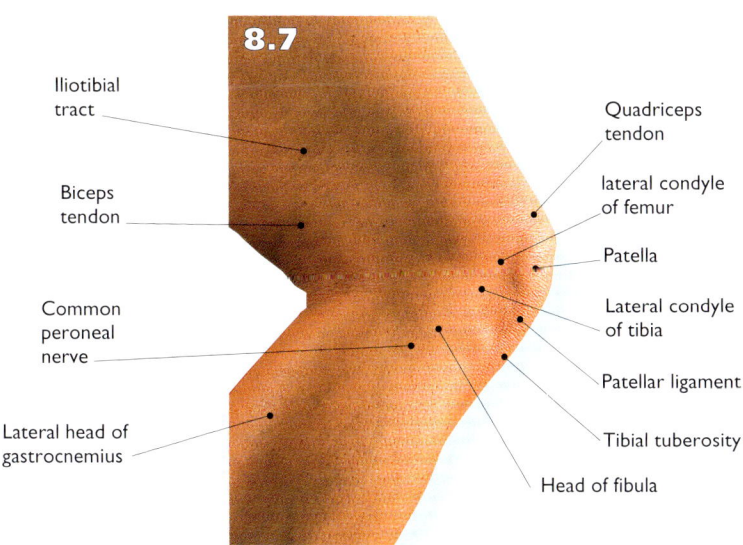

8.7. Surface features of the lateral side of the right knee, partly flexed

extrasynovial, with a sleeve-like extension of synovial membrane around it.

Lateral ligament – properly called the fibular collateral ligament, it is a rounded cord-like structure, about 5 cm long, and is easily felt when 'put on the stretch' (e.g. when sitting down, bring the left ankle up to rest on the right knee, and feel the left lateral ligament running from the head of the fibula to the lateral epicondyle of the femur).

Medial ligament – properly called the tibial collateral ligament, it is a broad band-like structure, about 12 cm long, that passes from the medial epicondyle of the femur to a broad area of the tibia below the medial condyle. It is not easily felt.

Cruciate ligaments – named from their attachments to the tibia: the *anterior* cruciate (**8.8A**) passes from the *front* of the upper surface of the tibia to the inside of the lateral condyle of the femur, and the *posterior* cruciate from the *back* of the upper surface of the tibia to the inside of the medial condyle of the femur.

Medial and lateral menisci – the 'cartilages of the knee' are C-shaped structures attached to the upper surface of the tibia. The *medial meniscus is also firmly attached to the medial ligament,* but the lateral one is *not* attached to the lateral ligament. The medial meniscus is thus the more firmly anchored and so more liable to be trapped and torn during twisting movements of the knee than is the lateral meniscus (**8.8A** and **B**).

> In 'twisting' injuries of the knee the **medial meniscus** is 20 times more liable to damage than the lateral.

Bursae – numerous in the knee region, but the largest is the suprapatellar bursa (**8.8A**), which is continuous with the upper end of the synovial cavity and extends behind the quadriceps tendon for three finger-breadths above the upper border of the patella. Others include the semimembranosus bursa, behind the tendon, which may communicate with the joint, and the subcutaneous prepatellar bursa, in front of the lower part of the patella and upper part of the patellar ligament (the bursa of 'housemaid's knee').

> Effusions into the knee joint ('**water on the knee**') inevitably distend this bursa as well.

Principal muscles that produce movements of the knee joint:
Flexion – hamstrings, gastrocnemius, and popliteus.
Extension – quadriceps femoris.
Medial rotation (of tibia, when semi-flexed) – semimembranosus and semitendinosus.
Lateral rotation (of tibia, when semi-flexed) – biceps.

Flexion and extension of the knee are hinge-like movements between the femur and tibia, although the movements are not identical with those of a simple hinge, but are complicated by a slight rotation between the two bones. To begin flexion from the fully extended position (and assuming the tibia to be fixed), popliteus (p. 178), passing from the upper part of the back of the tibia to the side of the lateral epicondyle, first 'unlocks' the joint by laterally rotating the femur on the tibia, and then the other flexors carry on the movement. From the flexed position, there is medial rotation of the femur on the tibia towards the end of extension (due to the shape of the joint surfaces and tension in the ligaments) – hence the need for the 'unlocking' movement by popliteus as flexion begins. In the semiflexed position, the hamstrings can produce some rotation of one bone on the other (e.g. with the femur fixed, biceps can cause some lateral rotation of the tibia on the femur, and

> Even a few days of bed rest causes a measurable loss of size and power in the **quadriceps muscles**, hence the feeling of unsteadiness on getting up and walking again.

Lower limb

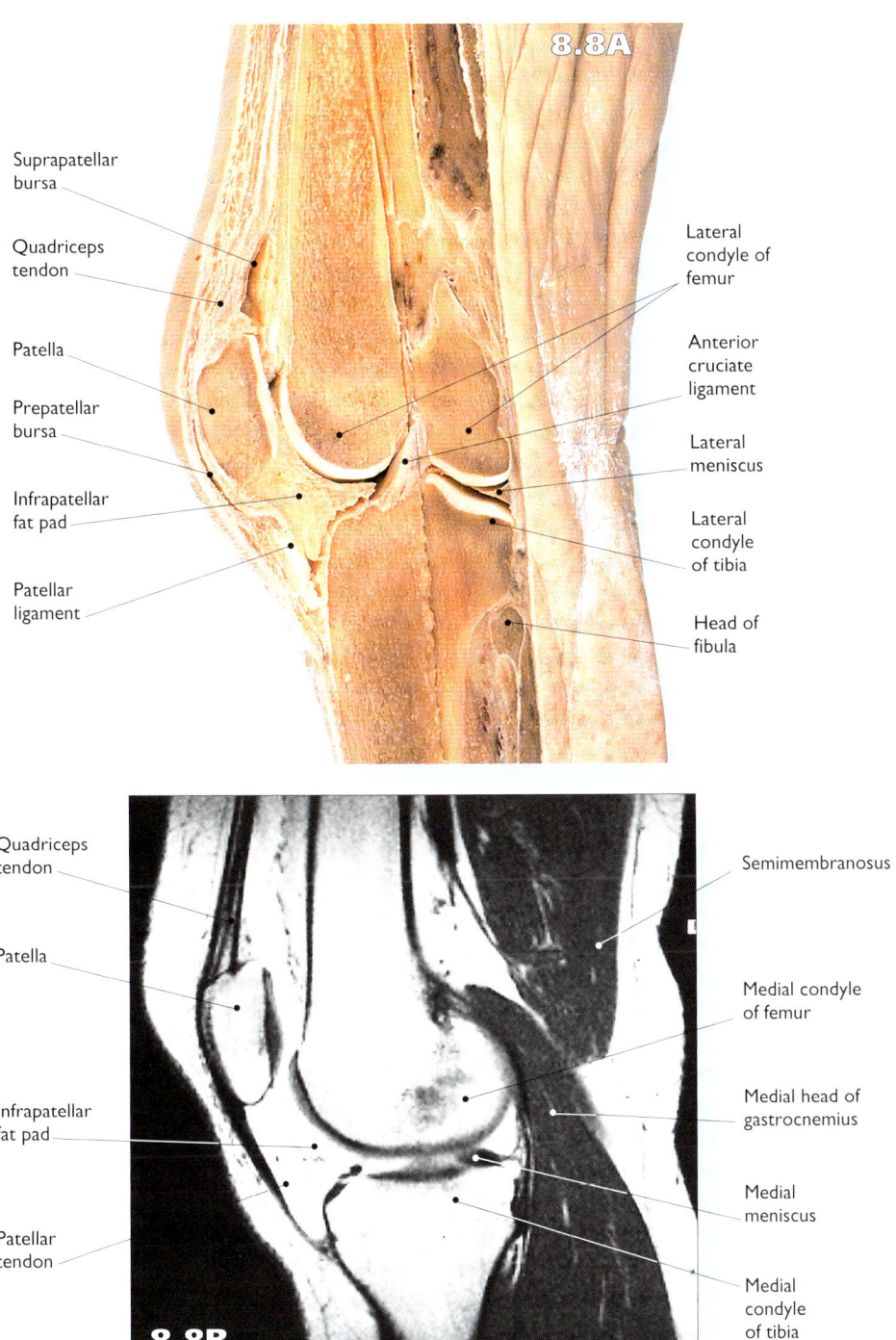

8.8. Sections of the left knee
A Combined coronal and sagittal section (anterior lateral quadrant removed), showing the lateral condyles of the femur and tibia
B Sagittal magnetic resonance image, showing the medial condyles of femur and tibia

Human Anatomy

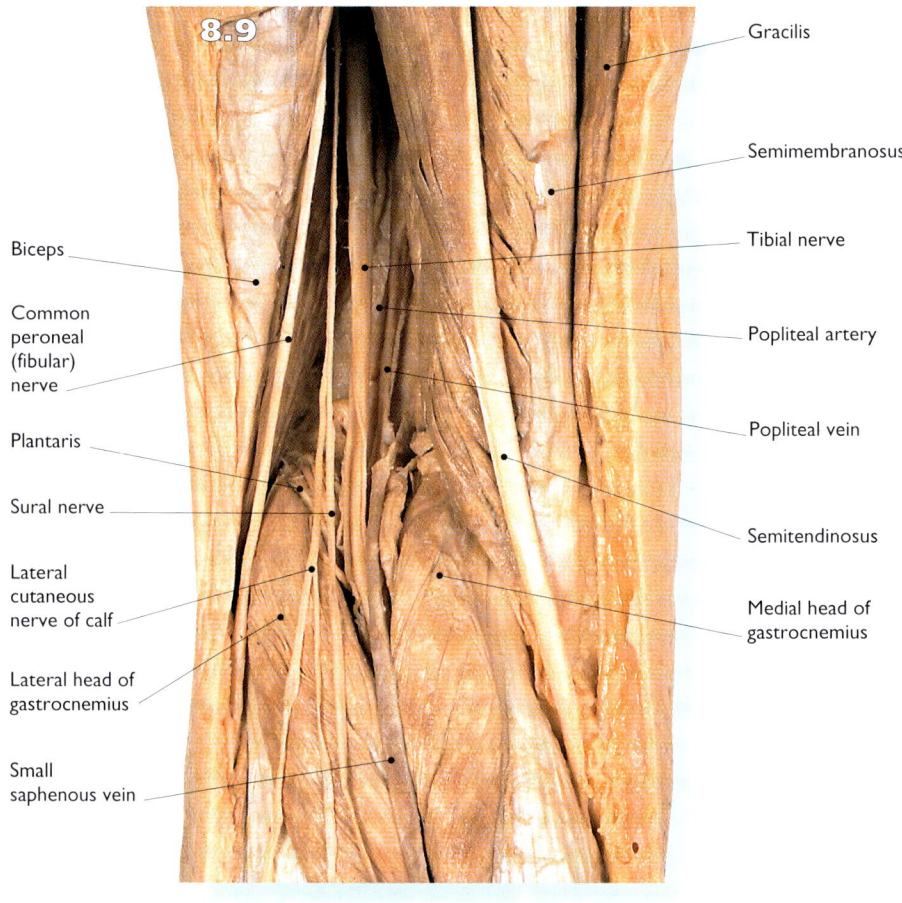

8.9. Dissection of the left popliteal fossa

the semimembranosus and semitendinosus some medial rotation). As part of quadriceps femoris, the lowest fibres of vastus medialis are of great importance for the last few degrees of extension.

Popliteal fossa – a diamond-shaped area behind the knee (**8.9**), its upper boundaries are the biceps, with the common peroneal nerve behind it on the lateral side, and the semimembranosus, with the tendon of semitendinosus behind it on the medial side; its lower boundaries are the lateral head of gastrocnemius and plantaris laterally, and the medial head of gastrocnemius medially. The three large structures in the fossa are the tibial nerve, popliteal vein, and popliteal artery, *in that order from superficial to deep.*

> Tearing of the muscular or tendinous fibres of **biceps** behind the knee is a common sports injury.

174

Tibial nerve – a direct continuation of the sciatic nerve that runs straight down the middle of the fossa (**8.9**) and disappears into the calf between the heads of gastrocnemius to run deep to the soleus. It supplies all the calf muscles and divides below the medial malleolus into the medial and lateral plantar nerves for the cutaneous and muscular supplies of the sole (**8.10**).

Popliteal vein – often double, it runs between the tibial nerve and popliteal artery, and receives the small saphenous vein, which pierces the fascial roof of the fossa (**8.9**).

Popliteal artery – a continuation of the femoral artery that enters the fossa through the opening in adductor magnus and enters the calf beneath the gastrocnemius. The depth of the artery (**8.9**) makes the popliteal pulse difficult to feel. The artery divides into the anterior and posterior tibial arteries, which supply the leg and foot.

> The **popliteal pulse** is best felt from the front with the knee flexed, with the examiner's thumbs on the front of the knee and the fingers of both hands pressing forwards into the middle of the fossa.

Anterior tibial artery – runs deeply between the extensor muscles of the leg, and at the ankle lies between the tendons of extensor hallucis longus and extensor digitorum longus. As it passes across the ankle joint it changes its name to the

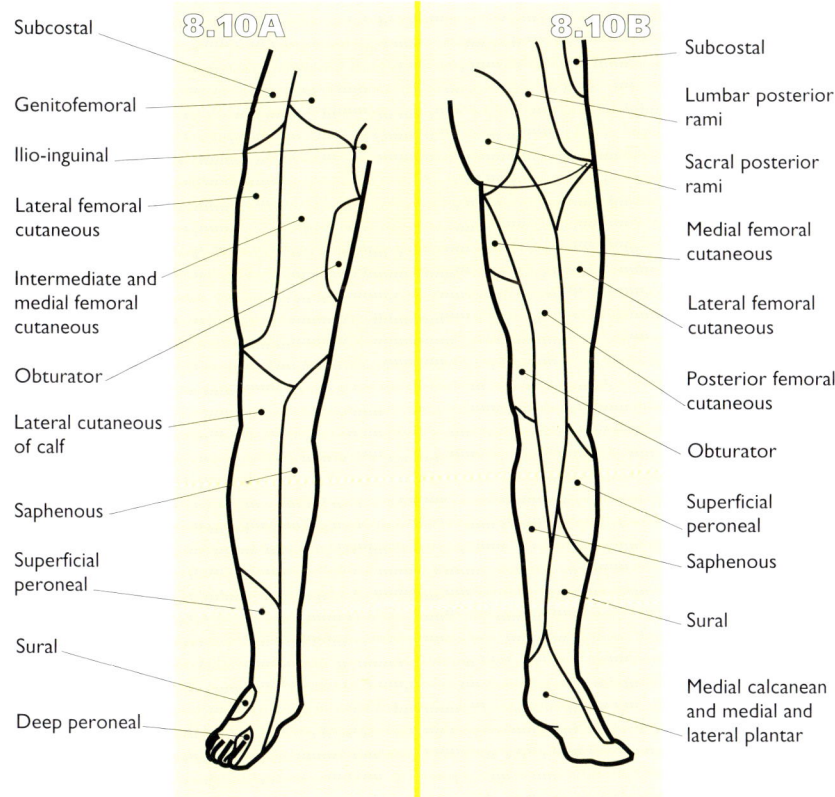

8.10. Cutaneous nerves of the right lower limb
A Front   **B** Back

The **dorsalis pedis pulse** can be felt along the upper part of a line from the midpoint between the malleoli towards the first toe cleft (but note that the artery is absent in about 12% of feet).

dorsalis pedis artery (**8.11**). Its metatarsal branches provide dorsal digital vessels for the sides of the toes.

Posterior tibial artery – runs deeply between the calf muscles on the tibial side, to reach the back of the medial malleolus (**8.12**). It gives off the peroneal artery that runs behind the fibula, and ends by dividing into the medial and lateral plantar arteries, which enter the sole. The lateral artery continues as the plantar arch (level with the bases of the middle metatarsal bones),

The **posterior tibial pulse** is felt behind the medial malleolus 2.5 cm in front of the medial border of the Achilles' tendon.

which anastomoses with the dorsalis pedis artery through the first intermetatarsal space. The metatarsal branches provide plantar digital vessels for the sides of the toes.

Common peroneal nerve – arising from the sciatic nerve at the top of the popliteal fossa, it runs down behind the biceps tendon and curls forwards around the neck of the fibula (**8.7**). Here it divides into the superficial peroneal nerve, which supplies skin on the front of the leg and dorsum of the foot and also the peroneus longus and brevis muscles, and the deep peroneal nerve, which runs with the anterior tibial artery and is the supply for the extensor muscles and a

It can be rolled against the bone and is liable to **injury** (e.g. by a tight plaster cast).

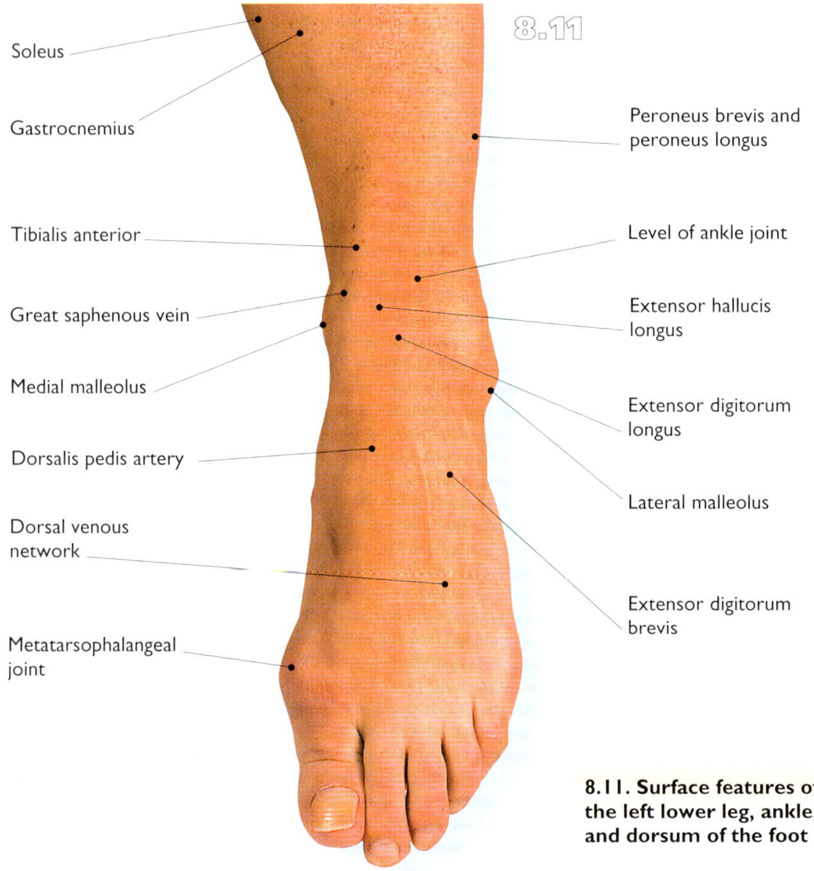

Soleus
Gastrocnemius
Tibialis anterior
Great saphenous vein
Medial malleolus
Dorsalis pedis artery
Dorsal venous network
Metatarsophalangeal joint

Peroneus brevis and peroneus longus
Level of ankle joint
Extensor hallucis longus
Extensor digitorum longus
Lateral malleolus
Extensor digitorum brevis

8.11. Surface features of the left lower leg, ankle, and dorsum of the foot

Lower limb

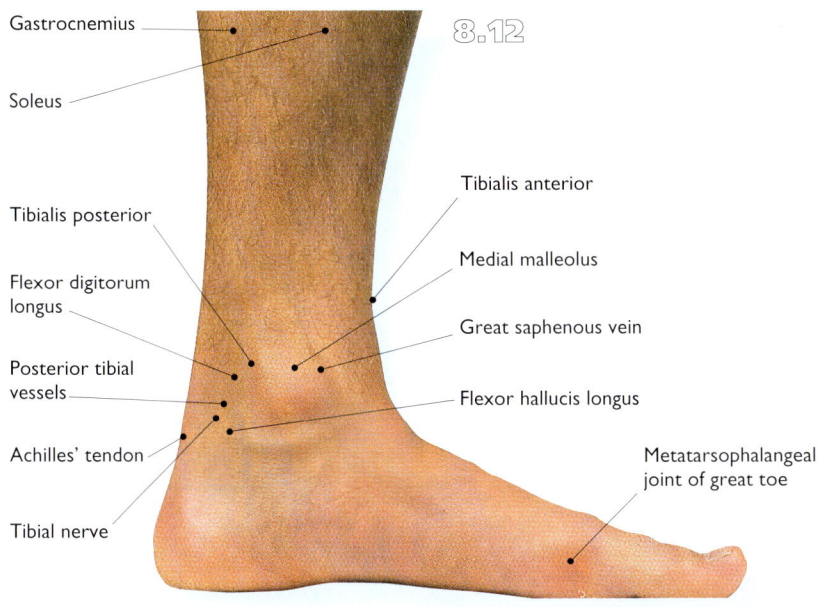

8.12. Surface features of the medial side of the left foot

small area of skin of the first toe cleft. (In modern terminology, 'peroneal' has been replaced by 'fibular'.)

Tibialis anterior – forms the bulge on the lateral side of the upper part of the shin. Its tendon passes across the front of the ankle joint (**8.11**) to be attached to the medial side of the medial cuneiform and base of the first metatarsal. It is supplied by the deep peroneal nerve.

Extensor hallucis longus and extensor digitorum longus – smaller muscles from the fibula and interosseous membrane. The tendons lie lateral to that of tibialis anterior (**8.11**) and pass to the great toe and other toes, respectively, to form dorsal digital expansions similar to those of the hand (p. 106). The lateral part of the digitorum muscle is peroneus tertius, which reaches the base and/or shaft of the fifth metatarsal. All are supplied by the deep peroneal nerve.

Superior and inferior extensor retinacula – thickenings of deep fascia at the ankle and on the dorsum of the foot, respectively, they prevent underlying tendons from bowing forwards. The order of the tendons at the ankle from medial to lateral is tibialis anterior, extensor hallucis longus, extensor digitorum longus (**8.11**). The anterior tibial vessels and deep peroneal nerve lie between the hallucis and digitorum tendons.

Extensor digitorum brevis – the only muscle of the dorsum of the foot, from the upper surface of the calcaneus, it gives tendons that join the hallucis and digitorum tendons to the four medial toes (the part going to the great toe is sometimes called the extensor hallucis brevis). It is supplied by the deep peroneal nerve.

Great saphenous vein – passing up from the medial side of the foot, it lies at

177

> The **great saphenous vein** runs in front of the medial malleolus; the **small saphenous vein** runs behind the lateral malleolus.

the ankle *in front of the medial malleolus* (**8.12**). This was formerly the common site for intravenous infusions, which may still be given here, but upper limb veins are now preferred since there is a greater risk of thrombosis in the leg veins. The vein runs upwards subcutaneously and at the knee lies a hand's breadth behind the medial border of the patella. Continuing upwards, it drains into the femoral vein (p. 166).

Small saphenous vein and sural nerve – passing up from the lateral side of the foot, the vein lies at the ankle behind the lateral malleolus and runs upwards subcutaneously to the popliteal fossa where it drains into the popliteal vein (**8.9**). It is accompanied by the sural nerve, a cutaneous branch of the tibial nerve.

Perforating veins – mostly behind the lower part of the tibia and medial malleolus, uniting deep and superficial veins. Some perforators are joined together by the posterior arch vein, which runs into the great saphenous at a higher level. These veins and their tributaries are the ones that may become dilated and tortuous – varicose veins. The perforating veins have valves which direct blood from superficial to deep, so that the 'muscular pump' of the muscles of sole and calf can help the return of blood to the top of the limb.

> **Varicose veins** are more common in females, and may lead to ulceration of the skin above the medial malleolus (venous ulcers).

When the valves become incompetent they allow blood to flow back into the superficial veins, so increasing pressure in them and causing them to enlarge.

Gastrocnemius – the most superficial calf muscle, with a medial head from the back of the femur above the medial condyle, and a lateral head from the *side* of the lateral condyle (**8.9**). It forms, with the tendon of soleus, the tendo calcaneus or Achilles' tendon, attached to the back of the calcaneus (**8.12, 8.13**). Gastrocnemius is supplied by the tibial nerve.

> A **ruptured tendon**, a painful injury, gives a palpable gap above the calcaneus.

Soleus – immediately deep to the gastrocnemius, with an arched origin from the back of the upper tibia and fibula, it becomes tendinous to unite with gastrocnemius. Viewed from behind it bulges slightly beyond the gastrocnemius at each side (**8.12**). It is supplied by the tibial nerve.

> In and around the soleus muscle is a plexus of veins in which, in those confined to bed, blood may stagnate and lead to **deep venous thrombosis**, with the possibility of pulmonary emboli (p. 120).

Plantaris – a very small muscle belly from the back of the femur above the lateral condyle, with a very long thin tendon running down between gastrocnemius and soleus to join the medial side of the Achilles' tendon. Rupture causes pain, but no palpable gap. It is supplied by the tibial nerve.

Popliteus – triangular-shaped muscle that arises from the upper posterior part of the tibia above the soleal line, and passes upwards and laterally to the lateral part of the lateral condyle of the femur, with an attachment also to the lateral meniscus. It plays the vitally important role of 'unlocking' the knee joint at the beginning of flexion (p. 172). It is supplied by the tibial nerve.

Tibialis posterior – deepest muscle of the calf, from the back of the *tibia and fibula* and interosseous membrane (which stretches between the two bones), with a tendon that lies immediately behind the medial malleolus (**8.12**) and runs to the tuberosity of the navicular bone. It is supplied by the tibial nerve.

Flexor digitorum longus – from the back of the *tibia*, with a tendon that runs behind that of tibialis posterior at

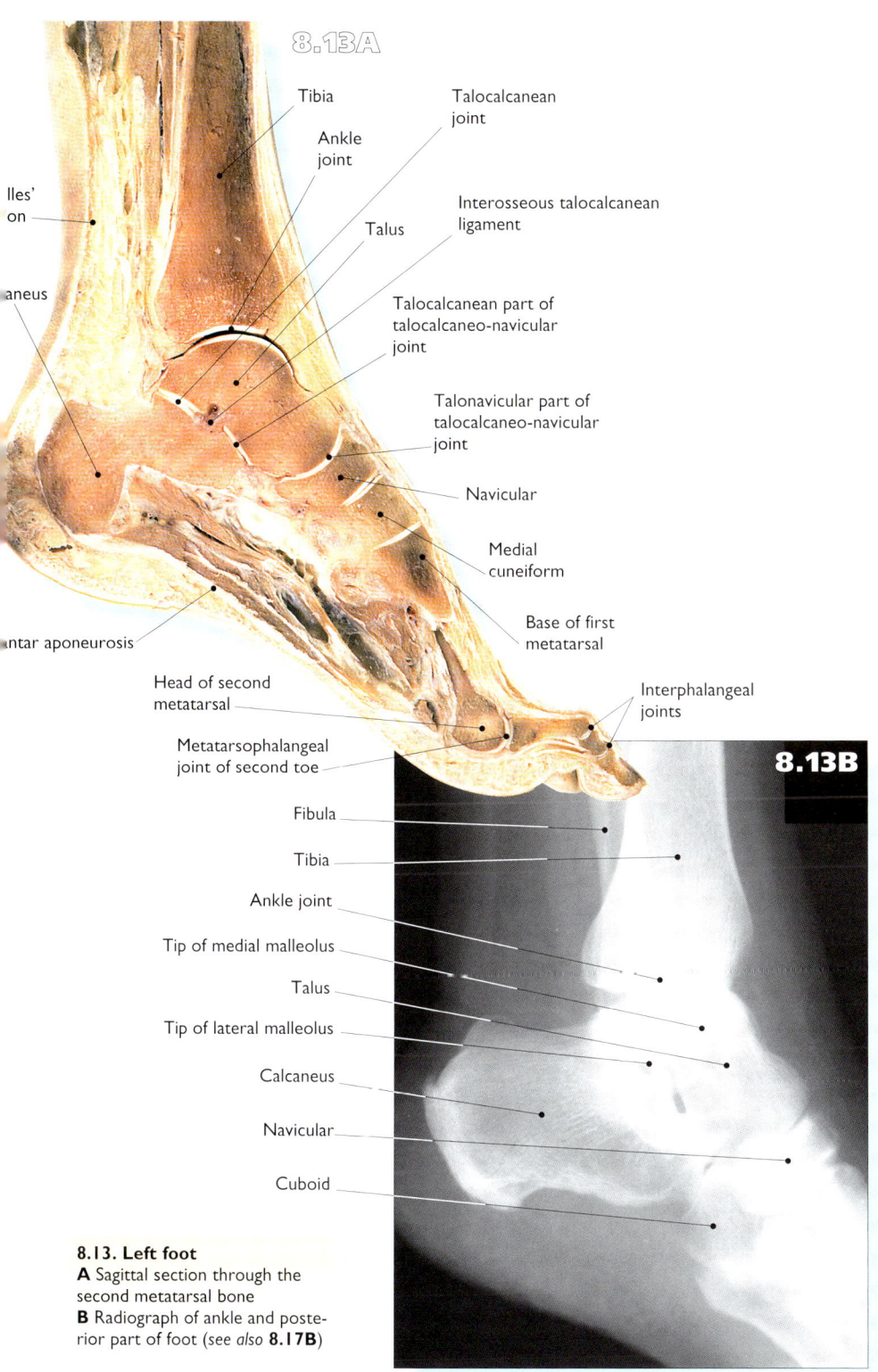

8.13. Left foot
A Sagittal section through the second metatarsal bone
B Radiograph of ankle and posterior part of foot (see also **8.17B**)

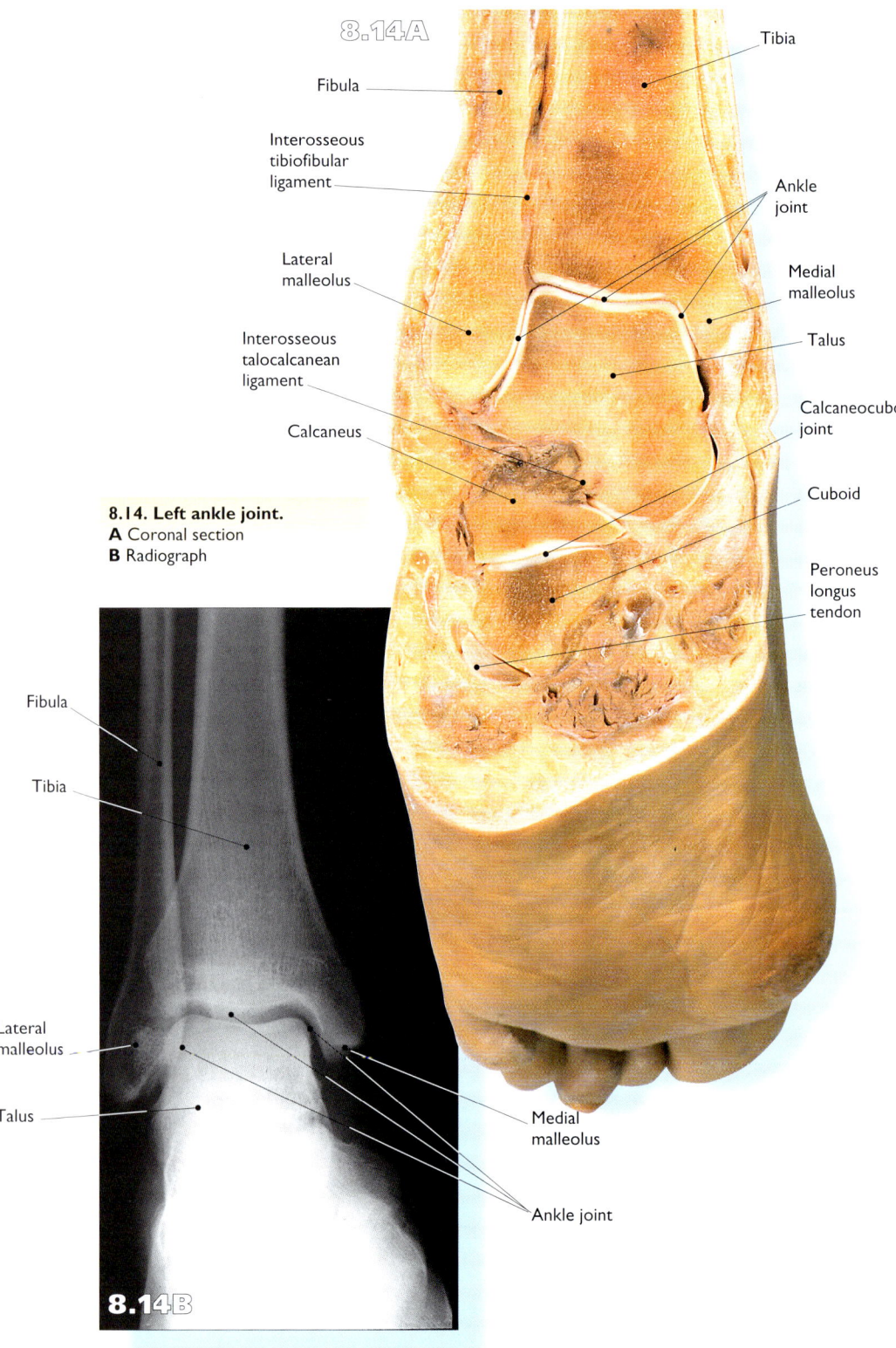

8.14. Left ankle joint.
A Coronal section
B Radiograph

the ankle (**8.12**) and forms in the sole tendons for the lateral four toes (corresponding to flexor digitorum profundus in the hand), where they are attached to the base of the distal phalanx. It is supplied by the tibial nerve.

Flexor hallucis longus – from the back of the *fibula*, with a tendon that grooves the back of the talus and then crosses medially in the sole to reach the base of the distal phalanx of the great toe (**8.16**). It is supplied by the tibial nerve.

Flexor retinaculum – from the medial malleolus to the side of the calcaneus, it keeps the flexor tendons in place. The order of tendons *behind the medial malleolus* from front to back is tibialis posterior, flexor digitorum longus, flexor hallucis longus (**8.12**). The posterior tibial vessels and tibial nerve lie between the digitorum and longus tendons and divide behind the malleolus into the medial and lateral plantar vessels and nerves, which supply the muscles and skin of the sole.

Peroneus longus and peroneus brevis – arising from the fibula, they form the muscles of the small lateral compartment of the leg. At the ankle the brevis tendon is in contact with the back of the lateral malleolus, and runs on to be inserted into the base of the fifth metatarsal. The longus tendon is behind that of brevis, and enters the sole where it lies in the groove on the cuboid bone (**8.14A**) and then attaches to the medial cuneiform and the base of the first metatarsal (on the sides of these bones opposite the attachment of tibialis anterior). Both muscles are supplied by the superficial peroneal nerve.

Superior peroneal retinaculum – from the lateral malleolus to the side of the calcaneus, it keeps the tendons of

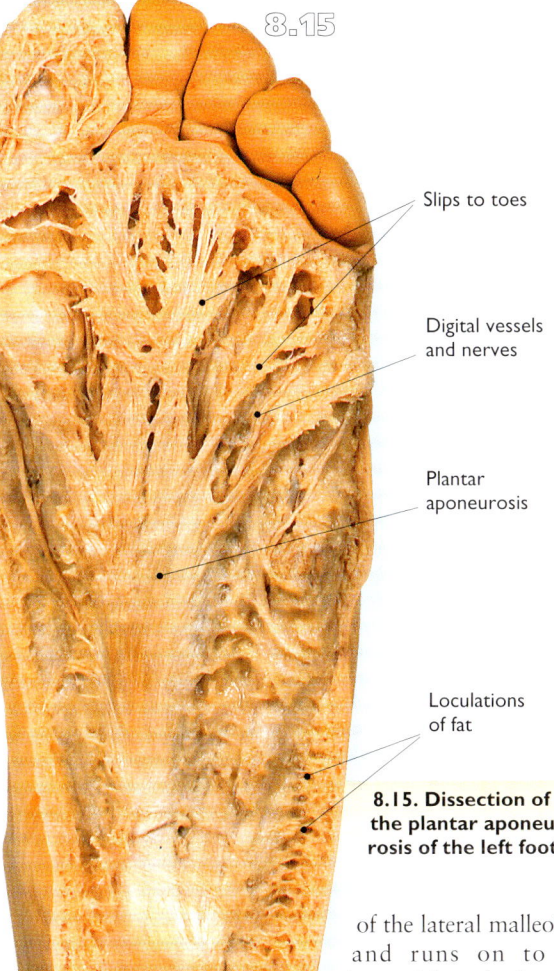

8.15. Dissection of the plantar aponeurosis of the left foot

- Slips to toes
- Digital vessels and nerves
- Plantar aponeurosis
- Loculations of fat

peroneus longus and brevis in place, with brevis in front of longus *behind the lateral malleolus,* where the small saphenous vein and sural nerve also lie.

Inferior peroneal retinaculum – holds the peroneus brevis and longus tendons against the side of the calcaneus, above and below the peroneal tubercle, respectively.

Ankle joint – between the lower ends of the tibia and fibula and the talus (**8.13**, **8.14**). The joint capsule is reinforced by the medial ligament (deltoid ligament), which runs from the medial malleolus to the side of the talus and the sustentaculum tali of the calcaneus. It is very strong; injuries usually fracture the medial malleolus rather than tear the ligament. On the lateral side there is not one ligament only, but three small ones: anterior and posterior talofibular, and calcaneofibular.

Principal muscles that produce movements at the ankle joint are:

Dorsiflexion (extension) – tibialis anterior, extensor hallucis longus, extensor digitorum longus, and peroneus tertius.

Plantarflexion (flexion) – gastrocnemius, soleus, tibialis posterior, flexor hallucis longus, flexor digitorum longus, peroneus longus, and peroneus brevis.

The way the talus is gripped between the tibia and fibula means that the only movements possible are dorsiflexion and plantarflexion (see below for other foot movements).

Subtalar joint – collective name for joints beneath the talus, which are the talocalcanean joint at the back (sometimes itself called the subtalar joint) and the talocalcaneonavicular joint (with two parts – talocalcanean and talonavicular) at the front (**8.13**, **8.14**). It is at these joints that most of the movements of inversion and eversion of the foot occur. The interosseous talocalcanean ligament (**8.13A**, **8.14A**), which passes between the adjacent grooves on the lower surface of the talus and upper surface of the calcaneus, is a strong band that holds the talus and calcaneus together. Imagine the talus gripped between the malleoli and the

8.16. Dissection of the sole of the left foot, after removal of the plantar aponeurosis and most of the flexor digitorum brevis

Labels: Flexor hallucis longus; Interosseus muscle; Lumbrical muscle; Abductor hallucis; Flexor digitorum longus; Medial plantar nerve and vessels; Flexor accessorius; Lateral plantar nerve and vessels; Flexor digitorum brevis

whole of the rest of the foot swivelling inwards (inversion) or outwards (eversion) underneath the talus.

Midtarsal joint – collective name for the calcaneocuboid joint and the talonavicular joint (front part of the talocalcaneonavicular joint), where a small amount of inversion and eversion occurs.

Principal muscles that produce movements at the subtalar and midtarsal joints are:
Inversion – tibialis anterior and tibialis posterior.
Eversion – peroneus longus and peroneus brevis.

Plantar aponeurosis – from the medial and lateral tubercles of the calcaneus, it divides at the front into five slips, one for each toe, and fuses with the fibrous flexor sheaths and the metatarsophalangeal joint capsules (**8.15**). It acts as a strong tie-beam that helps to preserve the longitudinal arches of the foot; it has numerous septa which run into the skin and subcutaneous tissue of the sole to give a firm union between these structures.

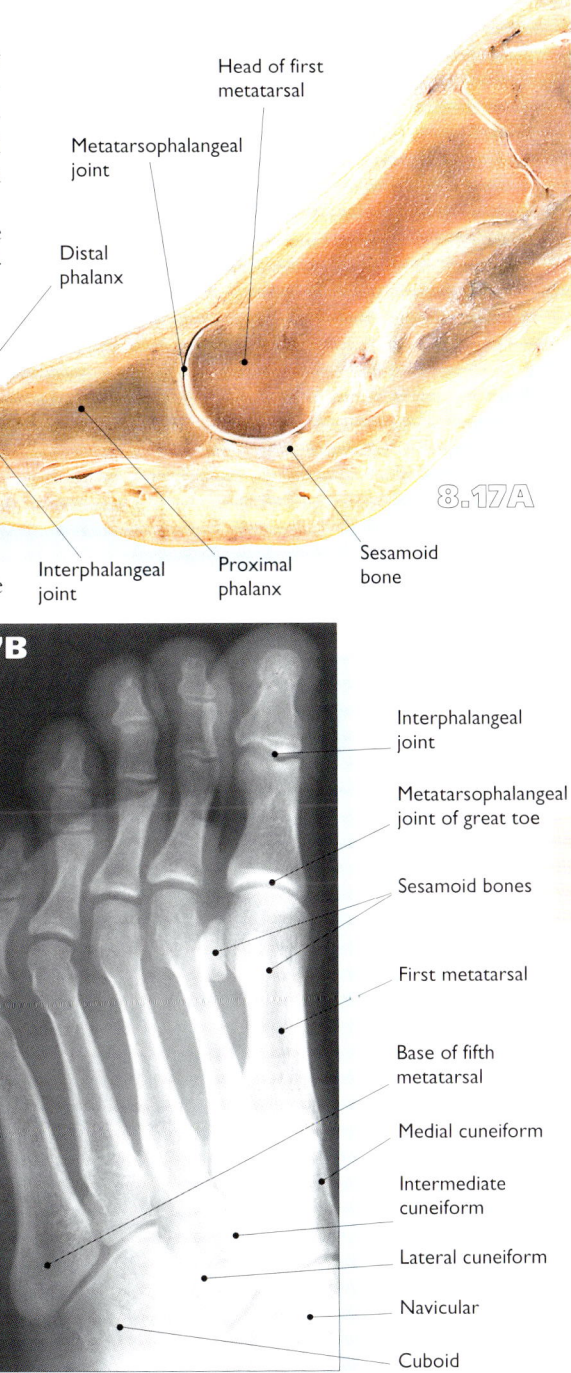

8.17. Left great toe
A Sagittal section
B Oblique radiograph of the left foot to show the sesamoid bones under the head of the first metatarsal

Muscles of the sole – like the palm of the hand, the sole has separate muscles for the great and little toes, as well as others with multiple tendons. Of the larger and more important, flexor digitorum brevis is the central superficial muscle of the sole, immediately below the plantar aponeurosis (it corresponds to flexor digitorum superficialis in the hand), with tendons to the middle phalanges of the four lateral toes splitting to allow the tendons of flexor digitorum longus to pass through to the distal phalanges (**8.16**). Flexor accessorius (sometimes called quadratus plantae) is under cover of brevis, attaches to flexor digitorum longus just before that muscle splits into its four tendons, and supposedly counteracts the slightly oblique pull of longus. The lumbrical and interosseus muscles have similar attachments to those of the hand, and are important in keeping the toes straight (i.e. flexing the metatarsophalangeal joints and extending the interphalangeal joints).

Medial and lateral plantar nerves – the nerves of the skin and muscles of the sole (**8.16**). The medial plantar supplies abductor hallucis, flexor digitorum brevis, flexor hallucis brevis, and the first lumbrical; *all the others* are supplied by the lateral plantar nerve, mostly by its deep branch, which curls around the lateral border of flexor accessorius. Cutaneous branches from the lateral plantar nerve supply the lateral side of the sole and lateral one-and-a-half toes, with medial plantar branches going to the medial three-and-a-half toes and the medial part of the sole.

Ligaments of the foot – many ligaments unite the various foot bones; because of the arched shape of the foot, those of the sole are particularly strong. The interosseous talocalcanean ligament is mentioned above. Others of particular importance are the long and short plantar ligaments and the spring ligament.

Long plantar ligament – a strong band that runs from the calcaneus to the cuboid and the bases of the middle three metatarsals. It converts the groove on the cuboid into a tunnel for the peroneus longus tendon.

Short plantar ligament – (properly called the plantar calcaneocuboid ligament) is under cover of the long plantar ligament.

Spring ligament – (properly called the plantar calcaneonavicular ligament) runs from the sustentaculum tali of the calcaneus to the navicular, blending at the side with the medial ligament of the ankle and forming an important support for the head of the talus on its upper surface.

> Despite its common name it does not contain an unusual amount of elastic tissue.

Joints of the toes – structurally similar to those of the fingers, the most important is the metatarsophalangeal joint of the great toe (**8.17**), which is particularly involved in the 'push-off' phase of walking and running. Ill-fitting shoes can produce a lateral deformity of the toe, hallux valgus, which once begun is enhanced by the pull of the long flexor and extensor tendons, to cause undue prominence of the head of the first metatarsal – a bunion.

Maintenance of arches – in the static foot the maintenance of the arches (p. 33) depends largely on ligaments (which cannot change their tension, although they may become stretched), mainly on the long and short plantars and the spring ligament, and on the plantar aponeurosis. During movement (walking and running), muscles assume an important role since they can contract and vary the tension exerted by their tendons as required. The important muscles are the small muscles of the foot, together with tibialis anterior and tibialis posterior on the medial side, and peroneus longus and peroneus brevis on the lateral side.

Summary

Deep to gluteus maximus, the **piriformis muscle** is the key to structures in the gluteal region: of the vessels and nerves that emerge from the pelvis to enter the region, all do so by passing below piriformis except for the superior gluteal nerve and vessels which emerge above the muscle. The most important structure in the region is the **sciatic nerve**, the largest in the body. At the top of the back of the thigh it lies midway between the ischial spine and the greater trochanter of the femur, and then runs down the thigh deep to the hamstrings, which it supplies, to end at the top of the popliteal fossa by dividing into the tibial and common peroneal nerves.

- The front of the capsule of the **hip joint** is attached to the intertrochanteric line, but the back of the capsule does not reach as far as the intertrochanteric crest, being attached halfway along the back of the femoral neck. Fracture of the neck disrupts blood vessels that supply the head of the femur.

- The **iliofemoral ligament**, reinforcing the front of the hip joint capsule, is one of the strongest in the body. The flexors of the hip (psoas major, rectus femoris) are mainly supplied by the **femoral nerve**, the adductors by the **obturator nerve**, and the hamstrings by the **sciatic nerve**, with **gluteus maximus** assisting in the extremes of extension (as in running and climbing stairs) supplied by the inferior gluteal nerve. **Gluteus medius** and **minimus** which prevent tilting of the pelvis when the opposite foot is off the ground during walking are supplied by the superior gluteal nerve.

- At the front of the upper thigh, the **femoral nerve** lies lateral to the palpable **femoral artery**, with the **femoral vein** on the medial side of the artery and the femoral canal (the site of a possible femoral hernia) on the medial side of the vein. Other palpable arteries in the lower limb are the popliteal, dorsalis pedis and posterior tibial.

- The **quadriceps tendon** is attached to the upper end of the patella; the patellar ligament attaches the lower end to the tuberosity of the tibia.

- The **tibial nerve** passes down among the muscles of the posterior or flexor compartment of the leg, which it supplies, to divide below the medial malleolus into the medial and lateral plantar nerves that supply the foot.

- The **common peroneal nerve** divides at the neck of the fibula into the superficial peroneal nerve, supplying skin of the leg and dorsum of the foot and the lateral compartment muscles (peroneus longus and brevis), and the deep peroneal nerve which is the motor nerve of the muscles of the extensor compartment of the leg.

Continued overleaf ...

... Continued from previous page

- **Hinge movements** during flexion and extension of the knee are complicated by rotation between the femur and tibia; with the tibia fixed, the popliteus muscle (tibial nerve) is required to 'unlock' the joint before flexion can continue. The medial meniscus of the knee joint is firmly fixed to the medial ligament, and is more frequently damaged than the lateral meniscus, which has an attachment to the popliteus tendon.

- Lying in front of the **ankle** the order of structures from medial to lateral is: tibialis anterior, extensor hallucis longus, anterior tibial vessels, deep peroneal nerve, and extensor digitorum longus.

- Behind the **medial malleolus** the order of structures from front to back is: tibialis posterior, flexor digitorum longus, posterior tibial vessels, tibial nerve, and flexor hallucis longus.

- Behind the **lateral malleolus**, peroneus brevis lies in front of peroneus longus.

- The **great saphenous vein** lies in front of the medial malleolus and ends by joining the femoral vein, passing through the saphenous opening which lies 3.5 cm below and lateral to the pubic tubercle.

- The **small saphenous vein** lies behind the lateral malleolus and runs up the back of the leg to drain into the popliteal vein in the popliteal fossa, where the order of structures from superficial to deep is: tibial nerve, popliteal vein and popliteal artery.

- At the ankle joint only flexion and extension occur; inversion and eversion of the foot take place at the joints beneath the talus, with the two tibialis muscles (anterior and posterior) producing inversion and the two peroneal muscles (longus and brevis) producing eversion.

- The segments of the **spinal cord** mainly concerned in supplying major limb muscles are: L2 - psoas major; L3 - quadriceps femoris; L4 – tibialis anterior and posterior; L5 – peroneus longus and brevis; S1 – gastrocnemius; S2 – small muscles of the foot.

Glossary

Most anatomical (and medical) terms have Latin (L) or Greek (G) origins, and the following list indicates derivations and meanings

A
abdomen L – probably meaning to hide
abducent L – leading from
acetabulum L – little vinegar cup
acoustic G – related to hearing
acromion G – extremity of shoulder
adenoid L – gland-like
aditus L – opening or entrance
adrenal L – towards the kidney
afferent L – carrying to
ampulla L – globular flask
anastomosis G – towards a mouth; joining together
annulus L – ring
antrum L – cave
anus L or Anglo-Saxon – to sit
aorta G – to lift or heave
aponeurosis G – derived from a sinew
arachnoid G – spider-like
artery G – keeping air (arteries were thought to contain air)
arytenoid G – like a ladle
atlas G – Greek god, bearing the earth on his shoulders
axilla L – armpit
azygos G – unpaired, not yoked

B
basilic G – important or prominent
biceps L – two heads
brachium L – arm
brevis L – short
bronchus G – windpipe
buccal L – cheek
buccinator L – trumpeter
bulla L – large vesicle
bursa L – purse

C
caecum L – blind
calcaneus L – heel
calcarine L – spur-shaped
callosum L – thick
canaliculus L – little canal
canine L – dog-like
canthus G – niche or corner
capitate L – head-like
capitulum L – little head
cardiac G and L – heart
carotid G – heavy sleep (from the Greek belief that the carotid arteries caused drowsiness)
carpus G and L – wrist
caudate L – tail
cephalic G – head
cerebellum L – little brain
cerebrum L – brain
cervix L – neck
chiasma G – crossed lines, like the Greek letter chi, χ
choana G and L – funnel
choroid G – like a vascular membrane
cilia L – eyelashes
circumflex L – bending round
clavicle L – little key
clitoris G – shut up
clivus L – slope
cloaca L – sewer
coccyx G – cuckoo, whose beak the bone resembles
cochlea L – snail or snail-shell
coeliac G and L – belly
colliculus L – little hill
colon G and L – large intestine
concha L – shell
condyle L – joint or knuckle
conjunctiva L – join together
conoid G – cone-like
coracoid G – crow-like, beak like a crow's
cornea L – horn
coronary L – encircling like a crown
corpus L – body
cortex L – bark or shell
cranium G and L – upper part of head
cribriform L – sieve-like
cricoid G – ring-like
cruciate L – crossed
cruciform L – cross-shaped
cubital L – elbow
cuneate, cuneiform L – wedge-shaped
cusp L – pointed tip
cutaneous L – skin
cyst G and L – sac or bladder

D
decussation G – crossing like the letter χ
deferens L – carrying away
deltoid G – triangular like the capital fourth letter of the Greek alphabet, Δ
dens L – tooth
dermatome G – cutting skin
diaphragm G – through a fence; a partition
dorsum L – back
duct L – to lead
duodenum L – twelve (length of 12 fingerbreadths)
dura mater L – tough mother

E
efferent L – carrying out
ejaculation L – throwing out
embryo G – to swell
endocrine G – to secrete inside
endolymph G – water inside
epidermis L – upon skin
epididymis G – upon the testicle
epiglottis G – upon the tongue
epiploic G – floating
epithelium G – upon the nipple
erythrocyte G – red cell
ethmoid G – sieve-like

F
falciform L – sickle-shaped
fascia L – bandage or sash
femur L – thigh
fibula L – buckle or brooch
fissure L – cleft or groove
flexion L – bending
follicle L – leather ball or money bag
foramen L – small opening
fornix L – arch
fossa L – ditch

187

fovea L – small pit
fundus L – bottom of a cavity

G
galli L – cock
ganglion G – knot or swelling
gastric G – stomach
gastrocnemius G – stomach of the leg
genitalia L – reproductive organs, belonging to birth
genu L – knee
gingiva L – gum
glans L – acorn
glenoid G – socket-like
glomerulus L – little ball
glottis G – vocal apparatus
gluteus L – rump
gonad G – seed
gracile L – slender
gyrus G and L – ring or circle

H
hallux L – great toe
hamate L – hooked
hepatic G – liver
hernia L – protrusion through an opening
hiatus L – gape
hilum L – a small bit or trifle
hormone G – to excite
humerus L – shoulder
humour G – liquid
hyaline G – glassy
hydro G – water
hyoid G – U-shaped, from the Greek letter υ
hypophysis G – undergrowth
hypothenar G – under the palm

I
ileum G and L – small intestine, twisting
ilium L – loin
incisor L – cut into
index L – forefinger, point out
infundibulum L – funnel
inguinal L – groin
iris G and L – rainbow
ischium G and L – hip

J
jejunum L – empty, hungry
jugular L – neck, throat or collar bone

K
keratin G – horn

L
labium, labrum L – lip
labyrinth G – maze
lacerum L – jagged
lacrimal L – tear
lactation L – milk
lamina L – plate or layer
larynx G – upper windpipe
lateral L – side or flank
latissimus L – widest
lemniscus G and L – ribbon
leucocyte G – white cell
levator L – lifter
lienal L – spleen, splenic
lingual L – tongue
lumbar L – loin
lumbrical L – earthworm
lunate L – crescent-shaped
lutea L – yellow
lymph L – clear water

M
magnus L – great
malleolus L – little hammer
malleus L – hammer
mamillary L – nipple
mamma L – breast
mandible L – lower jaw; chew
manubrium L – handle
manus L – hand
masseter G – chewer
mastoid G – breast-like
maxilla L – jawbone
maximus L – biggest
meatus L – passage
medial L – towards the midline
median L – in the midline
mediastinum L – median partition
medius L – middle
medulla L – marrow
meninges G – membranes
meniscus G and L – crescent
mental L – chin
mesentery G – middle intestine
micturition L – desire to pass urine
minimus L – smallest
molar L – mill for grinding
motor L – mover
myenteric G – intestinal muscle

N
nares L – nostril
navicular L – small boat
nephron G – kidney
neuron G – nerve or sinew
node L – knot
nucleus L – kernel, small nut

O
obturator L – plug an opening
occiput L – back of the head
oculomotor L – eye mover
oesophagus G – carrying food
olecranon G – head of the elbow
olfactory G – make smell
omentum L – fatty membrane, to clothe
ophthalmic G – eye
opponens L – placing against
optic G and L – sight
oral L – mouth
os L – mouth (plural ora)
os L – bone (plural ossa)
otic G – ear
ovum L – egg

P
palate L – palate
palpebra L – eyelid
pampiniform L – tendril-shaped
pancreas G – all flesh
papilla L – nipple
paralysis G – loosen alongside
parietal L – wall
parotid G – near the ear
patella L – flat dish
pectinate L – like a comb
pectoral L – breast
pedicle L – little foot
peduncle L – stalk
pelvis L – basin
penis L – tail
perilymph G – water around
perineum G – evacuate around
periodontal G – around tooth
peripheral G – carry around
peritoneum G – stretch around
peroneal G – brooch
pes L – foot
petrous G – stony
phalanx G – line of soldiers

Glossary

pharynx G – throat
philtrum L – love charm
phrenic G – mind or heart as centre of emotions
pia mater L – soft mother
pineal L – pine cone
pituitary L – mucus (the gland was thought to secrete nasal mucus)
placenta L – cake
plantar L – sole of foot
platysma G – broad
pleura G – rib, side
plexus L – network
pollex L – thumb
pons L – bridge
popliteus L – ham
porta L – entrance
prepuce L – foreskin
profundus L – deep
pronation L – bend forward
proprioceptive L – take one's own
prostate G – stand before
psoas G – loin muscle
pterion G – wing
pterygoid G – wing-like
ptosis G – falling
pubis L – secondary sex hair
pudendal L – ashamed
pulmonary L – lung
punctum L – sharp point
pupil L – doll (from image reflected in cornea)
pylorus G – gatekeeper

Q

quadrate L – four-sided
quadriceps L – four-headed

R

radius L – a spoke
ramus L – a branch
raphe G – a seam
rectus L – straight
recurrent L – run back
renal L – kidney
retina L – net
rima L – cleft
rotundum L – round

S

sagittal L – arrow
salpinx G – tube, trumpet
saphenous G – apparent, not hidden
sartorius L – tailor (sitting cross-legged)
scala L – staircase
scalene G – triangle with unequal sides
scaphoid G – boat-shaped
scapula L – shoulderblade
sciatic G – hip
sclera G – hard
scrotum L – bag
sebaceous L – grease
sella L – saddle
seminiferous L – carrying seed
serratus L – toothed
sesamoid G – like a sesame seed
sigmoid G – like the letter S
sinus L – curve or hollow
spermatozoa G – seed animals
sphenoid G – wedge-like
sphincter G – tight binder
splanchnic G – organ
squamous L – scale-like
stapes L – stirrup
sternum G and L – breast, breast bone
stroma G – bed, framework
styloid G – pillar-like
sulcus L – groove
supination L – bend backwards
sural L – calf
suture L – seam
symphysis G – growing together
synovial G – with egg (like white of egg)

T

talus L – ankle
tarsus G – flat surface
temporal L – time (temples, where hair first goes grey)
tegmen L – covering
tendon G – stretch out
teres L – round and long
testicle L – diminutive of testis
testis L – witness
thalamus G – chamber, bedroom
thenar G – palm of hand
thorax G and L – breastplate
thrombus G – curd, clot
thymus G – sweetbread (like a bunch of thyme flowers)
thyroid G – shield-like
tibia L – flute
trachea G – rough air channel
tragus G – goat (goat-like hairs in front of the ear)
triceps G – three-headed
triquetral L – three-cornered
trochanter G and L – runner
trochlea G and L – pulley
tuber L – protuberance
turbinate L – child's top
tympanum G and L – drum

U

ulna L – elbow
umbilicus L – navel
uncinate L – hooked
ureter G and L – urinary canal
uvula L – little grape

V

vagina L – sheath
vagus L – wandering
vallecula L – little hollow
vas deferens L – vessel carrying away
ventricle L – little belly
vermiform L – worm-like
vertebra L – turning joint
vesicle L – little bladder
viscus L – internal organ
vomer L – ploughshare
vulva L – wrapper

X

xiphoid G – sword-like

Z

zygomatic G – yoke

Index

A
Abdomen 127
　anterior wall 128
　posterior wall 131
　surface features 129
　vessels and nerves 133
　viscera 136
Adam's apple (laryngeal prominence) 79
Adenoids 41
Air cells, mastoid 21
Ampulla, hepatopancreatic 138
Anaesthesia, dental 66
Anastomosis, portal-systemic 135
Anatomical terms 15
Angle of Louis 110
Antrum, pyloric 137
Aorta 113
Aperture, posterior nasal (choana) 21
Apex, of heart 121
Aponeurosis, plantar 183
Appendix 140
Aqueduct of midbrain 49
Arachnoid mater 49
Arch, aorta 113
　deep palmar 102
　superficial palmar 102
　zygomatic 63
Arches of foot 184
Area, auditory 46
　motor 46
　sensory 46
　speech (Broca's) 46
　visual 46
Arm 90
Artery, arteries
　anterior interventricular 122
　anterior tibial 175
　aorta 113
　axillary 95
　brachial 97, 99
　brachiocephalic trunk 113
　coeliac trunk 133
　common carotid 79
　common hepatic 133
　common iliac 133
　coronary 122
　dorsalis pedis 176
　external carotid 79
　facial 62
　femoral 166
　gastroduodenal 134
　gonadal 133
　hepatic 134
　ileocolic 134
　inferior mesenteric 133, 134
　inferior pancreatico-duodenal 134
　inferior phrenic 133
　inferior thyroid 82
　internal carotid 79
　internal pudendal 169
　jejunal and ileal 134
　left colic 134
　left gastric 134
　left gastro-epiploic 134
　lumbar 133
　maxillary 65
　middle colic 134

middle meningeal 20
　ovarian 133
　popliteal 175
　posterior tibial 175
　profunda femoris 166
　pulmonary 114, 120
　radial 101
　renal 133, 145
　right colic 134
　right gastro-epiploic 134
　short gastric 134
　sigmoid 134
　splenic 133
　superficial temporal 63
　superior mesenteric 133, 134
　superior pancreatico-duodenal 134
　superior rectal 134
　superior thyroid 82
　supra-orbital 62
　testicular 133
　ulnar 101
　vertebral 82
Atrium, of heart 118
Axilla 90, 95

B
Balance 77
Bladder, urinary 156, 158
Body, perineal 155
Bone(s) 17
　carpal 29
　hip 29
　hyoid 21, 78
　lower limb 29
　metatarsal XX
　scaphoid 29
　tarsal 33
　upper limb 25
Brain 44
Brainstem 47
Breasts 110
Bulb of vestibule 160
Bundle, atrioventricular 122
Bursa omental 137
　prepatellar 172
　semimembranosus 172
　suprapatellar 172

C
Caecum 140
Calcaneus 33
Canal, anal 155, 158
　carotid 41
　cervical 1159
　femoral 167
　hypoglossal 41
　inguinal 128
　Schlemm 70
　optic 41
　pudendal 155
Capsule, internal 46
Cartilage(s), costal 25
　cricoid 41, 83
　of knee 172
　of larynx 83
　thyroid 41, 83
Cauda equina 57
Cavity, abdominal 128
　cranial 36
　nasal 20, 8
　orbital 20
　pelvic 128

Centres, cardiac 48
　respiratory 48
Cerebellum 46
Cerebrum 44
Chambers, of eye 70
　of heart 118
Chordae tendineae 118
Choroid 69
Circle, arterial (of Willis) 50
Circulation, pulmonary 116
　systemic 116
Circumcision 158
Clavicle 25
Clitoris 160
Coccyx 25
Colon 131, 141
Columns, white 55
Cord(s) , brachial plexus 80, 95
　spermatic 157
　spinal 44, 53
　vocal 41, 84
Cornea 69
Corpus callosum 44
　cavernosum 158
　spongiosum 158
　striatum 44
Cortex, cerebral 44
Cranium 20
Crus of diaphragm 112, 131
Cystitis 158

D
Deafness 76
Dermatomes 59
Diaphragm 112
　pelvic 150
　urogenital 155
Disc, intervertebral 25
Duct, accessory pancreatic 138, 145
　bile 143
　cystic 142
　hepatic 142
　pancreatic 138, 145
　parotid 62
　right lymphatic 80
　submandibular 80
　thoracic 115
Ductus (vas) deferens 157
Duodenum 130, 138
Dura mater 36, 49

E
Ear 74
Ejaculation 158
Elbow 97
Eminence, hypothenar 107
　thenar 106
Epididymis 157
Epigastrium 130
Epiglottis 41, 83
Erection 158
Examination, bimanual of uterus 158
　rectal
　vaginal
Eye 69
Eyelids 69

F
Face 60

Falx cerebri 43
Fascia lata 166
Femur 33
Fibres, afferent 56
　corticonuclear 46
　corticospinal 46
　efferent 56
　nerve 14
　thalamocortical 46
Fibula 33
Fissure, superior orbital 41
Flexure, left colic 141
　right colic 141
Fluid, cerebrospinal 49, 132
　seminal (semen) 157
Fold, gluteal 168
　vocal 41, 84
Foot 171
Foramen, foramina
　epiploic 137
　greater sciatic 33
　interventricular 49
　intervertebral 21
　jugular 41
　lacerum 41
　lesser sciatic 33
　magnum 41
　mandibular 40, 64
　obturator 29
　ovale 41
　rotundum 41
　skull 41
　spinosum 41
　stylomastoid 41
　vena caval
Forearm 97
Forebrain 44
Fossa, iliac 130
　anterior cranial 36
　cubital 98
　ischio-anal (ischiorectal) 155
　mandibular 21, 64
　middle cranial 36
　pituitary 36
　popliteal 174
　posterior cranial 40
Fracture, Colles' 97

G
Gall bladder 130, 142
Gallstones 143
Ganglion, ganglia, basal 44
　cranial nerve 47
　parasympathetic 15
　posterior root (spinal) 56
　sympathetic 15
　trigeminal 52
Genital organs, female 158
　male 155
Gingivae (gums) 66
Girdle, hip 25, 164
　shoulder 25, 90
Gland(s), adrenal 145
　greater vestibular (Bartholin's) 160
　lacrimal 72
　mammary 110
　parathyroid 83
　parotid 62
　pituitary 36
　sebaceous 8
　sublingual 65
　submandibular 80

190

Index

sweat 8
thyroid 82
Goitre 82
Granulations, arachnoid 49
Gray matter, brain 44
 spinal cord 54
Groove, deltopectoral 94
Gyri 44
Gyrus, postcentral 46
 precentral 46
 superior temporal 46

H
Haemorrhage, cerebral 46
Hallux valgus 184
Hand 97
Hearing 76
Heart 116
Hemiplegia 46
Hemisphere, cerebral 44
Hernia, femoral 167
 inguinal 129
Hilum, of kidney 145
 of lung 123
Hip 164
Horns, of spinal cord 54
Hydrocele 157
Hymen 159
Hypochondrium 130
Hypothalamus 44

I
Ileum 139
Ilium 29
Injection, gluteal intra-
 muscular 169
Intestine, large 139
 small 138
Ischium 29
Islets of Langerhans 144

J
Jejunum 139
Joint(s) 17, 18
 acromioclavicular 92
 ankle 182
 cartilaginous 18
 cricothyroid 83
 distal radio-ulnar 106
 elbow 101
 facet 25
 fibrous 18
 first carpometacarpal 107
 hip 170
 interphalangeal of fingers 107
 interphalangeal of toes 184
 knee 171
 manubriosternal 109
 metacarpophalangeal 107
 metatarsophalangeal 184
 midcarpal 106
 midtarsal 183
 proximal radio-ulnar 106
 sacro-iliac 164
 shoulder 94
 sternoclavicular 90
 subtalar 182
 synovial 18
 talocalcanean 182
 talocalcaneonavicular 182
 temporomandibular 21, 64
 wrist 106

K
Kidney 131, 145
Knee 171
Knuckle, aortic 113

L
Labia majora 160
 minora 160
Lacrimal apparatus 69, 72
Laryngopharynx 41
Larynx 41, 83
Leg 171
Lemniscus, medial 55
Ligament(s), anococcygeal 155
 broad 159
 cervical (lateral) 159
 conoid 92
 coraco-acromial 94
 coracoclavicular 92
 costoclavicular 92
 inguinal 128
 interosseous talocal
  canean 182
 long plantar 184
 round 159
 sacrospinous 33
 sacrotuberous 33
 short plantar 184
 spring (plantar calcaneon
  avicular) 184
 suspensory of ovary 151
 trapezoid 92
 uterosacral 159
 See also individual
  Joints
Ligamenta flava 25
Ligamentum arteriosum 114
Line, mylohyoid 40
Linea alba 128
Liver 130, 141
Lobe(s), frontal 41
 of liver 142
 of lung 123
 parietal 46
 temporal 46
Lower limb 163
Lungs 123
Lymph nodes, axillary 97
 cervical 80
 facial 63
 nodes inguinal 167

M
Mandible 20, 21
Manubrium 25
Maxilla 21
Meatus, internal acoustic 40
 nasal 68
Mediastinum 109, 112
Medulla oblongata 43
Membrane, cricothyroid 83
Meninges 49, 53
Meniscus, medial and
 lateral 172
Mesentery 137
Mesocolon, sigmoid 141
 transverse 141
Mesovarium 158
Midbrain 43
Mons pubis 159
Mouth 41, 65
Movements, of fingers 107
 of thumb 107
Mumps 62
Muscle(s), abductor pollicis
 brevis 106
 abductor pollicis longus 106
 adductor of thigh 168
 adductor brevis 168
 adductor longus 168
 adductor magnus 168
 biceps brachii 97
 biceps femoris 170
 brachialis 97

brachioradialis 98
buccinator 62
coccygeus 151
constrictors of pharynx 85
coracobrachialis 97
deltoid 94
diaphragm 112
erector spinae 77
extensor digitorum brevis 177
extensor digitorum longus 177
extensor hallucis longus 177
extensor of forearm 106
extensor pollicis brevis 106
extensor pollicis longus 106
external oblique 128
extra-ocular 70
facial 60
flexor accessorius 184
flexor carpi radialis 103
flexor digitorium brevis 184
flexor digitorum longus 181
flexor digitorum
 profundus 103
flexor digitorum
 superficialis 103
flexor hallucis longus 181
flexor pollicis brevis 106
flexor pollicis longus 103
gastrocnemius 178
gluteus maximus 168
gluteus medius 168
gluteus minimus 168
gracilis 168
hamstrings 170
iliacus 168
infraspinatus 92
internal oblique 128
interosseus of foot 184
interosseus of hand 107
lateral pterygoid 63
latissimus dorsi 92
levator ani 151
lumbrical of foot 184
lumbrical of hand 107
masseter 63
mastication 64
medial pterygoid 64
obturator internus 151
opponens pollicis 106
orbicularis oculi 62
orbicularis oris 62
palatopharyngeus 85
palmaris longus 103
papillary 118
pectineus 168
pectoralis major 92
peroneus brevis 181
peroneus longus 181
piriformis 151, 168
plantaris 178
popliteus 172, 178
posterior crico-arytenoid 83
pronator quadratus 104
pronator teres 98
psoas major 132
puborectalis 151
quadratus lumborum 132
quadriceps femoris 167
rectus abdominis 128
rectus femoris 167
rotator cuff 92
salpingopharyngeus 85
sartorius 168

scalenus anterior 79
semimembranosus 170
semitendinosus 170
serratus anterior 92
small of hand 106
of sole 184
soleus 178
sternocleidomastoid 77
stylopharyngeus 85
subscapularis 92
supinator 99
supraspinatus 92
temporalis 63
tensor fasciae latae 168
teres major 92
teres minor 94
tibialis anterior 177
tibialis posterior 178
transversus abdominis 128
trapezius 92
triceps 97
vastus intermedius 167
vastus lateralis 167
vastus medialis 167

N
Nasopharynx 41
Neck 77
Nerve(s), abducent 52
 accessory 53, 82
 auriculotemporal 65
 axillary 96
 buccal 64
 chorda tympani 64
 common peroneal 176
 cranial 50
 cutaneous of face
  and scalp 61
 cutaneous of lower limb 175
 cutaneous of upper limb 102
 deep peroneal 176
 facial 52, 62
 femoral 136, 166
 glossopharyngeal 52
 hypoglossal 53, 82
 ilio-inguinal 136
 iliohypogastric 136
 inferior alveolar 64
 inferior gluteal 169
 lateral femoral cutaneous 135
 lateral plantar 184
 lingual 64
 mandibular 61
 maxillary 61
 medial cutaneous of arm 96
 medial cutaneous of
  forearm 96
 medial plantar 184
 median 96, 102
 musculocutaneous 96
 obturator 52
 obturator internus 169
 oculomotor 50
 olfactory 50
 ophthalmic 61
 optic 50
 pelvic splanchnic 151
 phrenic 79, 116
 posterior femoral
  cutaneous 169
 posterior superior
  alveolar 65
 pudendal 169
 radial 96
 recurrent laryngeal 82, 83
 sciatic 168
 segmental of muscles 60

191

spinal 56
superficial peroneal 176
superior gluteal 169
suprascapular 80
sural 178
tibial 175
trigeminal 52, 61
trochlear 50
ulnar 96, 103
vagus 52, 80, 116
vestibulocochlear 52
Neuron, lower motor 56
upper motor 56
Node, atrioventricular (AV) 122
sinuatrial (SA) 122
Nose 41, 67
Nosebleed (epistaxis) 67
Nucleus, nuclei,
basal 44
brain 44
caudate 44
cranial nerve 47
lentiform 44

O
Oesophagus 113
Omentum, greater 137
lesser 137
Opening, aortic oesophageal
saphenous 166
Os, external 159
Ossification 18
Ovary 158

P
Pain 55, 59, 122
Palate 66
hard 21, 66
soft 41, 66
Pancreas 31, 144
Papilla, major duodenal 138, 144
minor duodenal 138
Paralysis, flaccid 56, 57
spastic 55, 56, 57
Patella 33
Pathway, pain 55
temperature 55
touch 55
visual 72
Pelvis 149
bony 33, 145
renal 145
Penis 158
Perineum 149
Peritoneum 128
Phalanges, of fingers 29
of toes 33
Pharynx 83
Pia mater 50
Plate, cribriform of ethmoid bone 36
Pleura 123
Pleurisy 124
Plexus, brachial 59, 80
cardiac 122
cervical 59, 78
choroid 49
lumbar 59
sacral 59, 150

tympanic 75
Pons 43
Porta hepatis 142
Position (kinaesthetic) sense 55
Pouch, recto-uterine (of Douglas) 159
rectovesical 156
Process, mastoid 21
xiphoid 25
Prostate 156
Pterion 20
Pubis 29
Pulse, brachial 97
carotid 79
dorsalis pedis 176
facial 62
femoral 166
popliteal 175
posterior tibial 175
radial 101
superficial temporal 63
ulnar 101
Puncture, lumbar 132

R
Radius 29
Rami, of spinal nerves 59
Rectum 155, 158
Reflexes, spinal 54
Region(s), of abdomen 129
anal 151
genital 151
gluteal 168
lumbar 130
umbilical 130
Retina 70
Retinaculum, extensor 106
flexor (wrist) 104
flexor (ankle) 181
inferior extensor 177
inferior peroneal 181
superior extensor 177
superior peroneal 181
Ribs 25
Root(s), of brachial plexus 80
of lung 123
of median nerve 96
of spinal nerve 56

S
Sac, lesser 137
pleural 123
Sacrum 25
Scalp 60, 61
Scapula 25
Sclera 69
Scrotum 158
Septum, interatrial 121
interventricular 121
nasal 67
Sheath(s), femoral 166
fibrous flexor 104
rectus 128, 130
synovial 104
Shoulder 90
Sinus(es), coronary 118
paranasal 21, 67
venous 40
Skeleton 8
appendicular 25

axial 20
facial 20
Skin 8
Skull 20
Snuffbox, anatomical 106
Space, subarachnoid 49
Spermatozoa 157
Sphincter, external urethral 157
internal urethral 157
pyloric 137
Spine, anterior superior iliac 29, 128, 164
ischial 29
Spleen 131, 146
Sternum 25
Stomach 137
Stroke 46
Sulci 44
Sulcus, calcarine 46
central 46
lateral 46
Sutures 18
Symphysis, pubic 164
System, cardiovascular 8
conducting of heart 122
digestive 11
endocrine 13
genito-urinary 13
lymphatic 8
muscular 8
nervous 14
portal venous 118
reproductive 13
respiratory 10
skeletomuscular 8
urinary 13

T
Talus 33
Teeth 66
Temperature sensation 55
Tendon(s), Achilles' 178
flexor of forearm 103
Tentorium cerebelli 43
Testicle 157
Testis 157
Thalamus 44
Thigh 164
Thorax 109
Thrombosis, cerebral 46
Thymus 115
Tibia 33
Tongue 65
Tonsil(s), palatine 87
pharyngeal 41
Touch 55
Trachea 113
Tract, alimentary (digestive) 10
biliary 142
corticospinal 55
cuneate 55
extrapyramidal 56
gracile 55
pyramidal 55
spinocerebellar 56
spinothalamic 55
Trapezium 29
Triangle, femoral 164
Trunk, brachial plexus 80
brachiocephalic 113

coeliac 133
pulmonary 114, 120
sympathetic 82, 115, 136, 150
Tube, uterine 159
Tubercle, pubic 128, 164
Tunnel, carpal 104

U
Ulna 29
Umbilicus 130
Upper limb 89
Ureter 145, 156
Urethra female 158
male 156
Urinary bladder 131, 156
Uterus 158

V
Vagina 159
Vallecula 83
Valve, aortic 120
mitral 120
pulmonary 118
tricuspid 118
Varices, oesophageal 135
Vasectomy 157
Vault, cranial 20
Vein(s), basilic 99
brachiocephalic 80, 114
cardiac 122
cephalic 99
common iliac 135
external jugular 79
femoral 166
gonadal 135
great saphenous 166, 177
hepatic 135
inferior mesenteric 134
internal jugular 80, 114
lumbar 135
ovarian 135
perforating 178
popliteal 175
portal 134
posterior arch 178
pulmonary 120
renal 135, 145
small saphenous 178
splenic 135, 146
subclavian 80, 114
superficial of upper limb 99
superior mesenteric 134
testicular 135
thyroid 82
varicose 178
Vena cava inferior 135
superior 114
Ventricles of brain 48
of heart 118
Vertebrae 21
Vesicle, seminal 157
Vessels, great 118
Vestibule, of vagina 159
Vibration sense 55

W
White matter, of brain 44
of spinal cord 54